Advance Praise for *Handbook of Assessment and Treatment of Eating Disorders*

"Dr. Timothy Walsh is one of the world's leading authorities on eating disorders. This well-researched and thorough guide, which he coauthored, will not only help clinicians and researchers better understand the condition but will also enable sufferers to get the help they so desperately need and deserve."

Joy Bauer, M.S., RDN, nutrition and health expert for NBC's Today show, #1 New York Times best-selling author, founder of Nourish Snacks

"This book, written by experts on the various aspects of eating disorders, will be particularly useful for those interested in the diagnosis and assessment of eating disorders. Too many books skip lightly over these important areas. Here you will find much substance."

Stewart Agras, M.D., Professor of Psychiatry Emeritus, Stanford University School of Medicine, Stanford, California

HANDBOOK OF

Assessment and Treatment of Eating Disorders

HANDBOOK OF Assessment and Treatment of Eating Disorders

EDITED BY

B. Timothy Walsh, M.D.

Evelyn Attia, M.D.

Deborah R. Glasofer, Ph.D.

Robyn Sysko, Ph.D.

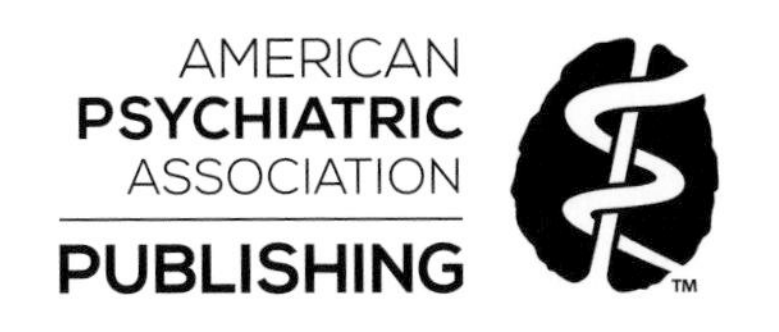

Note: The authors have worked to ensure that all information in this book is accurate at the time of publication and consistent with general psychiatric and medical standards, and that information concerning drug dosages, schedules, and routes of administration is accurate at the time of publication and consistent with standards set by the U.S. Food and Drug Administration and the general medical community. As medical research and practice continue to advance, however, therapeutic standards may change. Moreover, specific situations may require a specific therapeutic response not included in this book. For these reasons and because human and mechanical errors sometimes occur, we recommend that readers follow the advice of physicians directly involved in their care or the care of a member of their family.

Books published by American Psychiatric Association Publishing represent the findings, conclusions, and views of the individual authors and do not necessarily represent the policies and opinions of American Psychiatric Association Publishing or the American Psychiatric Association.

If you wish to buy 50 or more copies of the same title, please go to www.appi.org/specialdiscounts for more information.

Manufactured in the United States of America on acid-free paper
19 18 17 16 15   5 4 3 2 1
First Edition

Typeset in Adobe's Baskerville BE and HelveticaNeue LT Std.

American Psychiatric Association Publishing
1000 Wilson Boulevard
Arlington, VA 22209-3901
www.appi.org

Library of Congress Cataloging-in-Publication Data
Handbook of assessment and treatment of eating disorders / edited by B. Timothy Walsh, Evelyn Attia, Deborah R. Glasofer, and Robyn Sysko.–First edition.

p. ; cm.

Assessment and treatment of eating disorders

Includes bibliographical references and index.

ISBN 978-1-58562-509-3 (pb : alk. paper)–ISBN 978-1-61537-039-9 (eb)

I. Walsh, B. Timothy, 1946- , editor. II. Attia, Evelyn, editor. III. Glasofer, Deborah R., 1979- , editor. IV. Sysko, Robyn, editor. V. American Psychiatric Association, issuing body. VI. Title: Assessment and treatment of eating disorders.

[DNLM: 1. Eating Disorders–diagnosis. 2. Eating Disorders–therapy. WM 175]
RC552.E18
616.85'26–dc23

2015024909

British Library Cataloguing in Publication Data
A CIP record is available from the British Library.

Contents

PART II

Evaluation and Diagnosis of Eating Problems

PART IV
Treatment

Contributors

Evelyn Attia, M.D.
Professor of Psychiatry, Columbia University Medical Center; Professor of Psychiatry, Weill Cornell Medical College; Director, Eating Disorders Research Unit, New York State Psychiatric Institute, New York, New York

Anne E. Becker, M.D., Ph.D., S.M.
Maude and Lillian Presley Professor of Global Health and Social Medicine, Department of Global Health and Social Medicine, Harvard Medical School, Boston, Massachusetts

Kelly C. Berg, Ph.D., LP
Assistant Professor, Department of Psychiatry, University of Minnesota, Minneapolis, Minnesota

Allegra Broft, M.D.
Assistant Professor of Psychiatry, Columbia University Medical Center, New York State Psychiatric Institute, New York, New York

Amanda Joelle Brown, Ph.D.
Clinical Psychologist, Eating Disorders Research Unit, New York State Psychiatric Institute, New York, New York

Eva M. Conceição, Ph.D.
Research Fellow, School of Psychology, University of Minho, Braga, Portugal

Katherine Craigen, Ph.D.
Clinical Instructor, Eating and Weight Disorders Program, Icahn School of Medicine at Mount Sinai, New York, New York

Michael Devlin, M.D.
Professor of Clinical Psychiatry, Columbia University Medical Center, New York State Psychiatric Institute, New York, New York

Kamryn T. Eddy, Ph.D.
Co-director, Eating Disorders Clinical and Research Program, Massachusetts General Hospital; Assistant Professor of Psychology, Department of Psychiatry, Harvard Medical School, Boston, Massachusetts

Jo M. Ellison, Ph.D.
Psychologist, Neuropsychiatric Research Institute, Fargo, North Dakota

Scott G. Engel, Ph.D.
Research Scientist, Neuropsychiatric Research Institute; Associate Professor, Department of Psychiatry and Behavioral Science, University of North Dakota School of Medicine and Health Sciences, Fargo, North Dakota

Kelsie T. Forbush, Ph.D., LP
M. Erik Wright Assistant Professor, Department of Psychology, University of Kansas, Lawrence, Kansas

Eve Khlyavich Freidl, M.D.
Assistant Professor of Psychiatry, Columbia University Medical Center, New York, New York

Loren Gianini, Ph.D.
Postdoctoral Research Fellow, Columbia University Medical Center, New York State Psychiatric Institute, New York, New York

Deborah R. Glasofer, Ph.D.
Assistant Professor of Clinical Psychology in Psychiatry, Columbia University College of Physicians and Surgeons, New York State Psychiatric Institute, New York, New York

Neville H. Golden, M.D.
Professor of Pediatrics, and Chief, Division of Adolescent Medicine, Lucile Packard Children's Hospital, Stanford University School of Medicine, Stanford, California

Thomas Hildebrandt, Psy.D.
Program Director, Eating and Weight Disorders Program, Icahn School of Medicine at Mount Sinai, New York, New York

Marsha D. Marcus, Ph.D.
Professor of Psychiatry and Psychology, University of Pittsburgh School of Medicine, Pittsburgh, Pennsylvania

Laurel Mayer, M.D.
Associate Professor of Psychiatry, Columbia University Medical Center, New York State Psychiatric Institute, New York, New York

James E. Mitchell, M.D.
President and Scientific Director, Neuropsychiatric Research Institute; Chair, Department of Psychiatry and Behavioral Science, University of North Dakota, School of Medicine and Health Sciences, Fargo, North Dakota

Rollyn M. Ornstein, M.D.
Associate Professor of Pediatrics, and Interim Division Chief, Division of Adolescent Medicine and Eating Disorders, Penn State Hershey Children's Hospital, Hershey, Pennsylvania

Kathleen M. Pike, Ph.D.
Professor of Psychology in Psychiatry and Epidemiology, and Director, Global Mental Health Program, Columbia University, New York, New York

Christina A. Roberto, Ph.D.
Assistant Professor of Social and Behavioral Sciences and Nutrition, Harvard School of Public Health, Boston, Massachusetts

Janet Schebendach, Ph.D.
Assistant Professor of Neurobiology in Psychiatry, Columbia University Medical Center; Director of Research Nutrition, Eating Disorders Research Unit, New York State Psychiatric Institute, New York, New York

Natasha A. Schvey, Ph.D.
Postdoctoral Fellow, Department of Medical and Clinical Psychology, Uniformed Services University of the Health Sciences, Department of Defense, Bethesda, Maryland

Joanna Steinglass, M.D.
Associate Professor of Clinical Psychiatry, Columbia University Medical Center, New York State Psychiatric Institute, New York, New York

Robyn Sysko, Ph.D.
Assistant Professor of Psychiatry, Eating and Weight Disorders Program, Department of Psychiatry, Icahn School of Medicine at Mount Sinai, New York, New York

Marian Tanofsky-Kraff, Ph.D.
Associate Professor, Department of Medical and Clinical Psychology, Uniformed Services University of the Health Sciences, Department of Defense, Bethesda, Maryland

Jennifer J. Thomas, Ph.D.
Co-director, Eating Disorders Clinical and Research Program, Massachusetts General Hospital; Assistant Professor of Psychiatry, Harvard Medical School, Boston, Massachusetts

B. Timothy Walsh, M.D.
Ruane Professor of Pediatric Psychopharmacology in Psychiatry, Columbia University College of Physicians and Surgeons; Director, Division of Clinical Therapeutics, New York State Psychiatric Institute, New York, New York

Jennifer E. Wildes, Ph.D.
Assistant Professor of Psychiatry and Psychology, University of Pittsburgh School of Medicine, Pittsburgh, Pennsylvania

Stephen A. Wonderlich, Ph.D.
Chester Fritz Distinguished Professor, Associate Chairman, Department of Psychiatry and Behavioral Science, University of North Dakota School of Medicine and Health Sciences; Director, Clinical Research, Neuropsychiatric Research Institute; Chair, Eating Disorders, Sanford Health, Fargo, North Dakota

Disclosure of Competing Interests

The following contributors to this book have indicated a financial interest in or other affiliation with a commercial supporter, a manufacturer of a commercial product, a provider of a commercial service, a nongovernmental organization, and/ or a government agency, as listed below:

Evelyn Attia, M.D.–*Research support:* Eli Lilly and Company

Anne E. Becker, M.D., Ph.D., S.M.–*Honoraria:* John Wiley & Sons, Inc. for service as Associate Editor of the *International Journal of Eating Disorders*; *Book royalties:* University of Pennsylvania Press

Kelsie T. Forbush, Ph.D., LP–*Author and copyright holder:* Eating Pathology Symptoms Inventory (EPSI) and Iowa Eating Behaviors Questionnaire (IEBQ), which are free, publicly available self-report measures of eating disorder symptoms

Eve Khlyavich Freidl, M.D.–*Travel funds:* AACAP Annual Meeting (2014) as recipient of AACAP Pilot Research Award for junior faculty and child and adolescent psychiatry residents, supported by Lilly USA, LLC

Thomas Hildebrandt, Psy.D.–*Scientific advisor:* Noom, Inc.

Joanna Steinglass, M.D.–*Current support:* National Institute of Mental Health, Global Foundation for Eating Disorders, and New York state

Robyn Sysko, Ph.D.–*Common stock:* Pfizer Pharmaceuticals; *Book royalties:* Chapter on binge-eating disorder, UpToDate

B. Timothy Walsh, M.D.–*Research support:* AstroZeneca; *Royalties:* McGraw-Hill and UpToDate

Jennifer E. Wildes, Ph.D.–*Paid consultant:* McKesson Health Solutions, LLC

The following contributors to this book have indicated no competing interests to disclose during the year preceding manuscript submission:

Kelly C. Berg, Ph.D., LP
Allegra Broft, M.D.
Amanda Joelle Brown, Ph.D.
Eva M. Conceição, Ph.D.
Katherine Craigen, Ph.D.
Michael Devlin, M.D.
Kamryn T. Eddy, Ph.D.
Jo M. Ellison, Ph.D.
Scott G. Engel, Ph.D.
Loren Gianini, Ph.D.
Deborah R. Glasofer, Ph.D.
Neville H. Golden, M.D.
Marsha D. Marcus, Ph.D.
Laurel Mayer, M.D.
James E. Mitchell, M.D.
Rollyn M. Ornstein, M.D.
Christina A. Roberto, Ph.D.
Janet Schebendach, Ph.D.
Natasha A. Schvey, Ph.D.
Marian Tanofsky-Kraff, Ph.D.
Jennifer J. Thomas, Ph.D.
Stephen A. Wonderlich, Ph.D.

Foreword

In the words of Dr. Martin Luther King Jr., education has a twofold function. Education must first, "enable one to sift and weigh evidence, to discern the true from the false, the real from the unreal, and the facts from the fiction" (King 1947, p. 10). But education cannot stop here; it must further guide one's studies to ensure that "worthy objectives" are the targets of concentrated efforts (King 1947, p. 10).

The *Handbook of Assessment and Treatment of Eating Disorders* is masterful in achieving this twofold mission. It is a scholarly volume that provides thoughtful review and critical analysis of the state of the field. Each chapter grapples with complex and imperfect data; each chapter also provides practical and thoughtful integration of material to guide clinical practice and inform future research. It is easy to get bogged down by the lacunae in the empirical database, leading some mental health professionals to distance themselves from research and discount what is known. It is also easy to go into overdrive research mode to fill these gaps and lose sight of the priority clinical issues that should guide our work to maximize impact. This handbook has achieved the fine balance between research and clinical practice, between quantitative and qualitative ways of knowing, and between articulating clearly what we don't yet know and, nonetheless, working with what we do know to produce a useful text to guide clinical care and future research.

The impetus for the handbook was the publication of DSM-5 (American Psychiatric Association 2013), and this is most appropriate given that any study of eating disorders should begin with a careful consideration of our diagnostic system–what we call an eating disorder and the related phenomenology. Developed under the auspices of the American Psychiatric Association, the Diagnostic and Statistical Manual (DSM) system is an American classification system; however, it has been adapted to varying degrees in countries around the world, particularly with regard to research programs. As described in several chapters in the book, the success of DSM is variable in terms of its ability to accurately capture the clinical syndromes of eating pathology that cause suffering and propel individuals to seek treatment. DSM is further challenged in its ability to capture the most important aspects of eating disorders for diverse segments of the population (e.g., men) and across cultures. Around the globe, these are critical issues that will become more and more prominent in the near future as eating disorders become increasingly recognized in diverse cultural and economic contexts.

The Global Burden of Disease Study demonstrates that the health burden of eating disorders is steadily increasing (Vos et al. 2012), primarily because eating disturbances outside high-income, Western countries are rapidly growing in concert with rising rates of population weight. This is true in terms of both disability-adjusted life years and years lived with disability. In 81% of countries around the world, population weight has increased significantly over the past 30 years, with 36.9% of men and 38% of women falling in the overweight or obese categories today (Vandevijvere et al. 2015). In the United States, 39.96% of men and 29.74% of women are overweight, and an additional 35.04% of men and 36.84% of women are obese (Yang and Colditz 2015). Such demographic trends in eating and weight pathology call for global innovative interventions, including translation of assessment instruments, adaptation of treatment interventions, leveraging new technologies for assessment and treatment, and development of more aggressive treatments such as bariatric surgery.

Although the health consequences of eating disorders are well understood, the significance of the disability burden has largely been ignored within the global health field. Even more broadly, despite the fact that mental illness is the leading cause of disability around the world, mental health remains largely overlooked, if not invisible, within the health agendas and budgets of many nations around the globe. This failure might be considered unfortunate but understandable given the myriad health and other priorities that burden governments everywhere, until we consider the following: We have treatments for eating disorders that can reduce suffering for the majority of individuals; we have evidence of the successful implementation of psychotherapies for depression in low- and middle-income countries, suggesting that we can do the same for eating disorders; and we know that focusing on women's health has a multiplicative effect for families and communities. In the same way that focusing on women's education and empowerment has a positive impact on the educational achievement of the next generation, focusing on women's mental health must become a priority that is appreciated for the benefits accrued to the individual as well as the positive pay-it-forward benefits for the next generation.

The wisdom contained in the *Handbook of Assessment and Treatment of Eating Disorders* has the potential to guide both research agenda setting and clinical care for the field of eating disorders. Each chapter sifts and weighs evidence, discerns the true from the false, the real from the unreal, and the facts from the fiction. Each chapter provides incisive guidance on the worthy objectives for the field of eating disorders. Collectively, these chapters represent a volume of knowledge that promises to enhance every reader's education about eating disorders and better prepare us to carry forward the work of advancing understanding and care for individuals suffering from eating disorders around the world.

Kathleen M. Pike, Ph.D.
Professor of Psychology in Psychiatry and Epidemiology
Director, Global Mental Health Program
Columbia University, New York, New York

References

American Psychiatric Association: Diagnostic and Statistical Manual of Mental Disorders, 5th Edition. Arlington, VA, American Psychiatric Association, 2013

King ML Jr: The purpose of education. The Maroon Tiger, February 1947, p 10

Vandevijvere S, Chow CC, Hall KD, et al: Increased food energy supply as a major driver of the obesity epidemic: a global analysis. Bull World Health Organ 93:446–456, 2015

Vos T, Flaxman AD, Naghavi M, et al: Years lived with disability (YLDs) for 1160 sequelae of 289 diseases and injuries 1990-2010: a systematic analysis for the Global Burden of Disease Study 2010. Lancet 380(9859):2163–2196, 2012 23245607

Yang L, Colditz GA: Prevalence of overweight and obesity in the United States, 2007-2012. JAMA Intern Med June 22, 2015 26098405 [Epub ahead of print]

Preface

The major impetus for this book was the publication in the spring of 2013 of DSM-5 (American Psychiatric Association 2013). DSM-5 introduced both major and minor changes to the conceptualization of, and to the diagnostic criteria for, feeding and eating disorders. We felt it would be timely to review these changes and to embed them in a broader, up-to-date description of the assessment and treatment of individuals with eating disorders. In addition, in this new diagnostic era, there have been important developments in the technologies available to aid diagnosis, research, and treatment. Thus, this volume aims throughout the text to engage the reader (and the field in general) in thoughtful consideration of when, how, and why technology might be used to improve assessment and treatment.

The opening chapter in Part I ("Introduction") describes the evolution of the DSM-5 section on feeding and eating disorders. The rationale for making diagnoses is reviewed, including both advantages and disadvantages of the DSM approach. The specific alterations in the diagnostic criteria for each disorder are described, and guidance is provided for clinicians regarding how to apply criteria in practice. Two major changes in DSM-5 are highlighted, the official recognition of binge-eating disorder and the formulation of the newly named avoidant/restrictive food intake disorder.

Following Chapter 1, content is organized in three parts. Part II, "Evaluation and Diagnosis of Eating Problems," comprising six chapters, provides guidance for clinicians on the evaluation of individuals who have symptoms suggesting a possible eating disorder. The approaches to adults and to children and adolescents are described in Chapters 2 and 3; these chapters highlight the fundamental principles and practices necessary for careful assessments of individuals with eating disorders. Chapters 4–6 are guides to the assessment of individuals with more specialized problems, including overweight individuals, those considering bariatric surgery, and men and boys. Part II concludes with a description of the impact of culture on the manifestation and assessment of eating problems (Chapter 7).

Part III, "Assessment Tools," describes tools available to clinicians to assist in the assessment of eating disorders. The initial chapter of this section, Chapter 8, provides a critical review of the first assessment methods developed to assess eating disorders and the recent evolution of new instruments. Chapter 9 describes self-report measures; given the time pressures on modern clinical practice, such measures serve to enhance both the accuracy and the efficiency of patient care. Chapter 10 outlines how to use the Eating Disorder Assessment for DSM-5 (EDA-5), a semistructured interview developed by the group from the Columbia Center for Eating Disorders to rigorously but quickly determine whether DSM-5 criteria for a feeding or eating disorder are satisfied; this interview is available at www.eda5.org. Chapter 11 details methods to aid the assessment of children and adolescents, and Chapter 12 reviews the cutting edge of eating disorder assessments, namely, the use of handheld devices such as smartphones.

Part IV of the volume, "Treatment," consisting of three chapters, provides an overview of treatment. Chapter 13 focuses on restrictive eating disorders, such as anorexia nervosa and avoidant/restrictive feeding intake disorder. Chapter 14 reviews the treatment of binge eating, as seen in bulimia nervosa and binge-eating disorder. Chapter 15 addresses less commonly seen problems such as pica and rumination.

In association with the text, the authors have produced several short videos to highlight methods of patient assessment and diagnosis. The reader will find references to these videos in relevant chapters of the book. The videos may be accessed at www.appi.org/Walsh.

A critical part of our field's progress is an appreciation for all types of clinical expertise at all levels of experience. We ourselves represent different eras, and while each of us arrived at this project with a unique perspective on the past and present state of the assessment and treatment of eating disorders, our shared investment is certainly in its future. We greatly appreciate the equally diverse group of esteemed colleagues who have collaborated with us on this project. Among our authors are adult and child psychiatrists, psychologists, pediatricians, nutritionists, and postdoctoral fellows. Some of us have been devoted to this field for decades, while others have joined more recently with the hope of carrying the work forward for decades to come.

And we would be remiss not to mention Christine Call, A.B., our research assistant, without whom this project would not have gotten off the ground and certainly would never have landed safely!

Finally, we would especially like to thank our patients, from whom we continue to learn, for their courage in sharing their symptoms and struggles and for the privilege of allowing us to collaborate on their path to recovery.

We hope that whether you come to this text as a student or a seasoned professional, as a general practitioner or an eating disorders specialist, as a researcher or a clinician, our book will help to answer some of your questions and inspire new ones.

B. Timothy Walsh, M.D.
Evelyn Attia, M.D.
Deborah R. Glasofer, Ph.D.
Robyn Sysko, Ph.D.

Reference

American Psychiatric Association: Diagnostic and Statistical Manual of Mental Disorders, 5th Edition. Arlington, VA, American Psychiatric Association, 2013

Video Guide

The Video Learning Experience

The companion videos can be viewed at www.appi.org/Walsh.

Using the Book and the Videos Together

We recommend that readers use the boldface video prompts ▶ embedded in the text as indicators for viewing the associated clips. The cues identify the vignettes by number and title. Chapters 1, 2, 3, 4, 6, 7, 8, and 14 have associated videos.

Description of the Videos

The first video presents a brief roundtable discussion among clinicians. Each of the remaining four videos presents a brief interaction between a patient and a clinician; these videos aim to highlight general issues that can arise in the assessment of feeding and eating disorders and to illustrate some specific strategies for clinical intervention.

Video 1: Diagnostic issues in the age of DSM-5 (8:11)

For use with Chapters 1 and 8

This video, featuring clinical researchers involved in the development of DSM-IV and DSM-5, provides a window into the process of diagnostic changes described in DSM-5. Panelists discuss the rationale for the reorganization of DSM-5, including the developmental perspective now included in each diagnostic section. The discussion also highlights the new additions to the list of formally recognized conditions, including binge-eating disorder and avoidant/restrictive food intake disorder.

The clinical cases are fictional. Any resemblance to real persons is purely coincidental. The videos feature the work of volunteer clinicians and actor patients.

Video 2: Assessing eating problems in the primary care setting (3:24)

For use with Chapters 2, 3, and 14

This video depicts a clinical encounter between a primary care physician and a young woman who is reluctant to disclose the eating disorder behaviors that underlie her physical complaints. The discussion highlights ways to sensitively obtain critical clinical information in a primary care setting and how to engage a patient in next treatment steps.

Video 3: Assessing eating problems in overweight adults (5:52)

For use with Chapter 4

In this brief interaction, an eating disorder specialist (psychiatrist) meets with an overweight female patient to evaluate her eating behavior and associated psychological symptoms. The vignette demonstrates ways that a clinician can explain and assess a range of disturbances in eating behavior. It also models the importance of a nonjudgmental stance in the assessment of overweight individuals.

Video 4: Assessing eating problems in men (5:32)

For use with Chapter 6

In this vignette, an eating disorder specialist evaluates a male patient who presents with eating problems and preoccupation with body shape and weight, consistent with an eating disorder diagnosis. The video illustrates similarities and differences in the assessment of a male patient from that of a female patient. Examples of ways to ask questions about exercise habits, eating patterns, and compensatory behaviors, as well as the functional impairment of symptoms, are provided.

Video 5: Cultural considerations in the assessment of eating problems (6:10)

For use with Chapter 7

The video depicts a clinical encounter, exemplifying the assessment of an Asian woman with an eating disorder by a white clinician. The patient presents with somatic complaints and initially denies several commonly described eating disorder symptoms. In the interview, the clinician demonstrates how to probe for additional information sufficient to make a preliminary diagnosis and provides examples of some of what might be asked in the course of a comprehensive assessment.

Video Credits

We thank our wonderful video producer **Joe Faria** and the entire **Digital Communications Department of the New York State Psychiatric Institute** for their assistance in shooting, producing, and editing the videos accompanying the book. We also gratefully acknowledge the talented volunteer clinicians and actors without whom we could not have scripted or created this video content.

Evelyn Attia, M.D. (scriptwriter; videos 1 and 4), is Professor of Psychiatry at Columbia University Medical Center and Weill Cornell Medical College, and Director of the Eating Disorders Research Unit at New York State Psychiatric Institute.

Christine Call, A.B. (scriptwriter), is a doctoral candidate in clinical psychology in the Department of Psychology at Drexel University.

Wonda Clyatt (Video 5) is an actor.

Michael J. Devlin, M.D. (scriptwriter; videos 1 and 3), is Professor of Clinical Psychiatry at Columbia University College of Physicians and Surgeons and Associate Director of the Eating Disorders Research Unit at New York State Psychiatric Institute.

Michael First, M.D. (Video 1), is Professor of Clinical Psychiatry at Columbia University, and Research Psychiatrist at the Biometrics Department at the New York State Psychiatric Institute.

Deborah R. Glasofer, Ph.D. (scriptwriter; Video 5), is Assistant Professor of Clinical Psychology in Psychiatry at Columbia University College of Physicians and Surgeons, and a psychologist at the Eating Disorders Research Unit at New York State Psychiatric Institute.

Gabriella Guzman, A.B. (Video 2), is a research assistant at the Eating Disorders Research Unit at New York State Psychiatric Institute.

Matthew Shear, M.D., M.P.H. (Video 4), is Instructor in Psychiatry at Weill Cornell Medical College.

Karen Soren, M.D. (Video 2), is Associate Professor of Pediatrics and Public Health at Columbia University Medical Center and Director of Adolescent Medicine at New York Presbyterian Morgan Stanley Children's Hospital.

B. Timothy Walsh, M.D. (Video 1), is Ruane Professor of Pediatric Psychopharmacology in Psychiatry at Columbia University College of Physicians and Surgeons, and Director of the Division of Clinical Therapeutics at New York State Psychiatric Institute

Teresa Yenque (Video 3) is an actor.

We also thank **Professional Actors Training & Helping, LLC,** for their assistance.

PART I

Introduction

1 Classification of Eating Disorders

B. Timothy Walsh, M.D.
Evelyn Attia, M.D.
Robyn Sysko, Ph.D.

DSM-5 was published in the spring of 2013 (American Psychiatric Association 2013). Seven years in the making and almost 20 years since the publication of DSM-IV (American Psychiatric Association 1994), DSM-5 formalized significant changes in the official classification of eating disorders. The two biggest changes were the recognition of binge-eating disorder (BED) and the reconceptualization of feeding disorder of infancy or early childhood as avoidant/restrictive food intake disorder (ARFID). A number of important, but less far-reaching, changes were made to the diagnostic criteria for the other eating disorders. The purpose of this chapter is not only to review these changes, and the background and rationale justifying them, but also to provide a broad overview regarding the value of diagnostic categories. Video 1, "Diagnostic issues in the age of DSM-5," explores these changes in a roundtable discussion.

Introduction to the DSM Approach

Why Make a Diagnosis?

The thinking of Greek philosophers almost two millennia ago suggested to them that it was wise to define boundaries among phenomena where they naturally occurred, leading to the notion that science should "cleave nature at its joints." The work of the eighteenth-century Swedish botanist Carl Linnaeus, whose writings are cited as the basis for the distinctions "animal, vegetable, and mineral," is thought to be an excellent example of the utility of such an approach.

The application of this approach to the understanding of human diseases is of enormous potential value. If successful, it permits the identification of the cause or causes of a disease, eventually yielding major advances in improved knowledge of the pathological mechanisms underlying an illness and in the development of specific treatments targeting the underlying cause or causes. For example, the ability to go beyond the description of a patient's problem as "fever and a bad cough" to either "pneumonia secondary to infection with the pneumococcus bacterium" or "pneumonia secondary to infection with the influenza virus" is extremely useful for choosing the most effective treatment–an antibiotic for the former or an antiviral agent such as oseltamivir (Tamiflu) for the latter. Unfortunately, it has proven challenging to extend this model to the diagnosis of mental illness.

Diagnosis of Mental Illness

In 1960, Thomas Szasz, in *The Myth of Mental Illness* (Szasz 1960), argued that traditional psychiatric practice mislabeled individuals who were "disabled by living" as having a mental illness. Although this view has largely been relegated to the history books, there remain major challenges in knowing exactly where to draw the line between widely variable normal human behavior and the patterns of thinking and behaving that are generally conceived as illnesses.

The publication of DSM-III (American Psychiatric Association 1980) heralded a major shift in mainstream psychiatry from attempting to classify psychiatric illnesses based on theories of their etiology to a primarily descriptive approach. DSM-III grappled with the challenge inherent in Szasz's work: "How should a mental disorder be defined?" The authors of DSM-III and its successors, including DSM-5, recognized that there is no clear, strict, and universally accepted definition of a mental disorder. This is equally true of nonpsychiatric medical disorders; that is, perhaps surprisingly, there is no clear and universally accepted definition of what constitutes a disease (Allison et al. 2008). DSM-5 did not significantly alter the fundamental conceptualization of a mental disorder presented in DSM-III, and after considerable debate, the authors of DSM-5 settled on the following definition:

> A mental disorder is a syndrome characterized by clinically significant disturbance in an individual's cognition, emotion regulation, or behavior that

reflects a dysfunction in the psychological, biological, or developmental processes underlying mental functioning. (American Psychiatric Association 2013, p. 20)

DSM-5 also states that an expectable response "to a common stressor or loss…is not a mental disorder" (p. 20), thereby addressing the concerns of Szasz that socially deviant behavior and conflicts between the individual and society, of themselves, are not mental disorders. Finally, DSM-5 notes that mental disorders are usually associated with impairment of function or distress.

The goal of DSM-III was to provide clear and reliable diagnostic criteria for mental illnesses that would allow both clinicians and researchers to communicate accurately. DSM-III and its successors have largely met that goal. Although the reliability of diagnosis among different clinicians is certainly not perfect, agreement comparable to that of many nonpsychiatric medical diagnoses was achieved. A more ambitious goal of the DSM system beginning with DSM-III was to provide clear and reliable diagnostic criteria that would facilitate the identification of homogeneous groups of patients with identical problems. The hope was that studies of such groups would provide a foundation for the identification of causal factors underlying the illnesses. If almost all individuals with a particular form of depression had very similar symptoms, such as the degree to which they had lost the ability to enjoy life, developed insomnia, and lost their appetite, it would be possible for psychiatrists to distinguish the causes of that specific form of depression from other types of mood disturbance, much as physicians can distinguish between viral and bacterial pneumonia (as mentioned in the preceding subsection).

Problems With the DSM Approach

Unfortunately, except in rare instances, this goal has not been achieved. For example, there are few sharp dividing lines among the varied presentations of mood disturbance, and it increasingly appears that the genetic risks for developing many major psychiatric illnesses are not specific to a single disorder–even one that is very narrowly defined. Rather, multiple genes often exert small but cumulatively important effects for a range of disorders (e.g., Ruderfer et al. 2014). More generally, although many risk factors–environmental, genetic, and developmental–have been described, very few causes of specific mental disorders have been identified. In this regard, mental health continues to lag well behind areas such as cardiology and infectious disease, in which major strides have been made over the last several decades in identifying causative pathways for many disorders, thereby permitting the development of objective methods of diagnostic testing and of targeted treatment interventions.

The strategy employed in DSM-III and its successors also has had several unfortunate consequences. The articulation of many clearly but narrowly defined disorders and the understandable decision not to restrict the number of disorders that could be assigned to an individual have produced a high frequency of comorbidity. Individuals meeting criteria for one disorder often meet criteria for another. For example, many individuals meeting DSM criteria for an eating disorder also meet criteria for a depressive disorder, and current knowledge does not allow one disorder to be considered a result of or secondary to the other. In other words, it is generally difficult to know with certainty that an individual's bulimia nervosa is best attributed to her major depressive disorder or vice versa, or whether the two are independent.

A similar problem has been the high frequency of residual diagnoses, referred to in DSM-IV as "not otherwise specified" (NOS). Because diagnostic categories are narrowly defined in the DSM system, many individuals with a significant problem do not meet criteria for a specific DSM disorder. In the DSM-IV system, the eating disorders section provided a prime example of this problem. DSM-IV specifically defined only two eating disorders, anorexia nervosa (AN) and bulimia nervosa (BN). All other eating disorders of clinical significance received a formal diagnosis of eating disorder not otherwise specified (EDNOS), which included individuals with symptoms that barely missed the diagnostic threshold for AN or BN, along with individuals who met criteria for BED (a provisional diagnosis in DSM-IV). Despite the goals of DSM, the EDNOS moniker conveyed essentially no information beyond the fact that the individual had described a clinically significant eating problem. In some eating disorder programs, an EDNOS diagnosis was assigned to more than half of the patients presenting for treatment (Fairburn and Bohn 2005)!

Advantages of the DSM Approach

In light of these problems, why should the DSM approach be used at all? The short answer is that the DSM system, notwithstanding its significant limitations, is quite useful in communicating about the problem with the patient, with individuals close to the patient, and with other health care professionals. The DSM system is also useful in undertaking research to describe the development and course of mental disorders and to investigate treatment response. In short, the DSM categories have proven to have substantial clinical utility, even though their definitions are not based on fundamental knowledge of the causes of the disorders.

Path From DSM-IV to DSM-5

History

DSM-IV was published in 1994, 7 years after DSM-III-R (American Psychiatric Association 1987), which itself was published 7 years after the landmark promulgation of DSM-III in 1980. Planning for DSM-5 began in the early years of the new millennium with a series of conferences and edited volumes sponsored by the American Psychiatric Association (APA) to consider new ideas and approaches to the diagnostic system. One prominent example that had a significant impact on the DSM-5 development process was an emphasis on the dimensional nature of virtually all mental disorders (Helzer et al. 2008). This concept was most fully embraced in the proposed revisions of the personality disorders section, which suggested that individuals with such problems should first be characterized as having impairments in several broad areas of personality functioning, such as in developing and maintaining intimate interpersonal relationships, and then described in detail using a number of facets of personality function, such as emotional lability. This creative and carefully considered proposal provoked a storm of criticism from investigators and clinicians concerned about the magnitude of the change from the DSM-IV system and, in the end, was judged by the APA leadership to be too controversial to be officially recognized in DSM-5. The proposed new diagnostic approach for personality disorders is presented in DSM-5 in Section III, "Emerging Measures and Models." Regardless of the controversy, the dimensional perspective had a pervasive influence on DSM-5, leading, for example, to the incorporation of severity measures for many disorders, including the eating disorders.

Among the early and far-reaching decisions made by DSM-5 leadership was the elimination of the section of DSM-IV titled "Disorders Usually First Diagnosed in Infancy, Childhood, or Adolescence." Several important observations led to this decision. Among them was the fact that many disorders not included in this section of DSM-IV, such as anxiety disorders, mood disorders, and psychotic disorders, are *also* often recognized during childhood and adolescence. In the years since the publication of DSM-IV, it also became clear that many individuals with disorders listed in that section are first diagnosed later in life, including adults with attention-deficit and disruptive behavior disorders. Therefore, in DSM-5, the disorders previously included in the DSM-IV section on disorders usually first diagnosed in infancy, childhood, or adolescence were redistributed in DSM-5 to other sections, and a developmental perspective was incorporated throughout the text, including in the descriptions of each disorder. Pica, rumination disorder, and feeding disorder of infancy or early childhood joined the DSM-5 eating disorders section. Their inclusion led to the change in the title of this section to "Feeding and Eating Disorders," underlining the links to the two original sections of DSM-IV.

Approach and Process Leading to DSM-5

Work began in earnest on the eating disorders section of DSM-5 in 2006–2007 with the appointment of the 12 members of the Eating Disorders Work Group. This group comprised prominent clinical investigators from North America and Europe and included five psychiatrists, five psychologists, a nurse investigator, and a physician specializing in adolescent medicine. The work group continued work through the end of 2012 and achieved consensus on all recommendations regarding changes to the diagnostic criteria for feeding and eating disorders.

The initial review of the diagnostic landscape by the work group indicated that although the existing criteria for eating disorders had some problems, they were not completely "broken." In other words, the community of investigators and clinicians focused on eating disorders fundamentally agreed about the core diagnostic conceptualization of AN and BN. Furthermore, there was a clear consensus that the clinical features of these two disorders, while overlapping in some important regards, were sufficiently different to warrant their remaining distinct disorders. For example, it was clear that the course, complications, and treatment response of individuals with AN differed substantially from those of individuals with BN, emphasizing the clinical utility of separating the two groups diagnostically.

As noted, the major problem with the DSM-IV system for eating disorders was the unacceptably high frequency of the diagnosis of EDNOS in clinical populations. It was quickly apparent that from a logical perspective, there were only two ways to address this problem: to expand criteria for the existing disorders, allowing "near misses" to meet criteria for one of them, and to recognize new disorders. In the end, the work group recommended both. Several critical limitations restricted the breadth of changes considered. If the expansion of criteria was too radical, individuals now meeting the revised criteria for an existing diagnosis might not share the same core clinical characteristics captured by the original criteria. This could potentially be a major problem because it might invalidate decades of accumulated research and experience on the course, outcome, and treatment response of individuals with a disorder. A related and challenging issue throughout the process was a lack of good data to address the impact of many changes that might be considered. One of the standards employed by the work group was not to make significant changes without being reasonably confident of their impact on clinical utility. Therefore, despite the seeming appeal of a number of potential alterations to the diagnostic criteria, the work group endeavored to avoid recommendations not supported by evidence regarding the impact of the changes.

The first years of the work group's efforts were devoted to identifying specific possible options for change and to conducting a careful examination not only of existing literature but also of unpublished information in search of answers. Thirteen literature reviews, led by members of the work group, were published in 2009–2010 in the *International Journal of Eating Disorders*. These reviews were significantly augmented by several conferences jointly supported by the National Institute of Mental Health and the APA, culminating in an edited volume published in 2011 (Striegel-Moore et al. 2011). The work group's initial recommendations were presented in late 2010 on a Web site devoted to the DSM-5 effort and were discussed and debated at multiple international conferences over the next 3 years. The work group was fortunate to receive extensive comments from investigators and clinicians and from individuals who had experienced or were experiencing eating disorders, which led to important changes in the recommendations. A number of field trials, either sponsored by the APA or carried out by interested investigators who generously shared their results with the work group, provided concrete information on the utility and the problems of the recommended changes.

The final recommendations of the Eating Disorders Work Group were submitted to the DSM-5 Task Force by late 2012. After rigorous review by several internal committees and some minor text editing for consistency, the revised criteria were published in DSM-5 in the spring of 2013 largely as recommended.

Video 1, "Diagnostic issues in the age of DSM-5," features a roundtable discussion with B. Timothy Walsh, M.D., and colleagues involved in changes to feeding and eating disorder diagnoses in DSM-5.

Video Illustration 1: Diagnostic issues in the age of DSM-5 (8:11)

In the remainder of this chapter, we briefly describe the evolution of the feeding and eating disorders included in DSM-5.

Anorexia Nervosa

A Very Brief History

Although significant eating disturbances have presumably occurred since the dawn of human history, AN was the first to be clearly recognized as a clinical disorder. Richard Morton, in his *Treatise of Consumptions,* published in 1694, described an 18-year-old girl with what he termed "nervous consumption" (Morton 1694). Because Morton did not have the benefit of DSM, we cannot be certain that this young woman, who went on to die of her disorder, met today's formal criteria for AN. AN received its name almost 200 years later when, in 1873, Sir William Gull in England coined the term for the problems of three young women whose symptoms would clearly satisfy the DSM-III, DSM-IV, and DSM-5 definitions of this disorder (Gull 1997).

This brief history makes clear that the fundamental presentation and conceptualization of AN have remained impressively stable over centuries. The core features of the disorder are not in dispute. The challenge for DSM has been how best to capture them in a useful but concise set of diagnostic criteria.

DSM-IV to DSM-5

DSM-IV (pp. 544–545) required that individuals meet four criteria to merit a diagnosis of AN. The key features can be summarized as follows:

- Criterion A: "Refusal to maintain body weight at or above a minimally normal weight for age and height (e.g., weight loss leading to maintenance of body weight less than 85% of that expected...)"
- Criterion B: "Intense fear of gaining weight or becoming fat..."
- Criterion C: "Disturbance in the way in which one's body weight or shape is experienced, undue influence of body weight or shape on self-evaluation, or denial of the seriousness of the current low body weight"
- Criterion D: Amenorrhea

The work group reviewed these criteria and recommended changes to each. The DSM-5 criteria for AN are presented in Box 1–1, and the succeeding subsections describe the major changes from DSM-IV and the rationale supporting the revised criteria.

Box 1–1. DSM-5 Criteria for Anorexia Nervosa

A. Restriction of energy intake relative to requirements, leading to a significantly low body weight in the context of age, sex, developmental trajectory, and physical health. *Significantly low weight* is defined as a weight that is less than minimally normal or, for children and adolescents, less than that minimally expected.
B. Intense fear of gaining weight or of becoming fat, or persistent behavior that interferes with weight gain, even though at a significantly low weight.

C. Disturbance in the way in which one's body weight or shape is experienced, undue influence of body weight or shape on self-evaluation, or persistent lack of recognition of the seriousness of the current low body weight.

Low Body Weight

The salient physical characteristic of individuals with AN is low body weight. Although the DSM-IV Criterion A captured this feature, there were several problems.

The term *refusal* suggested that the individual's reluctance to consume sufficient calories to maintain a normal weight was a conscious and active decision and implied a degree of defiance. Although both of these characteristics are sometimes present, more frequently the basis of the inadequate calorie intake is complex, the individual's understanding of its persistence is poor, and his or her attitude about the problem is quite variable. *Refusal* also has a somewhat pejorative tone.

The example provided by DSM-IV in parentheses suggested that a low weight might be defined as one that was less than 85% of that expected, which was ultimately a source of significant confusion and controversy. Although intended only as an example, in many settings it became reified into a rigid rule. In addition, it was unclear what standard should be employed for the determination of the "expected" weight.

The DSM-5 Eating Disorders Work Group recommended that although the concept of low body weight was fundamental to AN, the wording of Criterion A should be substantially altered. The term *refusal* was eliminated in favor of a straightforward description of the behavior: "restriction of energy intake relative to requirements." The choice of *energy intake* as opposed to the more specific *food intake* reflected the work group's desire to make the definition broadly applicable, even to the very rare instances in which the individual's primary source of calorie intake was parenteral (e.g., via a gastric feeding tube or an intravenous line). The term "relative to requirements" encompasses situations in which the individual's caloric intake is statistically normal but inadequate based on unusual requirements, such as intense exercise.

To avoid the confusion that accompanied the inclusion of the example of "85% of expected" in DSM-IV, no numerical guidelines are provided within DSM-5 Criterion A; however, the text of DSM-5 reviews the diagnostic features in two paragraphs with detailed descriptions of standards that can be employed to assist the crucial judgment about whether an individual's weight is "significantly low." In the end, this judgment is made by the clinician on the basis of all the information available.

Fear of Gaining Weight

A small but significant fraction of individuals exhibiting other core characteristics of AN deny that they are afraid of gaining weight (Wolk et al. 2005). However, their overt behavior–classically, the steadfast avoidance of high-calorie foods and reluctance to consume foods outside a very narrow range–appears to belie their assertion. Therefore, in DSM-5, the phrase "persistent behavior that interferes with weight gain" was added to the DSM-IV Criterion B to include such presentations within full-threshold DSM-5 AN.

Distortion of Body Image

The work group's only concern about Criterion C focused on a single word, *denial*. This term might imply some underlying intrapsychic mechanism, which was not the intent. Therefore, the work group recommended that this term be changed to "persistent lack of recognition," which was thought to offer a more explicit description of the phenomenon.

Amenorrhea

The greatest change to the DSM-IV criteria for AN was the elimination of Criterion D, which had required amenorrhea. This decision was based on two observations. First, the DSM-IV criterion included a number of exceptions to this criterion, such as being male or being a woman who was taking oral contraceptives. Therefore, in practice, this criterion was often waived. Second, a literature review on this topic documented that there were a number of descriptions of women who met all the other criteria for AN but reported some menstrual activity (Attia and Roberto 2009). Therefore, to allow such individuals to receive the diagnosis of AN rather than EDNOS, the work group deleted this criterion.

The DSM-5 text, however, emphasizes that amenorrhea is a common physiological disturbance associated with AN, and its presence provides additional support for the diagnosis.

Bulimia Nervosa

A Very Brief History

The syndrome of BN was first clearly described and named in 1979 in a landmark paper by Professor Gerald Russell, a major figure in the eating disorders field at that time (Russell 1979). His clear summary of the symptoms of 30 patients captured the essential features of this disorder. DSM-III, published in 1980, included criteria for the syndrome, which was called simply "bulimia." In 1987, DSM-III-R refined those criteria and renamed the disorder "bulimia nervosa" in accordance with Russell. Only minor changes were made to the DSM-III-R criteria in DSM-IV and DSM-5 (presented in Box 1–2).

Box 1–2. DSM-5 Criteria for Bulimia Nervosa

A. Recurrent episodes of binge eating. An episode of binge eating is characterized by both of the following:
   1. Eating, in a discrete period of time (e.g., within any 2-hour period), an amount of food that is definitely larger than what most individuals would eat in a similar period of time under similar circumstances.
   2. A sense of lack of control over eating during the episode (e.g., a feeling that one cannot stop eating or control what or how much one is eating).

B. Recurrent inappropriate compensatory behaviors in order to prevent weight gain, such as self-induced vomiting; misuse of laxatives, diuretics, or other medications; fasting; or excessive exercise.

C. The binge eating and inappropriate compensatory behaviors both occur, on average, at least once a week for 3 months.

D. Self-evaluation is unduly influenced by body shape and weight.

E. The disturbance does not occur exclusively during episodes of anorexia nervosa.

DSM-IV to DSM-5

The DSM-IV criteria, closely mirroring those of DSM-III-R, required that individuals engage in both binge eating and inappropriate methods to avoid weight gain, such as self-induced vomiting; that both behaviors occur, on average, at least twice a week over the prior 3 months; and that shape or weight exert an undue influence on self-evaluation.

In the development of DSM-5, no data suggested the need for major changes to the DSM-IV criteria for BN. Only two, relatively small, alterations were suggested by the work group. A literature review (Wilson and Sysko 2009) found limited evidence to support the twice-weekly binge-eating and compensatory behavior frequency requirement; a small number of individuals presented for clinical care who met all the DSM-IV criteria but reported binge eating and purging only once a week. Therefore, in line with the effort to reduce the use of EDNOS, the work group recommended that the frequency criterion (Criterion C) be changed to "at least once a week." Another literature review found that the scheme in DSM-IV to classify individuals with BN as having either the purging or the nonpurging type was of limited utility and was frequently not employed (van Hoeken et al. 2009). Therefore, in DSM-5, the DSM-IV requirement that individuals be assigned to either the purging or the nonpurging type has been eliminated.

Binge-Eating Disorder

A Very Brief History

In 1959, the late Albert Stunkard, an eminent psychiatrist who was among the first mental health professionals to think carefully about the problems of individuals with obesity, published a paper on eating patterns among obese individuals that provided the first clear description of binge eating. These observations received surprisingly little attention until the development of DSM-IV was under way. Spearheaded by Robert Spitzer, the leader of the development of DSM-III, a major effort was made to develop criteria to capture the essential features of binge eating without the purging characteristic of BN. These efforts resulted in the first criteria for BED. Although there was significant interest in this disorder's being formally recognized in DSM-IV, in the end it was felt that sufficient data about its clinical characteristics, course, and outcome were unavailable, and the criteria were therefore included in DSM-IV in an appendix providing criteria sets for further study.

DSM-IV to DSM-5

A critical question considered by the DSM-5 work group concerning BED was whether to recommend that this disorder be formally recognized. To address this question, Stephen Wonderlich led a comprehensive review of the literature on BED that had emerged since DSM-IV (Wonderlich et al. 2009). This review documented the publication of over 1,000 articles in the medical literature since the preliminary criteria for BED were promulgated. These articles amply documented the breadth of clinical interest in this syndrome and provided detailed information on the characteristics of individuals meeting the provisional criteria. In particular, the data indicated that individuals with BED as defined by DSM-IV demonstrated an objective disturbance in eating behavior during meals observed in laboratory settings and had an increased frequency of mood and anxiety disturbance compared to similarly overweight or obese individuals without

BED. In addition, there were tentative indications that, to achieve the best clinical outcomes, individuals with BED should receive specific treatment interventions. For these reasons, the work group recommended that BED be formally recognized in DSM-5. After careful review by the DSM-5 Task Force, this recommendation was accepted (see Box 1–3 for criteria). Not surprisingly, this change contributed to a significant reduction in the frequency of use of EDNOS.

Box 1–3. DSM-5 Criteria for Binge-Eating Disorder

A. Recurrent episodes of binge eating. An episode of binge eating is characterized by both of the following:
   1. Eating, in a discrete period of time (e.g., within any 2-hour period), an amount of food that is definitely larger than what most people would eat in a similar period of time under similar circumstances.
   2. A sense of lack of control over eating during the episode (e.g., a feeling that one cannot stop eating or control what or how much one is eating).

B. The binge-eating episodes are associated with three (or more) of the following:
   1. Eating much more rapidly than normal.
   2. Eating until feeling uncomfortably full.
   3. Eating large amounts of food when not feeling physically hungry.
   4. Eating alone because of feeling embarrassed by how much one is eating.
   5. Feeling disgusted with oneself, depressed, or very guilty afterward.

C. Marked distress regarding binge eating is present.

D. The binge eating occurs, on average, at least once a week for 3 months.

E. The binge eating is not associated with the recurrent use of inappropriate compensatory behavior as in bulimia nervosa and does not occur exclusively during the course of bulimia nervosa or anorexia nervosa.

The work group also considered whether the draft criteria for the diagnosis of BED should be modified in any way. The available literature supported only a single small change. Specifically, to make the frequency requirement for BED identical to that for BN, the DSM-IV criterion was changed from a minimum of binge episodes occurring on at least 2 days per week, on average, over the last 6 months to a minimum of at least one episode of binge eating per week, on average, over the last 3 months (Wilson and Sysko 2009).

Avoidant/Restrictive Food Intake Disorder

As described in the section "Path From DSM-IV to DSM-5," an early and important decision in the development of DSM-5 was to combine, in a single section, the syndromes previously listed among the eating disorders and the feeding and eating disorders of infancy or early childhood sections of DSM-IV. The greatest challenge in doing so was presented by the DSM-IV diagnosis of feeding disorder of infancy or early childhood.

This diagnosis made its first appearance in the DSM system in DSM-IV and was intended to capture presentations of infants and young children who, for some reason, perhaps related to difficult interactions with their caregivers or other developmental issues, were not growing as they should. Members of the DSM-5 Eating Disorders Work Group performed a literature review to examine this diagnosis in detail and uncovered a number of problematic issues (Bryant-Waugh et al. 2010). Clinicians appeared to rarely use this diagnosis in practice, and virtually no scholarly research had focused on feeding disorder of infancy or early childhood. Furthermore, the work group became aware that there were a number of clinically significant eating problems particularly affecting young people that were not covered by this or any other DSM-IV diagnosis. Therefore, after extensive consultation with clinicians caring for young people with a range of eating problems, the work group recommended that the existing diagnosis of feeding disorder of infancy or early childhood be expanded and retitled avoidant/restrictive food intake disorder (ARFID). Studies initiated by a group of adolescent medicine specialists interested in eating disorders were generously made available to the work group during the final stages of DSM-5 development. Data from these studies indicated that in specialist practices focusing on eating problems of young people, the criteria for ARFID (presented in Box 1–4) successfully captured a significant number of individuals who did not meet criteria for any other eating disorder (Fisher et al. 2014; Ornstein et al. 2013).

Box 1–4. DSM-5 Criteria for Avoidant/Restrictive Food Intake Disorder

A. An eating or feeding disturbance (e.g., apparent lack of interest in eating or food; avoidance based on the sensory characteristics of food; concern about aversive consequences of eating) as manifested by persistent failure to meet appropriate nutritional and/or energy needs associated with one (or more) of the following:

1. Significant weight loss (or failure to achieve expected weight gain or faltering growth in children).
2. Significant nutritional deficiency.

3. Dependence on enteral feeding or oral nutritional supplements.
4. Marked interference with psychosocial functioning.

B. The disturbance is not better explained by lack of available food or by an associated culturally sanctioned practice.

C. The eating disturbance does not occur exclusively during the course of anorexia nervosa or bulimia nervosa, and there is no evidence of a disturbance in the way in which one's body weight or shape is experienced.

D. The eating disturbance is not attributable to a concurrent medical condition or not better explained by another mental disorder. When the eating disturbance occurs in the context of another condition or disorder, the severity of the eating disturbance exceeds that routinely associated with the condition or disorder and warrants additional clinical attention.

Excerpted from the *Diagnostic and Statistical Manual of Mental Disorders,* 5th Edition, Arlington, VA, American Psychiatric Association, 2013. Used with permission.

The final criteria for ARFID intentionally encompass a range of presentations. Individuals meeting the DSM-IV criteria for feeding disorder of infancy or early childhood are included in ARFID. In addition, individuals who have a problem with food intake associated with other problems may also meet criteria for this disorder. Common examples are individuals who have experienced a frightening or particularly difficult but transient gastrointestinal problem, such as an episode of acute vomiting after eating, and subsequently severely restrict their food intake to avoid another such episode. Another presentation is that of individuals who avoid foods of a certain texture or color. Minor variants of such problems occur commonly, especially among children, but the criteria for ARFID and the text of DSM-5 emphasize that the diagnosis should be assigned only in situations in which the food restriction leads to a clinically significant nutritional disturbance or to a serious impairment in psychosocial functioning. It is also critical to distinguish ARFID from AN. Although both disorders are associated with serious nutritional problems, individuals with AN, unlike those with ARFID, describe a marked overconcern about shape and weight and an intense fear of gaining weight or becoming obese.

Pica

Pica refers to persistent consumption of nonnutritive, nonfood items that is inappropriate for the individual's developmental age. Pica may occur in association with a number of medical conditions, including during normal pregnancy. The disorder should not be assigned if it is occurring in the context of another mental or medical condition or disorder unless it is so severe that it warrants additional clinical attention.

The only changes recommended to the DSM-IV criteria for pica were minor alterations to the wording of the criteria for clarification and to make clear that the disorder could be assigned to the behavior of adolescents and adults as well as children. The DSM-5 criteria for pica are presented in Box 1–5.

Box 1–5. DSM-5 Criteria for Pica

A. Persistent eating of nonnutritive, nonfood substances over a period of at least 1 month.
B. The eating of nonnutritive, nonfood substances is inappropriate to the developmental level of the individual.
C. The eating behavior is not part of a culturally supported or socially normative practice.
D. If the eating behavior occurs in the context of another mental disorder (e.g., intellectual disability [intellectual developmental disorder], autism spectrum disorder, schizophrenia) or medical condition (including pregnancy), it is sufficiently severe to warrant additional clinical attention.

Excerpted from the *Diagnostic and Statistical Manual of Mental Disorders,* 5th Edition, Arlington, VA, American Psychiatric Association, 2013. Used with permission.

Rumination Disorder

Rumination refers to the persistent, repeated regurgitation of food that has already been swallowed. Relatively little is known about this phenomenon. Rumination occurs among some individuals with AN and BN, but in such cases, an additional diagnosis of rumination disorder is not assigned.

As in the case of pica, the only changes recommended to the DSM-IV criteria for rumination disorder were for the purpose of clarification and to make clear that this disorder can be assigned to individuals across the life span. The DSM-5 criteria for rumination disorder are presented in Box 1–6.

Box 1–6. DSM-5 Criteria for Rumination Disorder

A. Repeated regurgitation of food over a period of at least 1 month. Regurgitated food may be re-chewed, re-swallowed, or spit out.
B. The repeated regurgitation is not attributable to an associated gastrointestinal or other medical condition (e.g., gastroesophageal reflux, pyloric stenosis).
C. The eating disturbance does not occur exclusively during the course of anorexia nervosa, bulimia nervosa, binge-eating disorder, or avoidant/restrictive food intake disorder.

D. If the symptoms occur in the context of another mental disorder (e.g., intellectual disability [intellectual developmental disorder] or another neurodevelopmental disorder), they are sufficiently severe to warrant additional clinical attention.

Conclusion

Virtually all of the diagnostic categories used to describe mental disorders, including the feeding and eating disorders, are based on descriptions of salient psychological and behavioral features but not on a detailed understanding of the underlying causes of the disorders. Nevertheless, the categories are of substantial clinical utility in facilitating accurate communication among patients, clinicians, and investigators. Changes to diagnostic criteria for feeding and eating disorders in DSM-5 should significantly reduce the use of residual categories ("not otherwise specified"), encourage continued research, including about ARFID and BED, and, it is hoped, provide a useful foundation for improved care of patients.

Key Clinical Points

- The fundamental features required for the diagnosis of anorexia nervosa (AN) and bulimia nervosa are unchanged in DSM-5.
- Binge-eating disorder was formally recognized in DSM-5.
- The avoidant/restrictive food intake disorder (ARFID) description includes a range of abnormal eating patterns that lead to significant nutritional or psychosocial problems.
- An important feature distinguishing ARFID from AN is the absence of fear of gaining weight or becoming fat.
- Although the feeding and eating disorders often develop during childhood or adolescence, they can occur throughout the lifetime and may present in adulthood.

References

Allison DB, Downey M, Atkinson RL, et al: Obesity as a disease: a white paper on evidence and arguments commissioned by the Council of the Obesity Society. Obesity (Silver Spring) 16(6):1161–1177, 2008 18464753

American Psychiatric Association: Diagnostic and Statistical Manual of Mental Disorders, 3rd Edition. Washington, DC, American Psychiatric Association, 1980

American Psychiatric Association: Diagnostic and Statistical Manual of Mental Disorders, 3rd Edition, Revised. Washington, DC, American Psychiatric Association, 1987

American Psychiatric Association: Diagnostic and Statistical Manual of Mental Disorders, 4th Edition. Washington, DC, American Psychiatric Association, 1994

American Psychiatric Association: Diagnostic and Statistical Manual of Mental Disorders, 5th Edition. Arlington, VA, American Psychiatric Association, 2013

Attia E, Roberto CA: Should amenorrhea be a diagnostic criterion for anorexia nervosa? Int J Eat Disord 42(7):581–589, 2009 19621464

Bryant-Waugh R, Markham L, Kreipe RE, et al: Feeding and eating disorders in childhood. Int J Eat Disord 43(2):98–111, 2010 20063374

Fairburn CG, Bohn K: Eating disorder NOS (EDNOS): an example of the troublesome "not otherwise specified" (NOS) category in DSM-IV. Behav Res Ther 43(6):691–701, 2005 15890163

Fisher MM, Rosen DS, Ornstein RM, et al: Characteristics of avoidant/restrictive food intake disorder in children and adolescents: a "new disorder" in DSM-5. J Adolesc Health 55(1):49–52, 2014 24506978

Gull WW: Anorexia nervosa (apepsia hysterica, anorexia hysterica). 1868. Obes Res 5(5):498–502, 1997 9385628

Helzer JE, Kraemer HC, Krueger RF, et al: Dimensional Approaches in Diagnostic Classification. Arlington, VA, American Psychiatric Association, 2008

Morton R: Phthisiologia, or, A Treatise of Consumptions. London, Smith & Walford, 1694

Ornstein RM, Rosen DS, Mammel KA, et al: Distribution of eating disorders in children and adolescents using the proposed DSM-5 criteria for feeding and eating disorders. J Adolesc Health 53(2):303–305, 2013 23684215

Ruderfer DM, Fanous AH, Ripke S, et al; Schizophrenia Working Group of Psychiatric Genomics Consortium; Bipolar Disorder Working Group of Psychiatric Genomics Consortium; Cross-Disorder Working Group of Psychiatric Genomics Consortium: Polygenic dissection of diagnosis and clinical dimensions of bipolar disorder and schizophrenia. Mol Psychiatry 19(9):1017–1024, 2014 24280982

Russell G: Bulimia nervosa: an ominous variant of anorexia nervosa. Psychol Med 9(3):429–448, 1979 482466

Striegel-Moore RH, Wonderlich SA, Walsh BT, et al (eds): Developing an Evidence-Based Classification of Eating Disorders: Scientific Findings for DSM-5. Arlington, VA, American Psychiatric Association, 2011

Szasz TS: The myth of mental illness. Am Psychol 15(2):113–118, 1960

van Hoeken D, Veling W, Sinke S, et al: The validity and utility of subtyping bulimia nervosa. Int J Eat Disord 42(7):595–602, 2009 19621467

Wilson GT, Sysko R: Frequency of binge eating episodes in bulimia nervosa and binge eating disorder: diagnostic considerations. Int J Eat Disord 42(7):603–610, 2009 19610014

Wolk SL, Loeb KL, Walsh BT: Assessment of patients with anorexia nervosa: interview versus self-report. Int J Eat Disord 37(2):92–99, 2005 15732073

Wonderlich SA, Gordon KH, Mitchell JE, et al: The validity and clinical utility of binge eating disorder. Int J Eat Disord 42(8):687–705, 2009 19621466

PART II

Evaluation and Diagnosis of Eating Problems

2 Eating Problems in Adults

Amanda Joelle Brown, Ph.D.
Janet Schebendach, Ph.D.
B. Timothy Walsh, M.D.

Eating problems and unhealthy weight-control behaviors are common to the point of being almost normative among adults in developed countries. In a U.S. population-based study (Neumark-Sztainer et al. 2011), 59% of young adult women reported currently dieting, 21% endorsed extreme weight-control behaviors (e.g., self-induced vomiting, inappropriate use of laxatives), and 14% reported binge eating with loss of control over a period of 1 year. Although the rates of diagnosable eating disorders are substantially lower, they are still notable, with lifetime prevalence rates of anorexia nervosa (AN), bulimia nervosa (BN), and binge-eating disorder (BED) ranging from 1% to 4% in epidemiological studies (Smink et al. 2012). Individuals with disordered eating often have complex histories and a range of symptoms that may not be easily observable or readily disclosed by the patient in the absence of direct questioning. The goal of any clinical assessment of eating problems in adults is to elicit sufficiently detailed information from the patient to facilitate the accurate description of his or her presenting symptoms and to guide appropriate treatment recommendations.

In this chapter, we describe an approach to the assessment of eating problems that is meant to be applicable in a variety of settings, including primary care and general psychiatric clinics. The approach includes an assessment of broad categories of eating-related symptoms, concerns about body shape and weight, medical and psychiatric comorbidities, social and occupational functioning, and treatment needs. Subgroups based on clusters of symptoms, including the diagnostic categories defined in DSM-5 (American Psychiatric Association 2013), are identified and described. We intend this approach to be useful for the early identification of feeding and eating disorders, the clinical management of early warning signs, and the identification of patients who should be referred for specialized care. We also comment on some of the potential challenges inherent in assessing individuals with eating disorders, including their tendency to minimize symptoms and frequent reluctance to admit the severity of their problems. The reader is encouraged to view Video 2, "Assessing eating problems in the primary care setting."

The Clinical Interview: An Overview

A variety of factors may prompt a clinician to conduct an in-depth evaluation of eating pathology. Significant increases, decreases, or fluctuations in weight over a relatively short period of time are clear signals for clinicians to ask a patient about his or her eating behavior. In addition, description of increasingly restrictive eating patterns, excessive concern with body shape and weight, and unexplained laboratory results (e.g., hypokalemia) may all be early warning signs of an eating disorder and should prompt follow-up questioning. The clinician conducting the interview may be the first treatment provider to assess the eating problem or may have received a referral from another provider who had reason to suspect an eating problem. When the patient has been referred, it may be helpful to start the interview by asking the patient to describe his or her understanding of why the referral was made, both to assess the patient's level of insight about the eating problem and to avoid "blindsiding" him or her with sensitive questions if the reasons for the referral were not previously clarified.

The primary goal of the clinical interview is to allow the patient to describe his or her current symptoms and to reflect on the development of these problems from his or her perspective. Patients with eating disorders are not always the most reliable reporters of their own struggles because of influences such as cognitive impairment from nutritional deprivation, the tendency to deny the potentially serious nature of their disorder, deliberate or unconscious minimization of symptoms, and ambivalence about treatment and/or recovery. Therefore, obtaining collateral information from the patient's family, other clinicians involved in his or her care, and previous treatment providers can be critically helpful and informative.

Given the aforementioned challenges to obtaining accurate self-reported information from patients with eating problems, it is essential that clinicians assume a collaborative, nonjudgmental stance during the clinical interview. The creation of a strong therapeutic alliance, through such tactics as asking open-ended questions and inquiring about the patient's understanding of his or her difficulties, facilitates the collection of accurate information and can be instrumental in strengthening patients' motivation for change. A patient may deny any understanding of the reason for the evaluation, may express annoyance at having to speak with a clinician, and may not feel that he or she has a significant clinical problem. In such instances, the clinician can assure the patient that the clinician is not making any value judgments about the patient's behavior and should aim to ally with the patient to help him or her better understand why other people might be concerned about his or her health and well-being. In many cases, the clinician's view of the patient's symptoms may differ from the patient's view; however, in all circumstances, open and empathic dialogue will assist in the formation of a therapeutic alliance and increase the likelihood of obtaining accurate information.

Video 2 presents a sample clinical assessment by a general practitioner.

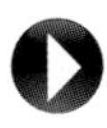

Video Illustration 2: Assessing eating problems in the primary care setting (3:24)

Assessment of Eating Behaviors

Development of Eating Problems

Once the patient understands the reason for the assessment, the focus of the interview should shift to a review of the development of the patient's eating symptoms. A history of changes in weight and eating behaviors should be obtained, beginning with open-ended questions about changes in the recent past or during the current disordered eating "episode." The patient should be encouraged to describe events or experiences (e.g., emotional or environmental) that he or she considers relevant to the development or exacerbation of the current eating problems. Because the onset of an eating disorder is frequently associated with a significant life change or interpersonal event, the clinician should ask the patient to describe the circumstances of his or her life at the time that symptoms began. Furthermore, while obtaining historical information about the evolution of eating symptoms, the clinician should be sensitive to information about personal life events that may have had a direct or indirect influence on illness progression.

A critical component of the assessment of individuals with disordered eating is obtaining a picture of the patient's current eating habits by asking the patient to describe the frequency and content of meals and snacks on a recent typical day. The clinician should also specifically inquire about several eating-related behaviors. The following sections outline categories of eating and eating-related symptoms that need specific attention in a clinical evaluation of a potential eating problem. Readers are referred to Table 2–1 for sample interview questions related to this approach.

Energy and Macronutrient Restriction

Individuals with eating disorders typically restrict their calorie intake; some do so consistently, whereas others eat normal amounts of food or binge eat between periods of restriction. Many patients attempt to adhere to a daily calorie limit. This amount should be ascertained by the clinician and assessed within the context of normal energy requirements. For example, a healthy adult female (age 25 years, height 64 inches, weight 120 pounds, body mass index 20.6 kg/m^2) requires about 2,000–2,400 kcal/day at low to moderate levels of physical activity for weight maintenance (U.S. Department of Agriculture and U.S. Department of Health and Human Services 2010). On average, patients with AN consume about 1,300 kcal/day (Forbush and Hunt 2014). Eating patterns outside of binge episodes are inconsistent in BN; some individuals restrict their food and energy intake, some eat normally, and others overeat (Forbush and Hunt 2014). Individuals with BED typically do not restrict their intake outside of binge episodes, often leading to substantial weight gain and obesity (American Psychiatric Association 2013).

Patients frequently monitor their food intake and count calories. It is noteworthy, however, that individuals with AN tend to overestimate their energy intake by approximately 20% (Schebendach et al. 2012). If the patient sets a daily calorie limit, the clinician should ask if there are consequences to exceeding that limit. For example, the individual may further decrease calorie intake, fast, increase exercise, or engage in purging behaviors on the following day.

In patients with AN, calorie restriction is typically accomplished by limiting fat intake (Forbush and Hunt 2014). Given that fat is the most energy-dense macronutrient (i.e., 9 kcal/g for fat vs. 4 kcal/g for carbohydrate and protein), there is logic to fat avoidance. Furthermore, with public health campaigns promoting low-fat, heart-healthy eating, patients can easily cloak their disordered eating behavior in the guise of a healthy lifestyle. Current U.S. dietary guidelines recommend that 20%–35% of total calorie intake be provided by fat; for a healthy, normal-weight female, this

TABLE 2–1. Sample questions to assess diet and eating behaviors

Energy and macronutrients	Do you limit your intake of calories, fat, carbohydrates, or protein?
	Do you have a specific daily limit or an acceptable range?
	Do you self-monitor your intake?
	What happens if you exceed your limit?
	Do you avoid any specific foods or food groups, such as added fats, red meat, fried foods, or desserts?
	Are you on a vegetarian or vegan diet?
Other dietary restrictions	Is your food choice limited by any condition or restriction?
	Food allergies?
	Food intolerances (e.g., lactose, gluten)?
	Religious or culturally based diet restrictions?
Meal patterns	How many meals and snacks do you eat each day?
	What are your typical mealtimes and snack times?
	Do you eat differently on different days of the week
	Workdays versus days off?
	Weekdays versus weekends?
Eating behaviors	Do you engage in any specific behaviors related to your food?
	Follow a strictly planned diet (i.e., calories, percentage of fat/carbohydrates/protein)?
	Weigh and measure your food intake?
	Use utensils to eat foods that are typically eaten by hand?
	Eat very slowly or very quickly?
	Prefer to eat alone and avoid others seeing you eat?
	Avoid eating foods prepared by others?
Binge eating	Do you ever feel a sense of loss of control over your eating?
	What are the contents of a typical binge-eating episode for you?
	Types of food consumed?
	Amounts (large vs. average/small)?
	How often do you binge eat in a given day, week, or month?
	Are your binge-eating episodes typically planned or impulsive?

TABLE 2–1. Sample questions to assess diet and eating behaviors *(continued)*

Purging	Do you do anything to purge food or "get rid of" calories?
	How often do you purge in a given day, week, or month?
	Do you use laxatives or enemas?
	Type/brand, dose, frequency?
	Do you take diuretics?
	Type/brand, dose, frequency?
	Do you exercise excessively and/or feel driven or compelled to exercise?
	Type/intensity/frequency of exercise?
	How do you feel if you are unable to exercise?

translates into 44–93 g/day of fat (U.S. Department of Agriculture and U.S. Department of Health and Human Services 2010). Patients with eating disorders often set a daily fat-gram limit and monitor their intake and derive a significantly lower fraction of their caloric intake from fat (Mayer et al. 2012). The evaluating clinician should therefore assess the degree of dietary fat restriction, as well as the inclusion or exclusion of added fats (e.g., oil, salad dressing, mayonnaise, butter) and fat-containing foods (e.g., dairy products, red meat, desserts).

Individuals with AN have also been described as carbohydrate avoidant (Russell 1967). However, carbohydrate restriction appears to be less pronounced than fat restriction. The U.S. dietary guidelines recommend carbohydrate intakes in the range of 45%–65% of calories; this translates into approximately 225–390 g/day for a female (U.S. Department of Agriculture and U.S. Department of Health and Human Services 2010). The fraction of calories from carbohydrates among individuals with AN is similar to or even a bit greater than that among healthy individuals (Mayer et al. 2012). Patients with restrictive eating typically avoid high-sugar foods, such as desserts, sweetened beverages, and added sugars, but they may also restrict their intake of natural carbohydrate sources, such as milk, fruit, fruit juice, and grains. In recent years, gluten-free diets have been adopted by many individuals for the purpose of weight loss, and patients with eating disorders may be similarly influenced by this dieting trend. Once again, the clinician should determine the presence and degree of dietary carbohydrate restriction, as well as self-monitoring (i.e., carbohydrate counting) behaviors.

Total protein intake may also be inadequate. In general, patients are less likely to restrict or monitor their protein intake, and some may even take protein and amino acid supplements. However, in an effort to decrease fat intake, many individuals narrow their repertoire of high-protein food choices by excluding red meat, cheese, milk, eggs, and nuts. Some individuals adopt vegetarian and vegan (i.e., no animal products) dietary practices during the course of their illness. The clinician should determine the timeline for adoption of a vegetarian or vegan diet and ask whether other household members eat a similar diet.

Claims of food allergies, food intolerances (e.g., lactose, gluten), and religious or cultural dietary practices may complicate the clinical assessment of eating disorders. The clinician should determine whether the diagnosis of a food allergy or intolerance has been confirmed by broadly accepted objective testing. Food restriction due to cultural norms and religious practices should be assessed within the context of family and peer group practices. Meal patterns, mealtimes, and the amount of time needed to consume a meal or snack should be ascertained. Behaviors such as preplanning food intake, weighing and measuring foods, only eating alone, not eating foods prepared by others, unusual cutting and food-handling behaviors, blotting oil or fat off foods, and atypical handling of eating utensils should also be explored.

Avoidant/restrictive food intake disorder (ARFID) is a DSM-5 diagnosis characterized by a general lack of interest in food (i.e., a "picky" or "lazy" eater), sensory food aversions (e.g., to appearance, smell, color, texture/consistency, taste, or temperature), concern about an aversive consequence of eating (e.g., choking), and/or a diet that consists of a markedly limited range of foods and little day-to-day variation in food intake. ARFID-related eating behaviors may result in a persistent failure to meet energy and nutrient requirements, and enteral feedings or oral nutritional supplements may be necessary (American Psychiatric Association 2013). During the assessment interview, the patient should be asked about current food intake (i.e., range of choice, amounts); duration of avoidant/restrictive behaviors; use of dietary supplements; and the degree to which current eating behaviors cause distress or interfere with day-to-day functioning (Bryant-Waugh 2013).

Binge Eating

The occurrence (times of day), duration, and frequency (episodes per day and week) of binge-eating episodes should be explored with all patients undergoing an evaluation for disordered eating. Binge eating is a defining characteristic of BN and BED and is also seen among a subset of individuals with the binge-eating/purging subtype of AN. Although the DSM-5 definition of binge eating requires the consumption of an objectively large amount of food, many individuals refer to the consumption of a modest or even small amount of food they had not intended to eat as a binge (i.e., a subjective binge). A shared characteristic of objective and subjective binge-eating episodes is a sense of loss of control over what or how much is eaten. The clinician should ascertain what is consumed during a typical episode of binge eating, as well as whether binge episodes tend to be planned or impulsive. Potential binge "triggers," such as emotional precipitants (e.g., stress, anxiety, depression, sadness), particular settings (e.g., restaurants, buffets, bakeries, supermarkets, social gatherings), and food cravings, should also be explored.

Purging Behaviors

The occurrence and frequency of purging behaviors, such as self-induced vomiting and laxative or diuretic misuse, should also be determined. Vomiting may be induced by stimulating the gag reflex with a finger, pencil, toothbrush, eating utensil, and so forth. Dental erosion, parotid gland hypertrophy, and Russell's sign (scarring of the dorsum of the hand) may suggest a longer duration of vomiting behavior. Use of an instrument to induce vomiting warrants exploration because of the potential risk of swallowing the device during the process. Syrup of ipecac is less commonly used to induce vomiting than in the past. Where the vomiting occurs (e.g., in a private vs. public bathroom, into a trash receptacle) may suggest how entrenched the purging behavior is for a given individual. If laxatives and diuretics are used, the type and brand, amount taken, and frequency of use should be ascertained. In addition to exploring the actual behavior, the clinician should question the patient's beliefs about the efficacy of purging methods. For example, the patient may believe that vomiting eliminates all calories consumed during a binge or that laxatives interfere with calorie absorption; inquiries into the patient's assumptions and beliefs provide an opportunity for psychoeducation about the relative inefficacy of purging (see Kaye et al. 1993).

Rumination

Patients with eating disorders may engage in rumination behavior–that is, regurgitating, re-chewing, and re-swallowing or spitting out of food. This behavior should be specifically queried. If the rumination behavior occurs exclusive of another eating disorder (i.e., AN, BN, BED, ARFID) or a medical condition and the severity of the behavior necessitates clinical attention, then a DSM-5 diagnosis of rumination disorder is warranted (American Psychiatric Association 2013).

Pica

Patients should be queried regarding *pica*, the consumption of nonfood items. The diagnosis of pica is characterized by a persistent ingestion of one or more nonnutritive, nonfood substances (e.g., chalk, soap, cloth, nails, paper, soil) over a period of at least 1 month. Although this behavior may occur in patients with other psychiatric disorders (e.g., developmental disorders, autism, schizophrenia) or medical conditions (e.g., pregnancy), a separate DSM-5 diagnosis of pica is made when the severity of the eating behavior warrants specific clinical management (American Psychiatric Association 2013).

Assessment of Shape and Weight Concerns

In addition to obtaining detailed information about the patient's current eating habits and the development of restricting, binge-eating, and purging behaviors, it is essential to the proper characterization of eating problems for the clinician to assess the patient's experience of his or her body shape and weight. Regardless of the patient's likely diagnosis, any assessment of eating-related pathology should include documentation of changes in weight and body size, including lifetime highest and lowest weights and any significant weight fluctuations. The clinician should also inquire about the patient's ideal weight, the patient's view of his or her current weight (e.g., too high, too low, tolerable, unacceptable), and the importance of shape or weight in the patient's self-evaluation.

Shape and weight concerns are important to both the onset and maintenance of eating-disordered thoughts and behaviors, and they play an essential role in differential diagnosis. Pica, rumination disorder, and ARFID are not associated with significant disturbances in the perception or evaluation of body shape and weight (American Psychiatric Association 2013). Individuals whose restrictive eating behaviors lead to significantly low body weight may meet DSM-5 diagnostic criteria for either AN or ARFID; shape and weight concerns distinguish these diagnoses from one another. Shape and weight concerns are a salient distinguishing feature of these diagnoses. Disturbances in the experience of body shape or weight, undue influence of body weight or shape on self-evaluation, and persistent lack of recognition of the seriousness of the current low body weight are characteristic of individuals with AN, whereas there is no evidence of a disturbance in the way in which one's body weight or shape is experienced among individuals with ARFID.

Furthermore, many individuals with AN report an intense fear of gaining weight or becoming fat. Explicit endorsement of this fear was a diagnostic requirement for AN in DSM-IV, but the criterion has been expanded in DSM-5 to include persistent behavior that interferes with weight gain despite the patient being at a significantly low weight. Focused inquiry regarding what foods the patient actually consumes and his or her emotional reaction to weight gain may elucidate the patient's level of concern about body shape and weight. Family members and treatment providers familiar with the patient's eating attitudes and behaviors may offer additional evidence to support or refute strong fears of weight gain.

DSM-5 also requires that individuals with BN endorse overconcern with body shape and weight. Although it is normal for body image to play a role in the regulation of self-esteem, individuals with BN overvalue shape and weight compared to individuals without eating disorders. Individuals with BED also typically endorse shape and weight concerns to a higher degree than individuals of a similar body size who do not binge eat, but such concern is not required for the diagnosis of BED according to DSM-5 criteria. Notably, overvaluation of shape and weight plays a key role in the transdiagnostic model of AN, BN, and BED and informs cognitive-behavioral therapy for eating disorders (Fairburn et al. 2003).

Assessment of Medical and Psychological Features Associated With Eating Problems

Physical Assessments

An essential component of the assessment of adults with eating problems is obtaining objective measures of current physical health status. Measuring height and weight, taking vital signs (e.g., pulse, blood pressure), performing a general physical examination, and obtaining laboratory tests are all important and can be done either by the clinician assessing the history, if he or she has the requisite training and experience, or by a physician who serves a general medical role. The nature of the presenting problem and the clinician's observations of the patient should inform the necessity for and extensiveness of the physical examination. For example, a patient with a history of substantial weight loss or of frequent purging is in more urgent need of a full medical workup than one with a normal, stable weight whose main presenting problem is psychological overconcern with body size.

Medical Complications

In addition to conducting an extensive assessment of the patient's current physical health status, the clinician should ask whether the patient has experienced any physical problems as a consequence of his or her eating disturbance. Specific inquiry should be made about emergency room visits, less acute medical and dental care, and the existence of physical or medical complications such as changes to skin, hair, or nails; dental complications, including dental caries and/or enamel erosion; and stress fractures or other evidence of osteoporosis. Medical complications associated with AN and BN are listed in Table 2–2. The medical complications associated with BED are those associated with overweight and obesity, including hypertension, cardiovascular disease, and diabetes.

Laboratory assessments, including blood tests for hemoglobin, white blood cell count, and a chemistry panel, should be included in a comprehensive physical assessment, because blood cell counts may be low in the context of undernutrition, and metabolic and electrolyte disturbances are common. One of the most dangerous electrolyte disturbances is low potassium, or hypokalemia, which often is a result of recurrent vomiting but may also occur secondary to severe and prolonged food restriction. Hypokalemia can result in cardiac arrhythmias and therefore must be regularly monitored, especially in high-risk cases (e.g., individuals with purging behaviors). Prolongation of QT and QTc (rate corrected) intervals is also possible, even in the absence of electrolyte abnormalities, and this risk may rise with decreasing weight (Takimoto et al. 2004). Electrocardiograms are essential to further evaluate the acuity of the hypokalemia and assess for signs of arrhythmias. Hypomagnesemia may also occur with hypokalemia and if left untreated will prevent sustained normalization of potassium.

Low sodium, or hyponatremia, may be present and is commonly accompanied by low chloride levels, or hypochloremia. The hyponatremia associated with eating disorders generally results from one of two possible mechanisms (Bahia et al. 2011). The more common is that related to increased water intake. Through normal homeostatic processes, patients lose sodium and water through sweat and urine. Drinking water alone is insufficient to replace these losses, and the sodium concentration in the blood is ultimately diluted. A second potential etiology of hyponatremia is the development of the syndrome of inappropriate antidiuretic hormone secretion (SIADH). In both cases, water restriction is usually the treatment of choice for clinically significant hyponatremia. If fluid restriction is insufficient to fully restore electrolyte balance (sodium levels), medical consultation should be obtained. Although the low sodium in patients

TABLE 2–2. Some physical and laboratory findings associated with anorexia nervosa and bulimia nervosa

	Anorexia nervosa[a]	Bulimia nervosa
Skin/extremities	Lanugo (fine hair on trunk/face)	Callus on back of hand
	Red/blue fingers	
	Edema	
Cardiovascular	Low pulse rate	
	Low blood pressure	
Gastrointestinal	Salivary gland enlargement	Salivary gland enlargement
	Slow stomach emptying	
	Constipation	Dental erosion
	Liver abnormalities	
Hematopoietic	Anemia	
	Low white blood cell count	
Fluid/electrolyte	Decreased kidney function	Low blood potassium
	Low blood potassium	Low blood sodium
	Low blood sodium	Reduced blood acidity
	Low blood phosphate	
Endocrine	Low blood sugar	
	Low estrogen or testosterone	
	Low-normal thyroid hormone levels	
	Increased cortisol	
Bone	Decreased bone density	

[a]Patients with the binge-eating/purging subtype of anorexia nervosa are at risk for the physical and laboratory findings associated with bulimia nervosa in the context of frequent purging.
Source. Adapted from Walsh and Attia 2011.

with AN is often the result of a gradual and chronic state, acute hyponatremia can precipitate seizures, and thus regular monitoring of electrolytes is indicated.

Signs of dehydration are common and can include tachycardia, orthostatic hypotension, and laboratory abnormalities suggestive of prerenal azotemia, including elevated creatinine and blood urea nitrogen levels. These issues generally resolve with resumption of regular food and fluid intake. However, the patient with symptoms of dehydration (e.g., lightheadedness, syncope) may require intravenous hydration, which will normalize these physical and laboratory abnormalities more quickly.

Refeeding syndrome, which can occur during the initial stages of weight recovery, is marked by metabolic disturbances and volume overload manifesting as edema (pedal and/or pulmonary) and cardiac failure. Reports indicate that early hypophosphatemia is a harbinger of refeeding syndrome (Ornstein et al. 2003; Trent et al. 2013). The mechanism of refeeding syndrome is thought to be related to changes in insulin-glucose functioning and the requirements for phosphorus, magnesium, and other elements in the catabolic process. Despite normal serum levels of phosphorus on initial evaluation, phosphorus levels may fall upon initiation of refeeding, with the nadir often occurring 3–4 days following the initiation of refeeding. Thus, phosphate levels should be monitored regularly during initial resumption of regular food intake and repleted as necessary.

In cases of significant food restriction, specific nutrient or vitamin deficiencies may be present, even if absolute weight is close to normal. For example, individuals who avoid fruits and vegetables or who eat a limited range of foods may need vitamin supplements. Those who refuse to swallow a recommended multivitamin supplement because of its feel or smell should be monitored for vitamin deficiencies.

Almost all of these medical complications are reversible with adequate nutrition. Supportive measures such as careful monitoring of cardiac function or electrolyte levels may be necessary for successful and safe refeeding. Slowed gastric motility becomes important during nutritional rehabilitation (see Chapter 13, "Treatment of Restrictive Eating and Low-Weight Conditions, Including Anorexia Nervosa and Avoidant/Restrictive Food Intake Disorder"); fullness and possible constipation may cause the refeeding process to be physically uncomfortable.

Comorbid Conditions

Because of the frequent occurrence of mood disturbance and substance abuse among individuals with eating disorders, symptoms of these and other psychiatric disorders should be reviewed during the clinical assessment of concerns related to eating and weight. Specific questions about the use of drugs and alcohol, both currently and in the past, should be asked directly in a nonjudgmental fashion. The clinician should be mindful of patients' potential reluctance to disclose such information and should assume an open, curious stance. Individuals at significantly low weight almost invariably endorse depressive symptoms, because such symptoms are associated with the pathophysiology of starvation and malnutrition (Keys et al. 1950, as cited in Kalm and Semba 2005). A detailed assessment of the course of mood symptoms and eating pathology may elucidate the relationship between these two domains, such as if a mood disorder was present prior to the onset of eating disorder symptoms or if mood disturbance developed solely in the context of weight loss or malnutrition.

Anxiety disorders, obsessive-compulsive and related disorders, and trauma- and stressor-related disorders may also be comorbid with eating disorders. Once again, it may be difficult to accurately attribute symptoms to one disorder or another, and clinicians should be aware that eating disorders, particularly AN, often involve heightened obsessionality and anxiety, both in the domain of food and eating and in other domains. The clinician should also be alert for indications of personality disorders, which are relatively common among individuals with eating disturbances. Personality traits commonly associated with eating disorders include perfectionism, impulsivity, and novelty seeking (Cassin and von Ranson 2005).

Differential Diagnosis

Before concluding that a patient's difficulties are best attributed to the existence of an eating disorder, the clinician should consider whether the eating disturbances are better accounted for by another psychiatric disorder or whether the symptoms may be secondary to a general medical condition. For example, binge-eating episodes may occur in association with major depressive disorder, and many medical illnesses can lead to substantial weight loss. Clinicians should consider the possibility that another medical or psychological issue accounts for the patient's eating or weight symptoms, particularly when the history is unclear or the features are unusual.

Differential diagnosis when the primary symptoms are restrictive eating and/or low weight involves assessment of the underlying assumptions and motivations for the abnormal eating behavior. Mood, anxiety, and psychotic disorders may occasionally be associated with weight loss and disturbances in eating behavior, but the concerns about shape and weight that are characteristic of AN are not present in these illnesses. Similarly, some of the psychological characteristics of individuals with social anxiety disorder, obsessive-compulsive disorder, or body dysmorphic disorder resemble those of patients with AN; however, individuals with these disorders do not exhibit the unrelenting drive for thinness seen in patients with AN.

Overeating with loss of control, a defining feature of BN and BED, may sometimes occur in association with major depressive disorder with atypical features and with borderline personality disorder. These disorders may be comorbid with BN or BED, and if a patient meets criteria for both BN or BED and another mental disorder, both diagnoses should be given. However, if the patient does not endorse overconcern with body shape and weight, a diagnosis of BN should not be given. Also, if binge eating does not occur at an average frequency of at least one episode a week, an alternative diagnosis should be considered. In this case, if no other psychological disorder is warranted and the eating symptoms are significant enough to cause distress or impairment, the diagnosis should be other specified feeding or eating disorder (e.g., BN or BED of low frequency and/or limited duration).

Many serious medical illnesses are associated with substantial weight loss, including gastrointestinal illnesses such as Crohn's disease and celiac disease, brain tumors and other malignancies, and AIDS. Some medical and neurological conditions, such as Kleine-Levin syndrome, are associated with binge eating. These and other medical illnesses should be considered in the differential diagnosis. Occasionally, an eating disorder and a medical illness occur together and multiple diagnoses are warranted. Key features are the intense psychological reward associated with losing weight and the fear of weight gain in AN and the use of compensatory behaviors to control weight and the overconcern with shape and weight that characterize BN.

Assessment of Family History and Social and Occupational Functioning

Two other areas warranting attention are the familial history of eating disorders and the patient's occupational and social history. Regardless of whether other family members have been formally diagnosed with eating disorder, the family's attitudes toward eating and accompanying behaviors (e.g., dieting), especially if taken to an extreme, can play a significant role in the formation of patients' attitudes and behaviors. The clinician should inquire about these family patterns, if not already volunteered by the patient, and the effect on his or her relationship to food. Similarly, the emphasis on shape and weight within the family structure and its influence on the patient's perceptions of shape and weight should be discussed.

A standard assessment of social, interpersonal, and occupational difficulties should be conducted, specifically noting the impact of the eating problem on the formation and maintenance of interpersonal relationships (e.g., loss of friendships due to avoidance of social eating) and on work or academic performance. Individuals with eating disturbances frequently engage in occupations in which shape and weight are highly emphasized (e.g., personal trainer) or food is the focal point (e.g., waitress). Whether the pursuit of such careers is a contributing factor to or a by-product of the eating disturbance undoubtedly varies, but the relationship of these occupations to the chronology of changes in eating and dieting practices should be reviewed. Such information may prove valuable in treatment planning when a consideration of career plans can be more thoroughly evaluated.

Assessment of Treatment Needs

The final step in the clinical evaluation of eating problems in adults is the assessment of treatment needs and the formulation of a plan for follow-up care. Various treatment settings (e.g., inpatient, partial hospitalization, outpatient), modalities (e.g., behavioral, cognitive, interpersonal, family oriented, psychopharmacological, medical), and intensities are currently employed in the treatment of eating disorders (see Part 4, "Treatment," in this volume). The nature of the patient's past treatments should be assessed, with the caveat that these treatments may be difficult for the patient (or clinician) to characterize accurately. Furthermore, for a patient with a long history of illness, a complete history of treatment may be too lengthy to obtain in a single assessment. The clinician should strongly consider, with the patient's permission, speaking with past treatment providers and obtaining a copy of important historical documents (e.g., hospital discharge summaries). It is important to ascertain whether and how often the patient has been hospitalized for treatment of an eating disorder or its complications, what psychological strategies and medication interventions have been attempted, and what the patient has found to be most and least helpful. It is also useful to determine the reason for termination of past treatment (e.g., expiration of insurance coverage, the patient's leaving treatment against medical advice).

The severity of the patient's current eating problems is the most important factor to consider in determining a recommended level of care. Medical instability, including such disturbances as low heart rate (e.g., <40 beats per minute), low blood pressure (e.g., <90/60 mmHg), electrolyte imbalance, dehydration, and organ failure requiring acute treatment, requires inpatient hospitalization. In addition, suicidal ideation with a specific plan or intent is a clear indicator of a need for hospitalization and should be assessed during the clinical interview. Maintenance of a body weight below 80% of expected weight for age, sex, and height or acute weight loss in the context of food refusal also suggests that a higher level of care (e.g., inpatient, residential) may be warranted. If a high degree of structure seems necessary for the patient to eat and gain weight, partial or full hospitalization should be considered. Success or failure in less intensive treatments may be the best indicator of this necessity (Yager et al. 2006).

A patient's motivation for change, cooperativeness, insight, and ability to control obsessive thoughts about food and eating should be at least fair if outpatient treatment is to be considered. Patients with severe symptoms but poor insight, little motivation, and constant preoccupation with eating-related obsessions require a higher level of care. In addition, any comorbid psychiatric illness requiring hospitalization (e.g., psychotic illness, severe obsessive-compulsive disorder) precludes the recommendation of outpatient or day programs. Finally, severe environmental stress, including family conflict, absent or inadequate social support, or unstable living arrangements, may influence clinical decision making about the proper level of care (Yager et al. 2006).

Patients for whom highly structured treatment programs are recommended should be aware that such programs represent only the beginning step in what is likely to be a lengthy process of treatment and recovery. The least restrictive environment that provides adequate support for the patient to practice making healthier eating choices should always be recommended, because practicing new behaviors in a familiar environment has the greatest potential to effect substantive and lasting change.

Challenges and Obstacles in the Assessment of Eating Problems

Cognitive Impairment

The clinician should be aware that severe malnutrition is associated not only with serious physical problems but also with significant psychological and cognitive disturbances. Underweight patients may exhibit delays in speech, illogical thought patterns, and difficulty concentrating. These disturbances may interfere with a patient's ability to reflect on his or her condition or to accurately report on his or her symptoms. It may be clinically useful to gently, without blame or judgment, draw the patient's attention to these psychological consequences of starvation in order to foster greater insight. At the same time, it is important to recognize that malnourished patients may misremember autobiographical information, experience intrusive thoughts during the course of the interview, and have difficulty answering more complex questions. Framing questions simply and directly will help patients maintain their focus and provide the most accurate information.

Patient Reluctance to Provide Information

For a variety of reasons, patients may be reluctant to provide accurate information about their difficulties. In some instances, patients are ashamed of beliefs or behaviors that they recognize as abnormal but feel unable to control. Patients may deny that they purge, may overreport their daily calorie consumption, or may consume excessive amounts of liquids or carry concealed objects when they are weighed. No approach to such denial and subterfuge is universally effective; however, it may be useful for the clinician to note that individuals with eating problems commonly have difficulties being open about all aspects of their disorder and therefore to ask, in a nonconfrontational manner, whether there are symptoms the patient has difficulty admitting. The clinician should avoid criticizing the patient for not being open, because such maneuvers are unlikely to yield more accurate information and will undermine the development of a therapeutic alliance.

Minimization of Symptom Severity and/or Need for Treatment

The final challenge in obtaining information from patients with eating disorders is their difficulty admitting that their behaviors are problematic or potentially harmful (Vitousek et al. 1990). Many deny that they have a psychiatric illness and decline offers for help. Individuals with AN, in particular, often vehemently deny that their weight is dangerously low or that their eating behaviors are not healthy, and many report extreme distortions in body image, often using words such as "obese," "enormous," and "whalelike" to describe their perception of their emaciated bodies. Individuals with BN and BED, particularly those seeking treatment, typically do not describe such drastic differences between their internal experience and the observations of others, but they may minimize the severity of aspects of their eating disorder they consider shameful or embarrassing, such as binge eating, purging, or laxative misuse. Furthermore, patients of any diagnosis who tend toward perfectionism and agreeableness may show overcompliance during the interview, answering questions in the way that he or she interprets as being "right."

We reiterate that there is no one way to deal with minimization, denial, or distortion in a clinical interview. The clinician can reflect back inconsistencies and discrepancies in the information provided by the patient in an open, curious manner, without assuming that the patient is deliberately trying to mislead. Efforts to normalize symptoms may increase patients' willingness to disclose information; for example, the clinician might ask, "Some people who try to keep their weight down do so by cutting out certain food groups–have you ever done that?" or "How many times would you say you binge eat in a given day or week?" By assuming a relatively high degree of symptom frequency or severity, the clinician can communicate to the patient that the symptoms are within the realm of what is typically encountered and may also engender the patient's trust in the clinician as someone who has experienced other individuals with similar struggles.

Conclusion

In this chapter, we have attempted to summarize the essential components of a thorough clinical assessment of individuals with suspected eating disorders. The clinician should obtain a comprehensive description of the patient's eating behavior and the psychological and emotional concomitants of that behavior. The clinician should also attempt to understand how these disturbances began and how they have evolved over time and should assess the patient's commitment to change. Physical assessments should be conducted to identify any medical complications of the disordered eating behavior. Other psychiatric disorders and general medical conditions that involve disturbances in eating and weight should be considered as alternative explanations of the presenting concern. Although the assessment of eating pathology in adults can be challenging because of the shame and secrecy typically involved in these disorders, carrying out the assessment in a thorough but empathic fashion should facilitate the formation of a strong therapeutic alliance with the patient.

Finally, it should be noted that the assessment approach described in this chapter is a semistructured method that can be used in most general clinical settings. A range of more structured assessment methods are available, including the Eating Disorder Assessment for DSM-5 (EDA-5; Sysko et al. 2015), as discussed in Part 3 ("Assessment Tools") of this volume. Such structured and semistructured assessments are routinely used in research settings, and they may also be usefully employed in routine clinical practice to obtain objective measures of the patient's symptoms.

Key Clinical Points

- The overarching goal of the clinical assessment of eating problems in adults is to elicit sufficiently detailed information from the patient to facilitate the accurate description of his or her presenting symptoms and to guide appropriate treatment recommendations.
- The assessment approach described in this chapter is a method that can be used in most general clinical settings. A range of more structured assessment methods are also available.

- The assessment of eating problems should begin with a thorough evaluation of eating behaviors. Once the nature of the eating problem has been established, further information should be obtained to contextualize the eating problem in terms of medical complications, comorbid conditions, social and occupational functioning, and treatment history and needs.
- Physical assessments, including measurement of height and weight, physical examination, and laboratory assessments as indicated, should be routinely included in the assessment of eating disorders in adults.
- The assessment of eating pathology in adults can be challenging because of the shame, secrecy, and ambivalence about change that are often involved in these disorders. A collaborative, nonjudgmental stance will facilitate the collection of accurate information and strengthen patients' motivation for change.

References

American Psychiatric Association: Feeding and eating disorders, in Diagnostic and Statistical Manual of Mental Disorders, 5th Edition. Arlington, VA, American Psychiatric Association, 2013 pp 329–354

Bahia A, Chu ES, Mehler PS: Polydipsia and hyponatremia in a woman with anorexia nervosa. Int J Eat Disord 44(2):186–188, 2011 20127934

Bryant-Waugh R: Avoidant restrictive food intake disorder: an illustrative case example. Int J Eat Disord 46(5):420–423, 2013 23658083

Cassin SE, von Ranson KM: Personality and eating disorders: a decade in review. Clin Psychol Rev 25(7):895–916, 2005 16099563

Fairburn CG, Cooper Z, Shafran R: Cognitive behaviour therapy for eating disorders: a "transdiagnostic" theory and treatment. Behav Res Ther 41(5):509–528, 2003 12711261

Forbush KT, Hunt TK: Characterization of eating patterns among individuals with eating disorders: what is the state of the plate? Physiol Behav 134:92–109, 2014 24582916

Kalm LM, Semba RD: They starved so that others be better fed: remembering Ancel Keys and the Minnesota experiment. J Nutr 135(6):1347–1352, 2005 15930436

Kaye WH, Weltzin TE, Hsu LKG, et al: Amount of calories retained after binge eating and vomiting. Am J Psychiatry 150(6):969–971,1993 8494080

Mayer LE, Schebendach J, Bodell LP, et al: Eating behavior in anorexia nervosa: before and after treatment. Int J Eat Disord 45(2):290–293, 2012 21495053

Neumark-Sztainer D, Wall M, Larson NI, et al: Dieting and disordered eating behaviors from adolescence to young adulthood: findings from a 10-year longitudinal study. J Am Diet Assoc 111(7):1004–1011, 2011 21703378

Ornstein RM, Golden NH, Jacobson MS, et al: Hypophosphatemia during nutritional rehabilitation in anorexia nervosa: implications for refeeding and monitoring. J Adolesc Health 32(1):83–88, 2003 12507806

Russell GFM: The nutritional disorder in anorexia nervosa. J Psychosom Res 11(1):141–149, 1967 6049025

Schebendach JE, Porter KJ, Wolper C, et al: Accuracy of self-reported energy intake in weight-restored patients with anorexia nervosa compared with obese and normal weight individuals. Int J Eat Disord 45(4):570–574, 2012 22271488

Smink FRE, van Hoeken D, Hoek HW: Epidemiology of eating disorders: incidence, prevalence and mortality rates. Curr Psychiatry Rep 14(4):406–414, 2012 22644309

Sysko R, Glasofer DR, Hildebrandt T, et al: The Eating Disorder Assessment for DSM-5 (EDA-5): development and validation of a structured interview for feeding and eating disorders. Int J Eat Disord Jan 30, 2015 [Epub ahead of print] 25639562

Takimoto Y, Yoshiuchi K, Kumano H, et al: QT interval and QT dispersion in eating disorders. Psychother Psychosom 73(5):324–328, 2004 15292631

Trent SA, Moreira ME, Colwell CB, et al: ED management of patients with eating disorders. Am J Emerg Med 31(5):859–865, 2013 23623238

U.S. Department of Agriculture, U.S. Department of Health and Human Services: Dietary Guidelines for Americans, 7th Edition. Washington, DC, U.S. Government Printing Office, 2010

Vitousek KB, Daly J, Heiser C: Reconstructing the internal world of the eating-disordered individual: overcoming denial and distortion in self-report. Int J Eat Disord 10:647–666, 1990

Walsh BT, Attia E: Eating disorders, in Harrison's Principles of Internal Medicine, 18th Edition. Edited by Longo DL, Fauci AS, Kasper DL, et al. New York, McGraw-Hill, 2011, pp 636–641

Yager J, Devlin MJ, Halmi KA, et al: Practice Guideline for the Treatment of Patients With Eating Disorders, 3rd Edition. Washington, DC, American Psychiatric Association, 2006

3 Eating Problems in Children and Adolescents

Neville H. Golden, M.D.
Rollyn M. Ornstein, M.D.

Medical professionals, including pediatricians, adolescent medicine specialists, and primary care practitioners, are uniquely suited for the early identification of eating problems in children and adolescents because patients in this age group are usually seen at regular intervals. However, the diagnosis of an eating disorder in this age group can be particularly challenging because these patients frequently fail to endorse cognitions typically associated with eating disorders (e.g., feeling fat, fearing weight gain, concern about body shape or weight) but may instead present with vague physical complaints such as nausea, difficulty swallowing, or abdominal pain after eating. Physicians working with youths would therefore benefit from additional information about the unique presentation of children and adolescents with feeding and eating problems. In particular, physicians would be helped by understanding the changing nosology of feeding and eating disorders as described in DSM-5 (American Psychiatric Association 2013) that may affect the diagnostic labels applied to eating problems in youths. Especially notable in DSM-5 is the development of a revised diagnostic category now entitled avoidant/restrictive food intake disorder (ARFID) and the inclusion of rumination disorder and pica in feeding and eating disorders in DSM-5.

The aim of this chapter is to provide a practical approach for pediatricians, adolescent medicine physicians, primary care practitioners, and other professionals who may need to assess children and adolescents with potential feeding or eating disorders. Given the aforementioned challenges of differing presentations in youths and the recently updated diagnostic scheme, this chapter provides assistance in the assignment of the diagnosis of a feeding or eating disorder in a child or adolescent. Guidance is offered for conducting a careful history and physical examination, and suggestions are offered for the exclusion of other medical and psychiatric conditions as part of this evaluation. The reader is encouraged to view Video 2, "Assessing eating problems in the primary care setting."

Epidemiology and Nosology of Eating Disorders

Although eating disorders have historically been considered diseases of affluent white adolescent females, data on epidemiology suggest changes over the past few decades (Pike et al. 2013). Increased prevalence rates have been identified among ethnic and racial minorities (Alegria et al. 2007; Marques et al. 2011; Nicdao et al. 2007; Taylor et al. 2007) and in countries where eating disorders were traditionally not reported (Chandra et al. 2012; Chisuwa and O'Dea 2010; Eddy et al. 2007; Jackson and Chen 2010; Lee et al. 2010). Although the onset of eating disorders was previously more common during middle to late adolescence, more recent studies indicate that the age at onset for both anorexia nervosa (AN) and bulimia nervosa (BN) has been decreasing (Favaro et al. 2009; van Son et al. 2006), with a significant increase in the numbers of individuals under age 12 presenting for treatment (Madden et al. 2009; Nicholls et al. 2011; Pinhas et al. 2011) and a notable increase in females ages 15–19 presenting with AN (van Son et al. 2006). Data also suggest an increase in the identification of males with eating disorders (Swanson et al. 2011) and a reduced female-to-male ratio in younger patients with restrictive eating disorders (Madden et al. 2009; Nicholls et al. 2011; Pinhas et al. 2011), highlighting the importance of broadening perceptions with relation to the sex and the presentation of individuals with feeding and eating disorders.

Under the DSM-IV diagnostic classification scheme, more than 50% of children and adolescents with eating disorders were assigned the diagnosis of eating disorder not otherwise specified (EDNOS), because they did not meet full criteria for either AN or BN, or they had an entirely different disorder (Eddy et al. 2008; Peebles et al. 2010). A goal of DSM-5 was to improve the clinical utility of the eating disorder diagnostic categories and decrease the need to employ the EDNOS category. Early studies demonstrated that application of the DSM-5 criteria leads to significant decreases in the proportion of EDNOS diagnoses and modest increases in both AN and BN diagnoses in children, adolescents, and young adults (Machado et al. 2013; Ornstein et al. 2013; Stice et al. 2013). In clinical samples of younger patients referred to specialized eating disorder programs, 5%–23% meet criteria for ARFID (Fisher et al. 2014; Nicely et al. 2014; Norris et al. 2014; Ornstein et al. 2013).

Basic Screening for a Feeding or Eating Disorder

Physicians can play a key role in identifying early eating problems among children and adolescents during health maintenance visits or preparticipation sports physical examinations. A critical element in screening for a feeding or eating disorder is the measurement of height and weight to plot body mass index (BMI; weight in kilograms divided by height in meters squared [kg/m^2]), which should be examined at each visit, with close attention paid to any significant change in percentiles for height, weight, or BMI. The degree of change and current status are important in determining level of concern. Children and adolescents who fail to make expected weight gain during a period of growth, even if they have not lost any weight, should be assessed further. Parents of a preteen or adolescent should be asked specific questions about concerns they may have regarding their child's dietary intake (e.g., limited consumption, greatly decreased range of foods eaten), physical activity, excessive weight concerns, or inappropriate dieting. In girls, primary or secondary amenorrhea in the context of dieting or excessive exercise should be a red flag. Any suspicion of a possible eating disorder requires a more comprehensive assessment, which may or may not be possible given the time and resource constraints of the physician's practice and the patient's insurance plan. If additional time cannot be spent on evaluation, the clinician should refer the patient to an eating disorder specialist.

Initial Medical Assessment for a Suspected Eating Disorder in a Child or Adolescent

The initial medical assessment of the child or adolescent who may have an eating disorder may be performed by a pediatrician, adolescent medicine specialist, or primary care practitioner. This evaluation aims to establish current eating disorder symptoms, develop a preliminary diagnosis, exclude other causes of weight loss or vomiting, evaluate for any associated medical complications, and, as appropriate, initiate a plan for treatment and ongoing monitoring. A mental health professional may be needed to perform a psychological assessment to evaluate for common comorbid psychiatric illnesses such as affective or anxiety disorders.

History

When a child or adolescent initially presents for an evaluation of a possible feeding or eating disorder, the health care provider should usually start by obtaining a history with both parent and patient together. Observing the interaction between child and parent(s) can be informative. Subsequently, the physician should speak individually with the child or adolescent and the parent(s) to ask each party about specific related disordered behaviors, such as purging, compulsive exercising, and other habits. Skilled interviewing can reveal any "hidden agenda" and clarify any discrepancies in perspective between parent(s) and child. For example, the clinician can ask the child or adolescent what he or she has been told about the reason for the appointment; the physician can then observe whether the parent automatically answers for the child or interrupts and whether the child speaks freely or looks to the parent to answer. With regard to the presented problem, the chief complaint may be weight loss, but it also may be amenorrhea, weakness, dizziness, fatigue, abdominal pain, nausea, vomiting, or a combination of complaints. A detailed history can usually differentiate an eating disorder from another etiology for symptoms. Sample questions that might be asked in this interview are provided in Table 3–1 and illustrated in Video 2.

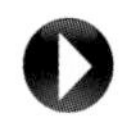

Video Illustration 2: Assessing eating problems in the primary care setting (3:24)

Physical Examination

A thorough physical examination is an essential component of the assessment of a child or adolescent suspected of having an eating disorder. Height should be obtained using a wall-mounted stadiometer, and post-voiding weight should be measured with the patient wearing only a hospital gown. The physician should calculate BMI, plot it on the Centers for Disease Control and Prevention charts (www.cdc.gov/growthcharts/clinical_charts.htm), and determine the percentage of median BMI (patient's BMI/median BMI × 100). It is important to review the patient's previous weights and heights on the growth chart to determine whether growth arrest has occurred. Particular attention should be paid to obtaining vital signs, including oral temperature and orthostatic measurements

TABLE 3–1. Eating disorders evaluation: sample questions and issues to explore in obtaining history

History of present illness

When did your eating habits change? Why did they change?

What is the most you ever weighed? How tall were you then? When was that?

What is the least you ever weighed in the past year? How tall were you then? When was that?

What would you like to weigh? Are there specific body parts you would wish to change?

What have you eaten in the last 24 hours?

Calorie counting? Fat-gram counting? Carbohydrate counting?

Food restrictions? Recent vegetarianism? Excessive noncaloric fluid intake?

Do you eat with others? Do you eat outside of your home?

Do you exercise? How much, how often, and what level of intensity? How do you feel if you miss exercising?

Have you engaged in binge eating? Frequency?

Have you purged by self-induced vomiting? Frequency?

Do you use laxatives, diuretics, or diet pills?

Have you ever had any previous treatment for an eating disorder or other mental health issue?

If there is a suspicion of avoidant/restrictive food intake disorder, may add these questions:

Do you have any fears about vomiting or choking? Have you ever experienced or witnessed episodes where someone choked on food?

Have you ever used oral nutritional supplementation or tube feedings? When?

Would you describe yourself/your child as a picky eater?

Are you bothered by characteristics of food related to smell, taste, texture, or color?

Past medical history

Birth history, neonatal course, feeding history, episodes of gagging or other intolerances to food, and texture/sensory issues

Medical or mental health problems, hospitalizations, and surgeries

Menstrual history (girls)

At what age did you have your first period (if applicable)?

Were your menstrual cycles regular prior to the eating disorder?

When was your last menstrual period?

Family history

Medical problems, recent illnesses, or deaths (e.g., obesity, diabetes, cardiovascular disease)

Family members with weight loss efforts, possible eating disorder

Mental health history, alcoholism, and/or substance abuse

TABLE 3–1. Eating disorders evaluation: sample questions and issues to explore in obtaining history *(continued)*

Review of systems
General: weight changes, sleep habits, fevers, night sweats, heat/cold intolerance, hair loss
Cardiovascular: chest pain, heart palpitations
Respiratory: shortness of breath, cough with or without exertion
Gastrointestinal: abdominal pain, fullness/bloating, early satiety, nausea, dyspepsia, reflux symptoms, vomiting, diarrhea, constipation
Musculoskeletal: weakness, numbness/tingling, pain, swelling
Neurological: headaches, dizziness, syncope
Psychiatric: symptoms of depression, anxiety, obsessive-compulsive disorder, substance abuse, physical and/or sexual abuse

of heart rate and blood pressure (measured when the patient is lying down and again 2 minutes after standing). It is not uncommon for significant bradycardia, hypotension, and hypothermia to be present. Physical examination may reveal loss of subcutaneous fat, prominence of bony protuberances, and lanugo hair on the back, trunk, and arms. Dental enamel erosion and enlargement of the parotid and salivary glands may be present in those who purge. Russell's sign, or calluses on the dorsum of the hand that are caused by the central incisors when the fingers are used to induce vomiting, may be evident. Examination of the heart may reveal a midsystolic click or murmur from mitral valve prolapse. Assessment of sexual maturity rating (Tanner staging for development of breasts and pubic hair for girls or for genitals and pubic hair for boys) is important to evaluate for pubertal delay or arrest. Common physical signs noted in children and adolescents with eating disorders are listed in Table 3–2, and conditions that would suggest a need for inpatient medical hospitalization are listed in Table 3–3.

Laboratory Investigations

Recommended laboratory tests are shown in Table 3–4. Laboratory tests are not diagnostic per se, but they may help confirm an eating disorder diagnosis by excluding other causes of weight loss or vomiting. Despite a patient's significant weight loss and severe dietary restriction, laboratory tests are usually normal.

TABLE 3–2. Physical findings associated with anorexia nervosa and bulimia nervosa in children and adolescents

	Anorexia nervosa	Bulimia nervosa
General	Low weight Loss of subcutaneous fat Proximal and intercostal muscle wasting Prominence of bony protuberances Hypothermia	Weight usually normal
Skin	Dry skin with hyperkeratotic areas Yellowish discoloration (carotenemia) Lanugo Acrocyanosis Hair loss or thinning Pitting and ridging of nails	Russell's sign (calluses on dorsum of hand caused by self-induced vomiting)
Cardiovascular	Bradycardia Hypotension Orthostasis Peripheral edema Systolic murmur sometimes associated with mitral valve prolapse Electrocardiographic abnormalities–bradycardia, low voltages, prolonged QTc	Electrocardiographic abnormalities, particularly QTc prolongation
Gastrointestinal	Scaphoid abdomen with stool palpable in left-lower quadrant Elevated transaminases	Parotid and salivary gland enlargement Dental enamel erosion Loss of gag reflex Dental caries, gingivitis, stomatitis, glossitis Abdominal distension after meals

TABLE 3–2. Physical findings associated with anorexia nervosa and bulimia nervosa in children and adolescents *(continued) (continued)*

	Anorexia nervosa	Bulimia nervosa
Metabolic/endocrine	Amenorrhea	Oligomenorrhea or normal menses; amenorrhea also possible
	Cold intolerance, hypothermia	
	Growth retardation	
	Delayed puberty	
Musculoskeletal	Muscle wasting	Usually normal weight
	Low bone mineral density with pathological fractures	Usually normal bone mineral density
Neurological	Cognitive and memory dysfunction	Cognitive and memory dysfunction
	Depression	Depression
	Anxiety	Anxiety
Hematological	Easy bruising, petechiae	
	Thrombocytopenia	
	Leukopenia	
	Anemia	

Medical Complications

Many of the medical complications of eating disorders are secondary to the effects of malnutrition and/or purging behavior. As described in the following subsections, almost every organ system may be involved.

Fluid and Electrolytes

Patients with eating disorders may present with dehydration and abnormal serum levels of sodium, potassium, chloride, phosphorus, magnesium, carbon dioxide, and blood urea nitrogen. Electrolyte disturbances, most commonly hypokalemia, are more likely in those patients who are vomiting and/or abusing laxatives or diuretics. Hyponatremia can occur in those who "water load" (i.e., consume large amounts of water to temporarily appear to weigh more) and can lead to seizures, coma, and death. Serum phosphorus levels may be normal on presentation but can drop during the process of refeeding, and careful monitoring is needed if physicians are overseeing an outpatient weight gain regimen for patients who are underweight. Hypophosphatemia may play a role in the development

TABLE 3–3. Indications for hospitalization in a child or adolescent with an eating disorder

≤75% median body mass index for age and sex
Dehydration
Electrolyte disturbance (hypokalemia, hyponatremia, hypophosphatemia)
Electrocardiographic abnormalities (e.g., prolonged QTc or severe bradycardia)
Physiological instability
Severe bradycardia (heart rate <50 beats/minute daytime; <45 beats/minute at night)
Hypotension (<90/45 mmHg)
Hypothermia (body temperature <96°F or 35.6°C)
Orthostatic increase in pulse (>20 beats/minute) or drop in blood pressure (>20 mmHg systolic or >10 mmHg diastolic)
Arrested growth and development
Failure of outpatient treatment
Acute food refusal
Uncontrollable bingeing or purging
Acute medical complications of malnutrition (e.g., syncope, seizures, cardiac failure, pancreatitis)
Comorbid psychiatric or medical condition that prohibits or limits appropriate outpatient treatment (e.g., severe depression, suicidal ideation, obsessive-compulsive disorder, type 1 diabetes mellitus)

Note. One or more of the indications justifies hospitalization.
Source. Adapted from Golden et al. 2015.

of cardiac arrhythmias and sudden unexpected death seen during refeeding (Katzman et al. 2014). Hypomagnesemia is more common among patients who purge (Raj et al. 2012).

Cardiovascular System

In patients with eating disorders, resting heart rates may be as low as 30–40 beats per minute, both systolic and diastolic blood pressures may be low, and there may be orthostatic changes in both pulse and blood pressure. These changes reflect an adaptive response to reduced energy intake and are generally seen in the restrictive eating disorders. Heart size is reduced and exercise capacity is diminished, but cardiac output and left ventricular function are usually preserved. A silent pericardial effusion may be present (Ramacciotti et al. 2003). Electrocardiographic abnormalities include sinus bradycardia, low voltage complexes, a prolonged QTc interval, increased QT interval dispersion, first- and second-degree heart block, and various

TABLE 3–4. Recommended laboratory and ancillary tests for the evaluation of a child or adolescent with a suspected eating disorder

Complete blood count and erythrocyte sedimentation rate
Urinalysis
Chemistry profile including blood urea nitrogen, creatinine, albumin, and electrolytes (sodium, potassium, calcium, phosphorus, and magnesium) and liver function tests
Serum amylase level (if patient is vomiting)
Triiodothyronine (T_3), thyroxine (T_4), and thyroid-stimulating hormone levels
Serum luteinizing hormone, follicle-stimulating hormone, estradiol, and prolactin (if patient is amenorrheic)
Serum 25-hydroxyvitamin D level
Electrocardiogram
Dual-energy X-ray absorptiometry (DXA)
Optional laboratory tests include
Celiac screen
Upper gastrointestinal tract series and small-bowel series
Magnetic resonance imaging of the head

atrial and ventricular arrhythmias. Congestive heart failure does not usually occur in the starvation phase but can occur during refeeding.

Gastrointestinal System

Among patients with eating disorders, bloating and constipation are frequent complaints and reflect delayed gastric emptying and decreased intestinal motility. Liver aminotransferases are elevated in 4%–38% of patients with AN and improve with nutritional rehabilitation (Narayanan et al. 2010). Weight loss can lead to the *superior mesenteric artery syndrome*, a condition that is characterized by pain and vomiting after eating and is caused by extrinsic compression of the duodenum by the superior mesenteric artery where it originates from the aorta. Rapid weight loss can also be associated with gallstone formation.

Recurrent vomiting results in erosion of dental enamel, esophagitis, Mallory-Weiss tears, and possibly esophageal or gastric rupture. Prolonged recurrent vomiting may cause Barrett's esophagus, which is a precancerous condition. Laxative abuse can be accompanied by bloody diarrhea. Serum amylase may be elevated in individuals who are bingeing or purging. Acute pancreatitis occasionally occurs. Total protein and serum albumin levels are usually normal in patients with eating disorders, in contrast to patients with other forms of malnutrition.

Endocrine System

Growth retardation and short stature can occur in children and adolescents who develop an eating disorder prior to completion of growth (Lantzouni et al. 2002; Modan-Moses et al. 2003). This is more likely to occur in adolescent boys with AN because they grow, on average, for 2 years longer than girls. Catch-up growth can occur with nutritional rehabilitation; however, even with intervention, these adolescents may not reach their genetic height potential (Lantzouni et al. 2002). Pubertal delay can occur in those who develop AN prior to completion of puberty. In girls, primary or secondary amenorrhea is common and usually follows weight loss but has been shown to precede weight loss in 20% of cases (Golden et al. 1997). Levels of luteinizing hormone, follicle-stimulating hormone, and estradiol are low, often in the prepubertal range. In males, testosterone levels can be low. In addition to suppression of the hypothalamic-pituitary-gonadal axis, hypothalamic dysfunction is evidenced by disturbances in satiety, difficulties with temperature regulation, and inability to concentrate urine. There is activation of the hypothalamic-adrenal axis with high levels of serum cortisol. The low T_3 (triiodothyronine) syndrome or sick euthyroid syndrome, is caused by an adaptive response to malnutrition or chronic illness and is frequently seen. Disturbances in thyroid function resolve with nutritional rehabilitation and should not be treated with thyroid replacement hormone. A serum 25-hydroxyvitamin D level that is below 30 ng/mL indicates vitamin D insufficiency and requires treatment to replenish vitamin D stores.

Musculoskeletal System

Because adolescence is a critical time for accrual of peak bone mass, reduced bone mineral density for age is a serious long-term complication of AN. It occurs in both boys and girls (Misra et al. 2008) and is associated with increased fracture risk even after patients recover from the eating disorder (Lucas et al. 1999; Vestergaard et al. 2002).

Hematological System

In patients with eating disorders, suppression of the bone marrow leads to leukopenia, anemia, and thrombocytopenia (Misra et al. 2004). Anemia is usually secondary to bone marrow suppression but may also be due to dietary deficiency of vitamin B_{12}, folate, or iron. The erythrocyte sedimentation rate is usually low secondary to decreased hepatic production of fibrinogen. The presence of an elevated sedimentation rate should arouse suspicion for another diagnosis.

Neurological System

The major neurological complications of eating disorders are syncope, seizures (secondary to electrolyte disturbances), and structural brain changes noted on imaging studies (Golden et al. 1996; Katzman et al. 1996). Muscle weakness and a peripheral neuropathy can also occur. Volume deficits of both gray and white matter have been identified in low-weight patients with AN, and neuropsychological testing has demonstrated impairment of attention, concentration, and memory, with deficits in visuospatial ability. These abnormalities improve substantially or disappear entirely with weight restoration.

Differential Diagnosis

The differential diagnosis of an eating disorder in a child or adolescent includes a variety of medical and psychiatric conditions that can be responsible for the presented symptoms. An outline of the differential diagnosis is shown in Table 3–5. It is important to exclude any other gastrointestinal conditions, such as inflammatory bowel disease or celiac disease, that can lead to pain and discomfort related to eating, weight loss, and growth retardation. However, it is also possible for an eating disorder to coexist with another condition.

Specific Eating Disorder Diagnosis and Associated Problems in Children and Adolescents

Anorexia Nervosa

Peak age at onset for AN is during mid-adolescence (ages 13–15 years), but children as young as 6–7 years may present with the classic syndrome. In older age groups, approximately 10% of patients with AN are male, but in those younger than age 14 years, one in six is male (Pinhas et al. 2011).

TABLE 3–5. Differential diagnosis for eating disorders

Medical conditions
Inflammatory bowel disease
Malabsorption: cystic fibrosis, celiac disease
Endocrine conditions: hyperthyroidism, Addison's disease, diabetes mellitus
Collagen vascular disease
Central nervous system lesions: hypothalamic or pituitary tumors
Malignancies
Chronic infections: tuberculosis, HIV
Immunodeficiency
Psychiatric conditions
Mood disorders
Anxiety disorders
Somatization disorder
Substance use disorders
Psychosis

Core features of AN include restriction of energy intake, leading to low body weight for age, sex, and development; fear of gaining weight or of becoming fat; and disturbance in the way in which one's body weight or shape is perceived. Children and younger adolescents frequently do not endorse fear of gaining weight or body image dissatisfaction, but with revisions to DSM-5, reliance on identifying behaviors that interfere with weight gain improves diagnostic utility in younger patients. In DSM-5, amenorrhea has been eliminated as one of the required diagnostic criteria for AN.

The medical findings associated with AN in children and adolescents are similar to those in adults, with a couple of exceptions. First, children and adolescents may become medically compromised much more rapidly than adults because of reduced nutritional reserves and increased metabolic demands for growth and development. Thus, significant medical complications can occur with a smaller relative amount of weight change or in the context of rapid weight loss. Second, certain complications such as growth retardation, interruption of puberty, and interference with peak bone mass acquisition and brain development have a greater impact in children and adolescents and are potentially irreversible. For children and adolescents with AN, ongoing medical monitoring in the primary care practitioner's office every 1–2 weeks is essential to ensure continued weight gain and to monitor for medical stability.

Bulimia Nervosa

Peak age at onset of BN is in late adolescence or early adulthood; however, BN does occur in children younger than age 14 years, and there is evidence that the age at onset for BN is decreasing (Favaro et al. 2009; van Son et al. 2006). Comorbidity of BN with affective disorders, anxiety disorders, personality disorders, and substance use disorders is high. The core features of BN include recurrent episodes of binge eating and recurrent compensatory behaviors (vomiting, laxatives, diuretics, fasting, exercising) to prevent weight gain, both occurring on average at least once a week for 3 months. The diagnosis of BN should be considered for any adolescent with weight and body image concerns and marked fluctuations in weight. On physical examination, particular attention should be paid to the three objective physical signs of BN: parotid hypertrophy, dental enamel erosion, and Russell's sign. Similar to AN, a multidisciplinary treatment approach is recommended. The role of the medical provider is to ensure medical stability and monitor for electrolyte disturbances associated with unhealthy weight-control practices.

Avoidant/Restrictive Food Intake Disorder

ARFID in DSM-5 is a revision and significant expansion of the DSM-IV diagnosis called "feeding disorder of infancy or early childhood." ARFID describes some individuals who previously were given a diagnosis of EDNOS and is frequently seen in younger patients but can occur at any age. The preponderance of males with ARFID is higher than with AN. Patients with ARFID may present with clinically significant restrictive eating, leading to weight loss or lack of weight gain, growth retardation, nutritional deficiencies, reliance on tube feeding or oral nutritional supplements, and/or disturbances in psychosocial functioning. Individuals with ARFID may have sensory problems related to the taste, smell, color, or texture of food, resulting in a limited variety of food consumed. Some have a fear of swallowing or an inability to swallow food, especially solid or lumpy foods, which often follows either a personal or witnessed choking episode. Others have a fear of vomiting, with resultant food refusal. Some patients with ARFID have symptoms of depression and/or anxiety and may offer somatic complaints as to why they are not eating (e.g., "my belly hurts"). To make a diagnosis of ARFID, avoidance or restriction of food cannot be better justified by another medical condition or psychiatric disorder; however, these disorders can coexist with the eating disorder, as long as the severity of abnormal eating behaviors necessitates further clinical attention (American Psychiatric Association 2013).

Because the criteria for ARFID are new in DSM-5, there is no validated assessment tool or formalized evaluation to aid clinicians in this diagnosis.[1] Recent studies have shown that the prevalence of ARFID in newly diagnosed patients presenting to adolescent medicine eating disorder programs ranges from 5% to 14% (Fisher et al. 2014; Ornstein et al. 2013; Norris et al. 2014).

Rumination Disorder

Rumination disorder is the repeated, unforced regurgitation of recently eaten food over at least a 1-month period, occurring multiple times per week and often daily. It is not associated with nausea or part of any medical illness (e.g., gastroesophageal reflux disease), but the diagnosis can be made concurrently with a medical condition, as long as the other condition is not the only reason for the behavior. Although rumination has been believed to occur most commonly in infants and individuals with developmental disabilities, it also occurs in children, adolescents, and adults of normal intelligence. It may be difficult to differentiate between regurgitation and self-induced vomiting; however, the behavior is effortless and does not serve as a method of weight control. Rumination may help to self-soothe or self-stimulate, especially in those with mental disabilities, whereas in others, it seems to be related to anxiety. The behavior can often be witnessed by clinicians (Chial et al. 2003).

Pica

The distinguishing feature of pica is the ingestion of one or more nonnutritive, nonfood substances on a continual basis for at least 1 month. The diagnosis of pica cannot be made before age 2, and the behavior cannot denote an endorsed cultural, religious, or social practice. Pica can be observed with other mental disorders (e.g., developmental disabilities, autism spectrum disorder, schizophrenia); it is only given as a separate diagnosis if the eating behavior is serious enough to warrant additional clinical management (American Psychiatric Association 2013).

Conclusion

Because eating disorders have recently become more prevalent among younger patients, it is incumbent upon pediatric health care providers to

---

[1] The Eating Disorder Assessment for DSM-5 (EDA-5; Sysko et al. 2015) does provide an assessment guide for ARFID, but no information about its performance is yet available. Refer to Part 3, "Assessment Tools," in this volume for additional information.

recognize the signs and symptoms and to make prompt diagnoses or refer to specialists as necessary. DSM-5 has the potential to improve clinical utility via more specific diagnostic categories.

Key Clinical Points

- When evaluating a child or adolescent with a possible eating disorder, the clinician needs to take a history from the patient and parents together, as well as from each individually.
- Skeletal growth retardation or growth in a prepubertal or early pubertal child without concomitant weight gain should be recognized as significant and akin to weight loss.
- Children and adolescents with eating disorders can become medically compromised much more rapidly than adults, and frequent monitoring for medical safety is recommended. Although amenorrhea has been removed as a diagnostic criterion for anorexia nervosa in DSM-5, it can still serve as a useful indicator of malnutrition and clinical severity.
- Although bulimia nervosa was often thought to occur primarily in older adolescents, younger patients are presenting with significant clinical symptomatology, which may represent a diagnostic continuum. The DSM-5 change in the minimum frequency criterion for binge eating and inappropriate compensatory behaviors to once weekly should help to include more patients in this category.
- Avoidant/restrictive food intake disorder is a newly articulated disorder in DSM-5 that is seen typically in younger patients, with a higher preponderance of males. More research is needed to elucidate its diagnosis, complications, and treatment.

References

Alegria M, Woo M, Cao Z, et al: Prevalence and correlates of eating disorders in Latinos in the United States. Int J Eat Disord 40(suppl):S15–S21, 2007 17584870

American Psychiatric Association: Diagnostic and Statistical Manual of Mental Disorders, 4th Edition. Washington, DC, American Psychiatric Association, 1994

American Psychiatric Association: Diagnostic and Statistical Manual of Mental Disorders, 5th Edition. Arlington, VA, American Psychiatric Association, 2013

Chandra PS, Abbas S, Palmer R: Are eating disorders a significant clinical issue in urban India? A survey among psychiatrists in Bangalore. Int J Eat Disord 45(3):443–446, 2012 22095676

Chial HJ, Camilleri M, Williams DE, et al: Rumination syndrome in children and adolescents: diagnosis, treatment, and prognosis. Pediatrics 111(1):158–162, 2003 12509570

Chisuwa N, O'Dea JA: Body image and eating disorders amongst Japanese adolescents: a review of the literature. Appetite 54(1):5–15, 2010 19941921

Eddy KT, Hennessey M, Thompson-Brenner H: Eating pathology in East African women: the role of media exposure and globalization. J Nerv Ment Dis 195(3):196–202, 2007 17468678

Eddy KT, Celio Doyle A, Hoste RR, et al: Eating disorder not otherwise specified in adolescents. J Am Acad Child Adolesc Psychiatry 47(2):156–164, 2008 18176335

Favaro A, Caregaro L, Tenconi E, et al: Time trends in age at onset of anorexia nervosa and bulimia nervosa. J Clin Psychiatry 70(12):1715–1721, 2009 20141711

Fisher MM, Rosen DS, Ornstein RM, et al: Characteristics of avoidant/restrictive food intake disorder in children and adolescents: a "new disorder" in DSM-5. J Adolesc Health 55(1):49–52, 2014 24506978

Golden NH, Ashtari M, Kohn MR, et al: Reversibility of cerebral ventricular enlargement in anorexia nervosa, demonstrated by quantitative magnetic resonance imaging. J Pediatr 128(2):296–301, 1996 8636835

Golden NH, Jacobson MS, Schebendach J, et al: Resumption of menses in anorexia nervosa. Arch Pediatr Adolesc Med 151(1):16–21, 1997 9006523

Golden NH, Katzman DK, Sawyer SM, et al; Society for Adolescent Health and Medicine: Position Paper of the Society for Adolescent Health and Medicine: medical management of restrictive eating disorders in adolescents and young adults. J Adolesc Health 56(1):121–125, 2015 25530605

Jackson T, Chen H: Sociocultural experiences of bulimic and non-bulimic adolescents in a school-based Chinese sample. J Abnorm Child Psychol 38(1):69–76, 2010 19707866

Katzman DK, Lambe EK, Mikulis DJ, et al: Cerebral gray matter and white matter volume deficits in adolescent girls with anorexia nervosa. J Pediatr 129(6):794–803, 1996 8969719

Katzman DK, Garber AK, Kohn M, et al; Society for Adolescent Health and Medicine: Refeeding hypophosphatemia in hospitalized adolescents with anorexia nervosa: a position statement of the Society for Adolescent Health and Medicine. J Adolesc Health 55(3):455–457, 2014 25151056

Lantzouni E, Frank GR, Golden NH, et al: Reversibility of growth stunting in early onset anorexia nervosa: a prospective study. J Adolesc Health 31(2):162–165, 2002 12127386

Lee S, Ng KL, Kwok K, et al: The changing profile of eating disorders at a tertiary psychiatric clinic in Hong Kong (1987–2007). Int J Eat Disord 43(4):307–314, 2010 19350649

Lucas AR, Melton LJ III, Crowson CS III, et al: Long-term fracture risk among women with anorexia nervosa: a population-based cohort study. Mayo Clin Proc 74(10):972–977, 1999 10918862

Machado PP, Gonçalves S, Hoek HW: DSM-5 reduces the proportion of EDNOS cases: evidence from community samples. Int J Eat Disord 46(1):60–65, 2013 22815201

Madden S, Morris A, Zurynski YA, et al: Burden of eating disorders in 5–13-year-old children in Australia. Med J Aust 190(8):410–414, 2009 19374611

Marques L, Alegria M, Becker AE, et al: Comparative prevalence, correlates of impairment, and service utilization for eating disorders across U.S. ethnic groups: implications for reducing ethnic disparities in health care access for eating disorders. Int J Eat Disord 44(5):412–420, 2011 20665700

Misra M, Aggarwal A, Miller KK, et al: Effects of anorexia nervosa on clinical, hematologic, biochemical, and bone density parameters in community-dwelling adolescent girls. Pediatrics 114(6):1574–1583, 2004 15574617

Misra M, Katzman DK, Cord J, et al: Bone metabolism in adolescent boys with anorexia nervosa. J Clin Endocrinol Metab 93(8):3029–3036, 2008 18544623

Modan-Moses D, Yaroslavsky A, Novikov I, et al: Stunting of growth as a major feature of anorexia nervosa in male adolescents. Pediatrics 111(2):270–276, 2003 12563050

Narayanan V, Gaudiani JL, Harris RH, et al: Liver function test abnormalities in anorexia nervosa–cause or effect. Int J Eat Disord 43(4):378–381, 2010 19424979

Nicdao EG, Hong S, Takeuchi DT: Prevalence and correlates of eating disorders among Asian Americans: results from the National Latino and Asian American Study. Int J Eat Disord 40(suppl):S22–S26, 2007 17879986

Nicely TA, Lane-Loney S, Masciulli E, et al: Prevalence and characteristics of avoidant/restrictive food intake disorder in a cohort of young patients in day treatment for eating disorders. J Eat Disord 2(1):21, 2014 25165558

Nicholls DE, Lynn R, Viner RM: Childhood eating disorders: British national surveillance study. Br J Psychiatry 198(4):295–301, 2011 21972279

Norris ML, Robinson A, Obeid N, et al: Exploring avoidant/restrictive food intake disorder in eating disordered patients: a descriptive study. Int J Eat Disord 47(5):495–499, 2014 24343807

Ornstein RM, Rosen DS, Mammel KA, et al: Distribution of eating disorders in children and adolescents using the proposed DSM-5 criteria for feeding and eating disorders. J Adolesc Health 53(2):303–305, 2013 23684215

Peebles R, Hardy KK, Wilson JL, et al: Are diagnostic criteria for eating disorders markers of medical severity? Pediatrics 125(5):e1193–e1201, 2010 20385643

Pike KM, Dunne PE, Addai E: Expanding the boundaries: reconfiguring the demographics of the "typical" eating disordered patient. Curr Psychiatry Rep 15(11):411, 2013 24122512

Pinhas L, Morris A, Crosby RD, et al: Incidence and age-specific presentation of restrictive eating disorders in children: a Canadian Paediatric Surveillance Program study. Arch Pediatr Adolesc Med 165(10):895–899, 2011 21969390

Raj KS, Keane-Miller C, Golden NH: Hypomagnesemia in adolescents with eating disorders hospitalized for medical instability. Nutr Clin Pract 27(5):689–694, 2012 22683565

Ramacciotti CE, Coli E, Biadi O, et al: Silent pericardial effusion in a sample of anorexic patients. Eat Weight Disord 8(1):68–71, 2003 12762627

Stice E, Marti CN, Rohde P: Prevalence, incidence, impairment, and course of the proposed DSM-5 eating disorder diagnoses in an 8-year prospective community study of young women. J Abnorm Psychol 122(2):445–457, 2013 23148784

Swanson SA, Crow SJ, Le Grange D, et al: Prevalence and correlates of eating disorders in adolescents. Results from the National Comorbidity Survey Replication Adolescent Supplement. Arch Gen Psychiatry 68(7):714–723, 2011 21383252

Sysko R, Glasofer DR, Hildebrandt T, et al: The Eating Disorder Assessment for DSM-5 (EDA-5): development and validation of a structured interview for feeding and eating disorders. Int J Eat Disord Jan 30, 2015 [Epub ahead of print] 25639562

Taylor JY, Caldwell CH, Baser RE, et al: Prevalence of eating disorders among blacks in the National Survey of American Life. Int J Eat Disord 40(suppl):S10–S14, 2007 17879287

van Son GE, van Hoeken D, Bartelds AI, et al: Time trends in the incidence of eating disorders: a primary care study in the Netherlands. Int J Eat Disord 39(7):565–569, 2006 16791852

Vestergaard P, Emborg C, Støving RK, et al: Fractures in patients with anorexia nervosa, bulimia nervosa, and other eating disorders–a nationwide register study. Int J Eat Disord 32(3):301–308, 2002 12210644

4 Eating Problems in Individuals With Overweight and Obesity

Marsha D. Marcus, Ph.D.
Jennifer E. Wildes, Ph.D.

Individuals with overweight or obesity constitute the majority of people in the United States. In general, the assessment of disordered eating in overweight or obese people does not differ from that in individuals at a healthy weight, but the presence of obesity requires clinical consideration. Therefore, we focus in this chapter on the clinical approach to the assessment of overweight and obese people with disordered eating; specifically, we discuss differential diagnosis, associated problems, physical assessment, and implications for treatment. Video 3, "Assessing eating problems in overweight adults," depicts the issues pertinent to overweight or obese patients.

Clinical Approach

It is crucial to define overweight and obesity to provide a context for the assessment of disordered eating and to provide some background for the perspective taken in this chapter. Simply stated, *obesity* refers to excess adiposity, but there is no specific threshold. Currently, the terms *overweight* and *obese* are defined using ranges of body mass index (BMI), a measure calculated using this formula: weight in kilograms divided by height in meters squared (kg/m^2). Specifically, a person with a BMI of 25–30 kg/m^2 is considered overweight, and one with a BMI of at least 30 kg/m^2 is considered obese (National Institutes of Health 1998). On the basis of BMI, 33.4% of U.S. adults currently are overweight and 34.9% are obese (Ogden et al. 2014); however, it is important to remember that BMI is a proxy for relative adiposity, and although BMI has been shown to correlate strongly with obesity-related health problems, it is an imperfect measure of body fat. Although it appears that the prevalence of overweight and obesity has stabilized in the United States, the overall prevalence remains high (Ogden et al. 2014).

The causes of excess adiposity are manifold, but there is little controversy about the fact that increases in obesity prevalence are associated with the widespread availability of highly palatable foods with high energy density as well as decreases in levels of physical activity. Indeed, available data from dietary surveys have documented that calorie intake in the United States has increased in a fashion parallel to the increased prevalence of obesity (Jeffery and Harnack 2007). However, the development of obesity is not simply a matter of persistent overeating. Rather, obesity develops in genetically vulnerable individuals as a consequence of an intricate cascade of interacting biological, psychological, family, community, and cultural factors. Thus, disordered eating in a given person must be evaluated in the context of the complex etiology of obesity in the current cultural milieu.

An issue of particular salience for clinicians working with obese individuals is weight bias or stigma. There is considerable evidence that negative appraisals of obese individuals are ubiquitous (Puhl and Heuer 2010) and are based on derisive stereotypes about the causes and correlates of obesity, which include gluttony, laziness, lack of discipline, self-indulgence, and slovenliness. Weight stigma leads to discrimination against obese individuals in social contexts, in the workplace, and, importantly, among health professionals, including those who specialize in the treatment of obesity (Schwartz et al. 2003). An increasing body of evidence indicates that stigma and discrimination are associated with significant negative health consequences, which may include promoting weight gain and the onset of obesity (Jackson et al. 2014).

Negative weight biases appear especially relevant for obese individuals with aberrant eating, because obesity-related stigma is complicated further by awareness that problematic eating behavior may contribute to unwanted weight gain. For example, Barnes et al. (2014) compared obese individuals with and without binge-eating disorder (BED) who sought treatment for weight and eating problems. Although all study participants had negative attitudes toward obesity, weight bias was significantly higher among individuals with BED and was associated with more depression and eating disorder psychopathology. It is not surprising that blame heaped on obese individuals may lead them to have intense feelings of shame, which, in turn, perpetuate a cycle of behaviors that promotes binge eating and excess weight gain. Given compelling evidence that the presence of weight bias and stigmatization among care providers and patients may pose significant barriers to effective treatment, it is imperative that clinicians treating eating disorders maintain awareness of their own attitudes and beliefs and that they ensure that patients' feelings about being larger than average size are recognized and validated during the assessment process.

Given the high levels of body shame and body dissatisfaction reported by obese people with disordered eating, clinicians need to appreciate that these individuals often are desperate to lose weight. As noted by Bulik et al. (2012), a mismatch between the patient's expectations (i.e., help for disordered eating *and* weight loss) and the goals of clinicians that focus on eating disorder treatment (mitigation of disordered eating) may lead to treatment dropout or failure. To enhance the likelihood of achieving congruence between the goals of patients and those of treating clinicians, the overall eating disorder assessment should include evaluation of both weight history and disordered eating. Optimally, a thorough assessment will validate patients' concerns regarding body weight, create a shared understanding, and establish a firm basis for treatment recommendations.

A list of assessment topics to guide the clinician in the evaluation of a patient's weight and eating behavior history appears in Table 4–1. The suggestions are not exhaustive but are presented to illustrate the interconnectedness of body weight, diet history, and eating behavior. For example, given that 40%–70% of the variance in body size is explained by genetic factors that affect obesity proneness (Barsh et al. 2000), it is important for the assessment clinician and the patient to understand personal obesity vulnerability by discussing family and personal weight history. Similarly, because duration of obesity is associated with the development of comorbidities, information about age at onset may provide some insight into the likelihood of the presence of obesity-related conditions that require independent medical attention.

Questions related to variation in body weight during adulthood allow for assessment of weight suppression or significant diet-induced weight loss that is sustained for a year or more (Lowe 1993). Weight suppression, which is calculated as the difference between the highest previous adult body weight (when not pregnant) and current weight, has been shown to

TABLE 4–1. Weight history assessment

Assessment topic	Rationale
Family and personal history of obesity	Obesity runs in families.
Duration of obesity/pediatric obesity	Medical comorbidity increases with duration of obesity.
Weight suppression (difference between the highest previous adult body weight [when not pregnant] and current weight)	Weight suppression predicts increases in body mass index, eating disorder psychopathology, and poorer treatment outcome.
History of weight loss efforts	It is crucial to identify history of significant dietary restriction, history of low weight, and contraindications for weight loss.
Personal ideal body weight	It is important to identify and discuss patient expectations.
Current weight loss goals	Understanding current expectations is salient for intervention recommendations.
Weight change during previous year	Many individuals gain weight in the period prior to seeking treatment.
Age at onset of disordered eating	Individuals who report loss-of-control or binge eating prior to their first diet may have different course.

predict increases in BMI (Stice et al. 2011), poor response to eating disorder treatment (Butryn et al. 2006), and increases in bulimic pathology (Thomas et al. 2011). Understanding the temporal relationship among dieting history, weight, and aberrant eating also may yield information that will help guide treatment planning. Evidence indicates that a significant proportion (38.7%–55%) of overweight and obese individuals report the onset of binge eating before the initiation of dieting (Abbott et al. 1998; Spurrell et al. 1997). This developmental pattern is associated with more eating disorder psychopathology and other psychiatric symptoms (Marcus et al. 1995; Spurrell et al. 1997) and suggests that dieting behavior may be a consequence rather than a cause of binge eating for a substantial proportion of individuals with binge-eating problems. Given the potential clinical implications, it is important for clinicians to include the discussion of weight history as part of a comprehensive assessment.

Video 3 illustrates the special considerations in the assessment and treatment of overweight patients.

Video Illustration 3: Assessing eating problems in overweight adults (5:52)

Differential Diagnosis

The differential diagnosis of disordered eating in individuals who are overweight or obese includes consideration of any DSM-5 (American Psychiatric Association 2013) feeding or eating disorder except anorexia nervosa (AN), which requires a significantly low body weight. In this section, we first discuss the assessment of disorders characterized by binge eating–that is, BED and bulimia nervosa (BN)–and then the assessment of other specified eating disorders. Finally, we describe avoidant/restrictive food intake disorder (ARFID), a new feeding disorder in DSM-5.

Before discussing BED and BN, it is important to note that *binge eating* is defined identically in both disorders as the intake of an unusually large amount of food given the circumstances (i.e., more than others would eat in a similar situation), accompanied by a sense of a lack of control during the episode (see also Chapter 10, "Use of the Eating Disorder Assessment for DSM-5"). Because BED is strongly associated with obesity (Marcus and Wildes 2009), much of the available data on aberrant eating among obese individuals is from the population with BED. Indeed, data from the National Comorbidity Survey Replication (Hudson et al. 2007), a population-based study of U.S. men and women, showed that 81.1% of individuals with a 12-month prevalence of BED were overweight or obese.

The DSM-5 diagnostic criteria for BED include persistent binge eating in the absence of the regular compensatory behaviors to prevent weight gain that are a cardinal feature of BN. For a BED diagnosis, binge-eating episodes must be associated with marked distress and three or more of the following correlates: eating much more quickly than normal; eating until feeling uncomfortably full; eating large amounts of food when not physically hungry; eating alone because of feeling embarrassed by the quantity that one is eating; and feeling disgusted with oneself, depressed, or very guilty afterward. Finally, the binge eating must occur at least once per week, on average, for 3 months (see the DSM-5 diagnostic criteria in Box 1–3 in Chapter 1, "Classification of Eating Disorders").

Although the cognitive correlates of disordered eating required for a diagnosis of AN or BN are not required for a BED diagnosis, there is evidence that the presence of an undue influence of body shape or weight on self-evaluation has prognostic significance. For example, Grilo et al. (2013) found that overvaluation of shape and weight in individuals with BED was strongly related to distress and eating-related psychopathology and negatively associated with treatment outcome. Therefore, clinicians should ask obese individuals routinely about overvaluation of weight and shape and other cognitive symptoms of disordered eating.

BN also should be included as a differential diagnosis in the assessment of individuals who are obese. BN is characterized by recurrent binge eating, accompanied by regular inappropriate compensatory behaviors (i.e., self-induced vomiting; misuse of laxatives, diuretics, or other medications; fasting; or excessive exercise) to prevent weight gain. The binge eating and inappropriate compensatory behaviors must occur, on average, at least once a week for a minimum of 3 months. A diagnosis of BN also requires that an individual's self-evaluation be unduly influenced by shape and weight (see the DSM-5 diagnostic criteria in Box 1–2 in Chapter 1).

Although long considered to be primarily a disorder of nonobese individuals, BN is also associated with adiposity. For example, Hudson et al. (2007) found that 84.2% of individuals with a 12-month diagnosis of BN were overweight or obese. Similarly, recent data from the World Health Organization World Mental Health Surveys, a population-based study of more than 24,000 men and women in 14 countries, documented the prevalence and correlates of BED using BN as a comparator (Kessler et al. 2013). Individuals with BN and BED both had higher BMIs than those without a history of eating disorders; 32.8% of individuals with BN and 41.7% of individuals with BED were obese. Moreover, there were no significant differences between BN and BED in proportions of underweight, healthy weight, overweight, or obese individuals, confirming the importance of considering both diagnoses in overweight and obese individuals who present with recurrent binge eating.

In DSM-5, individuals who have symptoms of disordered eating associated with distress and dysfunction but do not meet full criteria for a specific feeding or eating disorder may be diagnosed with other specified feeding or eating disorder (OSFED). One example provided in DSM-5 is atypical AN, in which the individual's body weight is normal or above normal despite persistent dietary restriction and significant weight loss but the person meets all of the other criteria for AN. Therefore, a previously obese individual who loses a significant amount of weight and develops all of the signs and symptoms of AN except a markedly low body weight may be given the diagnosis of atypical AN. Although this presentation is not uncommon in eating disorder specialty care settings, little is known about how or whether the course and outcome of atypical AN differ from those of full-syndrome AN.

Another example of OSFED is *night eating syndrome*, which is characterized by recurrent episodes of night eating (eating after awakening from sleep or excessive food consumption after the evening meal) with awareness and recall of the eating. This pattern of eating is not better explained by BED or another mental disorder and is not due to another medical disorder or the effects of medication. Criteria for night eating syndrome have evolved over time, and many studies have failed to control for the overlap between night eating syndrome and BED. Consequently, there has been uncertainty as to whether night eating syndrome is a distinct clinical entity (Runfola et al. 2014). Nevertheless, night eating syndrome appears to be more common in overweight and obese individuals and may lead to weight gain in vulnerable people (Gallant et al. 2012). Although a complete evaluation of disordered eating in overweight and obese individuals should include consideration of night eating syndrome, there is only preliminary evidence to suggest that a form of cognitive-behavioral therapy (CBT) adapted to incorporate sleep hygiene, relaxation, and consideration of either bright light or medication treatments may be helpful for these patients (Allison et al. 2010).

DSM-5 feeding and eating disorders also include pica, rumination disorder, and ARFID, any of which may be diagnosed in overweight and obese individuals. *Pica* (the persistent ingestion of nonnutritive food substances) and *rumination disorder* (the repeated regurgitation of food that is then re-chewed, re-swallowed, or spit out) have been studied in special populations, such as pregnant women and individuals with developmental disabilities, but, in general, they are poorly understood. A recent study of individuals in a residential program for eating disorders and an outpatient weight management program found that diagnosable pica and rumination disorder were rare, but reports of pica-like behaviors (e.g., eating uncooked pasta, chewing ice) and rumination were more common (Delaney et al. 2015). The authors suggested that questions regarding behaviors associated with pica and rumination should be included routinely in eating disorder assessment.

ARFID is a new feeding disorder in DSM-5. The criteria for feeding disorder of infancy or early childhood in DSM-IV (American Psychiatric Association 1994) were expanded and renamed in recognition that in addition to young children, there are older children, adolescents, and adults who habitually restrict food intake to a degree that they develop medical or psychosocial consequences (Attia et al. 2013). ARFID is characterized by a persistent failure to meet nutritional and/or energy needs associated with one or more of the following: significant weight loss (or failure to gain expected weight or faltering growth in children), significant nutritional deficiency, dependence on enteral feeding, or marked interference with psychosocial functioning. The food restriction cannot be due to a lack of available food or associated with a culturally sanctioned practice, and there is no disturbance in the experience of body shape or weight (i.e.,

ARFID is not diagnosed in addition to AN or BN). Finally, the eating disturbance cannot be better explained by a concurrent medical condition or another mental disorder (see the DSM-5 diagnostic criteria for ARFID in Box 1–4 in Chapter 1). Very little is known about ARFID, in general, and about the disorder in adults, in particular. Research is needed to determine the course, prognosis, and outcome of the disorder (Kreipe and Palomaki 2012). Nevertheless, given initial reports about preferences among highly selective eaters for highly palatable, nutrient-dense foods and indications that overweight and obesity rates in these individuals are comparable with those in the general population (Wildes et al. 2012), clinicians evaluating aberrant eating in obese individuals should assess significant dietary restriction associated with distress, dysfunction, or nutritional deficiency.

Finally, although not included in DSM-5 as a diagnosis, individuals who are overweight or obese may seek treatment for food addiction. The concept of food addiction has been the focus of extensive attention in the scientific literature and the lay press, and the notion that certain foods, particularly those that are highly palatable and high in calories, are addicting has considerable face validity. Briefly, the addiction model of obesity posits that substance use disorders and persistent overeating of highly palatable foods share a common phenomenology (e.g., escalation of use over time and continued misuse of the substance despite negative consequences). These observations are bolstered by animal studies and a growing number of human studies that have shown that repeated consumption of palatable foods results in behavioral and neurochemical changes analogous to those seen in chronic substance use (Marcus and Wildes 2014). The notion that the reinforcement from highly palatable food can override homeostatic eating and co-opt the dopaminergic neurocircuitry involved in reward sensitivity and incentive motivation has both research support (Volkow et al. 2013) and prominent critics (Ziauddeen and Fletcher 2013), and the topic continues to be controversial. Indeed, given mixed findings from studies comparing obese and lean individuals, there have been investigations focusing on binge eaters as the obesity phenotype characterized by food addiction (Dalton et al. 2013). As noted by Gearhardt et al. (2011), understanding the relationship between food addiction and BED may help explicate the etiology of aberrant eating or may offer neurobiological targets for treatment. At this point in time, however, the implications of food addiction for treatment, course, and outcome of disordered eating are unknown.

Associated Problems

Eating disorders and obesity are associated with other psychiatric comorbidities, suggesting that individuals with both conditions may have an increased mental health burden. There is robust evidence that BED and BN are associated with psychiatric comorbidity; data from the National Comorbidity Replication Study (Hudson et al. 2007) documented that 78.9% of individuals with BED and 94.5% of those with BN met criteria for at least one additional DSM-IV psychiatric disorder. Odds ratios indicated that the risk of a comorbid lifetime psychiatric disorder was higher in BN than in BED, but comorbid mood and anxiety disorders, in particular, were highly prevalent in both groups (e.g., 46.4% of individuals with BED and 70.7% of individuals with BN had a lifetime history of comorbid mood disorder). A population-based study of BED and BN in 14 countries (Kessler et al. 2013) mirrored findings from the United States (Hudson et al. 2007); that is, the majority of individuals with BED (79%) and BN (84.8%) met lifetime criteria for an additional DSM-IV psychiatric disorder. Moreover, BED and BN were associated with comparable levels of impairment in social and occupational functioning across countries, demonstrating the clinical significance of both disorders.

Obese individuals also are at elevated risk for psychiatric comorbidity. For example, in an analysis of data from 177,047 participants in the 2006 Behavioral Risk Factor Surveillance System (Zhao et al. 2009), rates of self-reported diagnoses of current depression, lifetime diagnosed depression, and anxiety were higher in women who were overweight or obese than among nonoverweight women and were higher in men with severe obesity than among nonoverweight men, after the authors controlled for multiple potential confounders, including medical illness and psychosocial factors. Similarly, a meta-analysis of longitudinal studies examining the association between obesity and depression confirmed a reciprocal link between depression and obesity, such that obesity increased the risk for depression and, to a lesser extent, depression predicted the development of obesity (Luppino et al. 2010). Finally, the risk of mood disorders, but not anxiety or substance use disorders, is markedly higher among individuals with severe obesity compared with overweight or moderately obese individuals (Petry et al. 2008).

Given the risk of psychiatric comorbidity in individuals with eating disorders and obesity, and the potential of an additive or interactive effect for individuals who are obese and have disordered eating, clinicians should conduct a complete psychiatric assessment and consider the role of psychiatric comorbidity in treatment planning.

Physical Assessment

The medical consequences of obesity are indisputable and affect virtually all aspects of human functioning (Hill and Wyatt 2013). Obesity is associated with cardiovascular and metabolic risk, kidney disease, several types of cancer, osteoarthritis, sleep apnea, and reduced quality of life (Eckel 2008; Vucenik and Stains 2012; Wang et al. 2011). Binge eating also may contribute to medical morbidity over and above that associated with obesity alone. For example, in a prospective 5-year study of individuals with and without BED matched for baseline BMI, investigators documented that BED conferred an increased risk for self-reported dyslipidemia and two or more components of the metabolic syndrome (Hudson et al. 2010). Another investigation documented that overweight and obese individuals with BED, when compared with those without BED, were significantly more likely to have irritable bowel syndrome and fibromyalgia (Javaras et al. 2008). Although additional research is needed to confirm that BED is an independent contributor to obesity-related medical comorbidity, assessment and management of obesity-related comorbidities are necessary for all overweight individuals.

It is likely that patients who are obese who do receive regular medical care have been advised to lose weight to mitigate the risk of developing comorbidities, particularly cardiovascular disease and diabetes. In this context, it is appropriate for mental health clinicians to communicate with primary care providers regarding the presence of disordered eating to enhance the likelihood that medical recommendations are consistent with the treatment of disordered eating (Bulik et al. 2012).

Mental health clinicians need to keep in mind that eating disorders in individuals of any body size are associated with medical sequelae that might require attention. Purging behaviors, especially self-induced vomiting and misuse of laxatives, and to a lesser extent binge eating, are associated with multiple medical complications (see Mehler et al. 2011 for review). Medical assessment prior to treatment is advisable, and depending on the severity of the eating disorder behaviors, routine medical monitoring may be indicated.

Implications for Treatment

Research on the treatment of overweight and obese individuals with disordered eating has focused primarily on BED. Although both disordered eating and excess adiposity may serve as the focus of treatment for overweight and obese individuals with BED, we recommend that the eating disorder should be the initial focus of intervention. Some studies have shown that behavioral weight loss interventions are effective in reducing binge eating and promoting modest weight loss in obese BED patients in the short term, but there now is solid evidence that addressing binge eating is more effective than behavioral weight loss in the treatment of BED. In the most compelling study to date, Wilson et al. (2010) randomly assigned more than 200 overweight or obese men and women with BED to 20 sessions of a behavioral weight loss program, interpersonal therapy (IPT), or CBT guided self-help (CBTgsh). Two-year follow-up data showed that both IPT and CBTgsh were more effective than behavioral weight loss in achieving remission from binge eating. Although weight loss was limited and similar across intervention conditions, remission from binge eating was associated with a greater likelihood of weight losses that were at least 5% of initial body weight.

Bolstering the recommendation for a primary focus on disordered eating, a study that examined patterns of weight change among treatment-seeking obese individuals with BED found that a significant minority (35.4%) had gained 10% of body weight or more in the year preceding treatment. Thus, although treatment focusing on disordered eating may not lead to weight loss, especially in the short term, findings suggest that eating disorder intervention may serve to stabilize weight and prevent increases in obesity severity (Masheb et al. 2013). In summary, clinicians are in a strong position to advise that the treatment of disordered eating should be the focus: successful intervention may stabilize weight, and long-term abstinence from binge eating may be associated with decreases in body weight.

Much less is known about the treatment of obese individuals with BN or other feeding or eating disorders. To our knowledge, there are no investigations comparing the treatment outcome of overweight and nonoverweight individuals with BN. Furthermore, it is not currently known whether the apparent increase in obesity among patients with BN is explained by demographic trends or if obese and nonobese individuals differ in salient clinical characteristics. Some evidence suggests that individuals with BN who report binge eating before the onset of dieting behavior, when compared with those who dieted before the onset of binge eating, have an earlier onset of aberrant eating, higher weights, and a lower frequency of vomiting in relation to binge eating; that is, they tend to resemble individuals with BED (Haiman and Devlin 1999). Future research is needed to clarify how obesity may affect treatment outcome of BN; however, at this point, CBT is the treatment of choice for BN and BED (Wilson et al. 2007). Finally, because the evidence base for the treatment of DSM-5 feeding disorders or other specified feeding and eating disorders is small, there is little to guide clinicians on the management of obese individuals presenting with these problems.

Although we recommend a primary focus on disordered eating for individuals with BED or BN, questions remain for clinicians and treatment-seeking obese individuals with binge-eating problems–whether and when patients can or should pursue weight loss. Although stabilization of eating behaviors through the successful treatment of BED may provide a better foundation for subsequent weight loss interventions, there also is substantial evidence that behavioral weight loss programs focusing on the achievement of even 3%–5% sustained decreases in initial body weight are associated with significant improvements in cardiometabolic risk factors, psychiatric symptoms, and quality of life. Indeed, guidelines for the management of adults who are overweight or obese (Jensen et al. 2014) advise that all patients with a BMI over 30 kg/m^2 and those with a BMI greater than or equal to 25 kg/m^2 with one or more additional risk factors (e.g., hypertension) should be referred for comprehensive behavioral lifestyle intervention. Furthermore, there is evidence that a significant percentage of participants in comprehensive behavioral weight loss programs are able to sustain at least some weight loss and associated decreases in cardiometabolic risk over a several-year period when there is continued contact with interventionists (Knowler et al. 2009).

Nevertheless, there are important caveats when considering behavioral weight management for obese individuals with binge-eating problems. First, many individuals with BED will not be satisfied with modest weight losses, and individual weight loss goals for those entering obesity treatment programs have been shown to be significantly greater than the reasonable weight losses suggested by health guidelines (Foster et al. 1997). Second, weight loss programs may not lead to sustained weight losses for most individuals, and data from a study by Gorin et al. (2008) suggest that long-term weight loss maintenance is more problematic for individuals with BED than for those without.

Despite these concerns, it also is important to note that there is little evidence showing that comprehensive behavioral weight management programs are associated with the exacerbation of eating-related psychopathology. For example, although Wilson et al. (2010) found that interventions that targeted binge eating were superior to behavioral weight management in achieving remission from binge eating, there was no evidence that comprehensive behavioral weight management was associated with exacerbation of eating-related psychopathology at any assessment point. Thus, consideration of weight management for obese individuals with BED should involve a detailed discussion of the pros and cons of pursuing weight loss at a given point in time.

Finally, in the context of considering the management of obesity, discussion of Health at Every Size (HAES; Miller and Jacob 2001) is warranted because this movement has gained increased traction in the eating disorders community. Briefly stated, the philosophy of HAES emphasizes shifting the focus from weight loss to promotion of healthy behaviors as a goal for people of all sizes. Proponents argue that weight loss programs do not lead to sustained improvements in health or weight and are associated with negative consequences such as increased body and food preoccupation, reduced self-esteem, disordered eating, and weight stigmatization (Bacon and Aphramor 2011; Miller and Jacob 2001). The effects of traditional weight loss programs are indeed modest, but the evidence offers meager justification for the proposition that HAES leads to superior outcomes. There have been few controlled trials of HAES interventions. In one randomized controlled trial comparing a 4-month HAES intervention with a social support intervention and a wait-list control group (Provencher et al. 2009), no differences were observed between the HAES and social support groups at 1-year follow-up, and neither of the intervention conditions was associated with improvements in weight, lipoproteins, blood pressure, self-reported energy intake, or physical activity.

In a second trial, Bacon et al. (2002, 2005) evaluated the relative efficacy of a behavioral weight management program and a HAES program. Weekly group sessions were offered for 6 months, and an additional six monthly sessions followed. Participants also were evaluated 1 year after completion of the 1-year intervention. There was a high rate of attrition in both groups (nearly 50%) at follow-up, and no significant between-group differences were observed in weight-related parameters or cardiovascular risk factors. Nevertheless, those in the HAES group, compared to the behavioral weight control participants, showed significant improvements in subscale scores on the Eating Disorder Inventory (Garner 1991). HAES also was associated with greater improvements in self-esteem, but both groups showed significant improvement over the 2-year period of observation.

In summary, results of the few extant studies provide initial evidence that HAES may have psychosocial benefits for some patients, but support for the idea that HAES improves weight-related or cardiovascular risk profiles is scant. Conversely, and consistent with other data about the effects of weight management on aspects of disordered eating, the one HAES study that used a behavioral weight management comparison condition (Bacon et al. 2002, 2005) did not document negative effects of the program on any measured variable, raising questions regarding the oft-stated HAES proposition that unsuccessful weight management is associated with significant harms.

In addition to a lack of evidence for the utility of HAES interventions, HAES advocates have argued that the strong associations between obesity and multiple medical comorbidities do not prove causality and that many studies fail to control for salient covariables that explain the obesity and medical illness relationship (Bacon and Aphramor 2011). Imperfect research may abound, but the contention that obesity-related health risks are overstated and unproven is inconsistent with an enormous amount of evidence and scientific consensus. Furthermore, the notion of metabolically healthy obesity (Lavie et al. 2015) has been questioned. Recent analyses have shown that individuals who are obese are at increased risk for unfavorable outcomes even when they have no current metabolic abnormalities and indicate that increased adiposity is not a benign condition (Kramer et al. 2013). Thus, although additional research may substantiate the utility of HAES interventions, there is no current justification for statements averring its efficacy.

Conclusion

In this chapter, we have outlined multiple and often interacting factors that are salient for the assessment of individuals who are obese and who have disordered eating. This population requires special consideration, especially in light of data suggesting that weight stigma and weight discrimination exist among health professionals, including specialists in the treatment of obesity (Schwartz et al. 2003). Available evidence indicates that binge eating should be treated first, but behavioral weight management may mitigate obesity-related risk and does not appear to be associated with eating disorder symptoms.

Key Clinical Points

- The majority of individuals in the United States are overweight or obese.
- The etiology of obesity is multifactorial, and most obese individuals do not report disordered eating.
- It is important for clinicians to understand how shaming and stigma affect treatment-seeking individuals and that body shame and body dissatisfaction often are associated with an intense desire to lose weight as well as to stop disordered eating.
- Overweight and obese individuals may be diagnosed with any DSM-5 feeding or eating disorder except anorexia nervosa, and thus the full range of feeding and eating disorders should be considered.
- Disordered eating among individuals who are obese is associated with marked psychiatric comorbidity and impairments.
- Obesity is associated with significant nonpsychiatric medical comorbidity, and the presence of binge eating may confer additional

risks. Thus, referral for comprehensive health assessments is recommended prior to the initiation of treatment.

- Eating disorder treatment, particularly cognitive-behavioral therapy, should be the first-line intervention for obese individuals with binge-eating problems, although cognitive-behavioral therapy is not usually associated with short-term weight loss.
- The pros and cons of behavioral weight management interventions for obese individuals should be considered carefully, but modest weight losses may improve cardiometabolic health without psychosocial harms, and therefore these interventions can be considered for selected individuals.

References

Abbott DW, de Zwaan M, Mussell MP, et al: Onset of binge eating and dieting in overweight women: implications for etiology, associated features and treatment. J Psychosom Res 44(3–4):367–374, 1998 9587880

Allison KC, Lundgren JD, Moore RH, et al: Cognitive behavior therapy for night eating syndrome: a pilot study. Am J Psychother 64(1):91–106, 2010 20405767

American Psychiatric Association: Diagnostic and Statistical Manual of Mental Disorders, 4th Edition. Washington, DC, American Psychiatric Association, 1994

American Psychiatric Association: Diagnostic and Statistical Manual of Mental Disorders, 5th Edition. Arlington, VA, American Psychiatric Association, 2013

Attia E, Becker AE, Bryant-Waugh R, et al: Feeding and eating disorders in DSM-5. Am J Psychiatry 170(11):1237–1239, 2013 24185238

Bacon L, Aphramor L: Weight science: evaluating the evidence for a paradigm shift. Nutr J 10:9, 2011 21261939

Bacon L, Keim NL, Van Loan MD, et al: Evaluating a 'non-diet' wellness intervention for improvement of metabolic fitness, psychological well-being and eating and activity behaviors. Int J Obes Relat Metab Disord 26(6):854–865, 2002 12037657

Bacon L, Stern JS, Van Loan MD, et al: Size acceptance and intuitive eating improve health for obese, female chronic dieters. J Am Diet Assoc 105(6):929–936, 2005 15942543

Barnes RD, Ivezaj V, Grilo CM: An examination of weight bias among treatment-seeking obese patients with and without binge eating disorder. Gen Hosp Psychiatry 36(2):177–180, 2014 24359678

Barsh GS, Farooqi IS, O'Rahilly S: Genetics of body-weight regulation. Nature 404(6778):644–651, 2000 10766251

Bulik CM, Marcus MD, Zerwas S, et al: The changing "weightscape" of bulimia nervosa. Am J Psychiatry 169(10):1031–1036, 2012 23032383

Butryn ML, Lowe MR, Safer DL, et al: Weight suppression is a robust predictor of outcome in the cognitive-behavioral treatment of bulimia nervosa. J Abnorm Psychol 115(1):62–67, 2006 16492096

Dalton M, Blundell J, Finlayson G: Effect of BMI and binge eating on food reward and energy intake: further evidence for a binge eating subtype of obesity. Obes Facts 6(4):348–359, 2013 23970144

Delaney CB, Eddy KT, Hartmann AS, et al: Pica and rumination behavior among individuals seeking treatment for eating disorders or obesity. Int J Eat Disord 48(2):238–248, 2015 24729045

Eckel RH: Clinical practice: nonsurgical management of obesity in adults. N Engl J Med 358(18):1941–1950, 2008 18450605

Foster GD, Wadden TA, Vogt RA, et al: What is a reasonable weight loss? Patients' expectations and evaluations of obesity treatment outcomes. J Consult Clin Psychol 65(1):79–85, 1997 9103737

Gallant AR, Lundgren J, Drapeau V: The night-eating syndrome and obesity. Obes Rev 13(6):528–536, 2012 22222118

Garner D: Eating Disorder Inventory-2: Professional Manual. Odessa, FL, Psychological Assessment Resources, 1991

Gearhardt AN, White MA, Potenza MN: Binge eating disorder and food addiction. Curr Drug Abuse Rev 4(3):201–207, 2011 21999695

Gorin AA, Niemeier HM, Hogan P, et al: Look AHEAD Research Group: Binge eating and weight loss outcomes in overweight and obese individuals with type 2 diabetes: results from the Look AHEAD trial. Arch Gen Psychiatry 65(12):1447–1455, 2008 19047532

Grilo CM, White MA, Gueorguieva R, et al: Predictive significance of the overvaluation of shape/weight in obese patients with binge eating disorder: findings from a randomized controlled trial with 12-month follow-up. Psychol Med 43(6):1335–1344, 2013 22967857

Haiman C, Devlin MJ: Binge eating before the onset of dieting: a distinct subgroup of bulimia nervosa? Int J Eat Disorder 25(2):151–157, 1999 10065392

Hill JO, Wyatt HR: The myth of healthy obesity. Ann Intern Med 159(11):789–790, 2013 24297199

Hudson JI, Hiripi E, Pope HG Jr, et al: The prevalence and correlates of eating disorders in the National Comorbidity Survey Replication. Biol Psychiatry 61(3):348–358, 2007 16815322

Hudson JI, Lalonde JK, Coit CE, et al: Longitudinal study of the diagnosis of components of the metabolic syndrome in individuals with binge-eating disorder. Am J Clin Nutr 91(6):1568–1573, 2010 20427731

Jackson SE, Beeken RJ, Wardle J: Perceived weight discrimination and changes in weight, waist circumference, and weight status. Obesity (Silver Spring) 22(12):2485–2488, 2014 25212272

Javaras KN, Pope HG, Lalonde JK, et al: Co-occurrence of binge eating disorder with psychiatric and medical disorders. J Clin Psychiatry 69(2):266–273, 2008 18348600

Jeffery RW, Harnack LJ: Evidence implicating eating as a primary driver for the obesity epidemic. Diabetes 56(11):2673–2676, 2007 17878287

Jensen MD, Ryan DH, Apovian CM, et al; American College of Cardiology/American Heart Association Task Force on Practice Guidelines; Obesity Society: 2013 AHA/ACC/TOS guideline for the management of overweight and obesity in adults: a report of the American College of Cardiology/American Heart Association Task Force on Practice Guidelines and the Obesity Society. Circulation 129(25) (suppl 2):S102–S138, 2014 24222017

Kessler RC, Berglund PA, Chiu WT, et al: The prevalence and correlates of binge eating disorder in the World Health Organization World Mental Health Surveys. Biol Psychiatry 73(9):904–914, 2013 23290497

Knowler WC, Fowler SE, Hamman RF, et al; Diabetes Prevention Program Research Group: 10-year follow-up of diabetes incidence and weight loss in the Diabetes Prevention Program Outcomes Study. Lancet 374(9702):1677–1686, 2009 19878986

Kramer CK, Zinman B, Retnakaran R: Are metabolically healthy overweight and obesity benign conditions? A systematic review and meta-analysis. Ann Intern Med 159(11):758–769, 2013 24297192

Kreipe RE, Palomaki A: Beyond picky eating: avoidant/restrictive food intake disorder. Curr Psychiatry Rep 14(4):421–431, 2012 22665043

Lavie CJ, De Schutter A, Milani RV: Healthy obese versus unhealthy lean: the obesity paradox. Nat Rev Endocrinol 11(1):55–62, 2015 25265977

Lowe MR: The effects of dieting on eating behavior: a three-factor model. Psychol Bull 114(1):100–121, 1993 8346324

Luppino FS, de Wit LM, Bouvy PF, et al: Overweight, obesity, and depression: a systematic review and meta-analysis of longitudinal studies. Arch Gen Psychiatry 67(3):220–229, 2010 20194822

Marcus MD, Wildes JE: Obesity: is it a mental disorder? Int J Eat Disord 42(8):739–753, 2009 19610015

Marcus MD, Wildes JE: Disordered eating in obese individuals. Curr Opin Psychiatry 27(6):443–447, 2014 25247456

Marcus MD, Moulton MM, Greeno CG: Binge eating onset in obese patients with binge eating disorder. Addict Behav 20(6):747–755, 1995 8820527

Masheb RM, White MA, Grilo CM: Substantial weight gains are common prior to treatment-seeking in obese patients with binge eating disorder. Compr Psychiatry 54(7):880–884, 2013 23639407

Mehler PS, Birmingham CL, Crow SJ, et al: Medical complications of eating disorders, in The Treatment of Eating Disorders: A Clinical Handbook. Edited by Grilo CM, Mitchell JE. New York, Guilford, 2011, pp 66–80

Miller WC, Jacob AV: The health at any size paradigm for obesity treatment: the scientific evidence. Obes Rev 2(1):37–45, 2001 12119636

National Institutes of Health: Clinical Guidelines on the Identification, Evaluation, and Treatment of Overweight and Obesity in Adults–The Evidence Report. Obes Res 6 (suppl 2):51S–209S, 1998 9813653

Ogden CL, Carroll MD, Kit BK, et al: Prevalence of childhood and adult obesity in the United States, 2011–2012. JAMA 311(8):806–814, 2014 24570244

Petry NM, Barry D, Pietrzak RH, et al: Overweight and obesity are associated with psychiatric disorders: results from the National Epidemiologic Survey on Alcohol and Related Conditions. Psychosom Med 70(3):288–297, 2008 18378873

Provencher V, Bégin C, Tremblay A, et al: Health-At-Every-Size and eating behaviors: 1-year follow-up results of a size acceptance intervention. J Am Diet Assoc 109(11):1854–1861, 2009 19857626

Puhl RM, Heuer CA: Obesity stigma: important considerations for public health. Am J Public Health 100(6):1019–1028, 2010 20075322

Runfola CD, Allison KC, Hardy KK, et al: Prevalence and clinical significance of night eating syndrome in university students. J Adolesc Health 55(1):41–48, 2014 24485551

Schwartz MB, Chambliss HO, Brownell KD, et al: Weight bias among health professionals specializing in obesity. Obes Res 11(9):1033–1039, 2003 12972672

Spurrell EB, Wilfley DE, Tanofsky MB, et al: Age of onset for binge eating: are there different pathways to binge eating? Int J Eat Disord 21(1):55–65, 1997 8986518

Stice E, Durant S, Burger KS, et al: Weight suppression and risk of future increases in body mass: effects of suppressed resting metabolic rate and energy expenditure. Am J Clin Nutr 94(1):7–11, 2011 21525201

Thomas JG, Butryn ML, Stice E, et al: A prospective test of the relation between weight change and risk for bulimia nervosa. Int J Eat Disord 44(4):295–303, 2011 21472748

Volkow ND, Wang GJ, Tomasi D, et al: Obesity and addiction: neurobiological overlaps. Obes Rev 14(1):2–18, 2013 23016694

Vucenik I, Stains JP: Obesity and cancer risk: evidence, mechanisms, and recommendations. Ann N Y Acad Sci 1271:37–43, 2012 23050962

Wang YC, McPherson K, Marsh T, et al: Health and economic burden of the projected obesity trends in the USA and the UK. Lancet 378(9793):815–825, 2011 21872750

Wildes JE, Zucker NL, Marcus MD: Picky eating in adults: results of a Web-based survey. Int J Eat Disord 45(4):575–582, 2012 22331752

Wilson GT, Grilo CM, Vitousek KM: Psychological treatment of eating disorders. Am Psychol 62(3):199–216, 2007 17469898

Wilson GT, Wilfley DE, Agras WS, et al: Psychological treatments of binge eating disorder. Arch Gen Psychiatry 67(1):94–101, 2010 20048227

Zhao G, Ford ES, Dhingra S, et al: Depression and anxiety among U.S. adults: associations with body mass index. Int J Obes (Lond) 33(2):257–266, 2009 19125163

Ziauddeen H, Fletcher PC: Is food addiction a valid and useful concept? Obes Rev 14(1):19–28, 2013 23057499

5 Assessment of Eating Disorders and Problematic Eating Behavior in Bariatric Surgery Patients

Eva M. Conceição, Ph.D.
James E. Mitchell, M.D.

Bariatric surgery procedures substantially alter the normal anatomy of the gastrointestinal (GI) tract, leading to significant changes in eating behavior. However, a number of bariatric surgery patients report problematic eating behaviors, as well as full and subthreshold eating disorders, both preoperatively and postoperatively, which have been associated with poor weight treatment outcomes (Conceição et al. 2013a, 2014). The notable heterogeneity in eating pathology documented in the literature and the lack of an identified nomenclature for these problems are serious challenges, and understanding disordered eating in candidates for bariatric surgery is important for clinicians attempting to devise and implement an effective therapeutic approach.

Currently, no diagnostic terms have been specifically developed to describe eating disorders and problematic eating in individuals before or after bariatric surgery. The criteria used for diagnosis in these populations have been the standard *Diagnostic and Statistical Manual* criteria, but important differences should be considered when assessing eating disorders and problematic eating behaviors in bariatric surgery patients, both preoperatively and in the postoperative period. In this chapter, we focus on the assessment of eating disorders before and after surgery and in the application of DSM-5 criteria for eating disorders in bariatric surgery patients (American Psychiatric Association 2013). We also address problematic eating behaviors and GI syndromes that play an important role in bariatric surgery outcomes, such as grazing, emotional eating, and dumping syndrome. Finally, we provide specific guidelines for the clinical assessment of eating disorders and problematic eating behaviors.

Special Considerations for the Clinical Assessment

It is strongly recommended that mental health professionals assessing individuals before and after bariatric surgery possess specialized interest in and knowledge about obesity, weight control, and weight loss surgery. The clinical assessment of eating disorders and problematic eating behaviors in bariatric surgery patients requires not only specific knowledge of the different surgical procedures, the associated nutritional requirements, and the variations in eating that these patients must implement over time, but also attention to subsyndromal presentation of symptoms and atypical behaviors not often seen in nonbariatric surgery patients with eating disorders. Additionally, clinicians need to have open communication with the rest of the multidisciplinary bariatric team to exchange information particularly regarding adherence to nutritional requirements, as well as other factors affecting surgical outcomes. These factors may result in less weight loss or greater weight regain and also may dictate the need for additional clinical attention. The remainder of this chapter focuses on the specific types of information relevant to the assessment of eating disorders and problematic eating among individuals having bariatric surgery.

When a bariatric surgery candidate or postoperative patient is referred for evaluation, standard assessments for the DSM-5 diagnostic criteria for eating disorders should be used. The assessment of eating pathology is often intended to identify patients who are engaging in behaviors that may increase the risk for poor outcomes, including attenuated weight loss, excessive regain, or impaired psychological functioning. Because interviews typically occur during what is often a mandatory psychiatric assessment, there is a risk that participants will deny problematic behaviors to avoid delay or denial of surgery. With postsurgery patients, assessment should take place at critical postoperative time points, particularly after the weight loss nadir is reached at about 1–2 years after surgery, when eating behavior may potentially deteriorate (Magro et al. 2008). Like other individuals with symptoms of an eating disorder, post–bariatric surgery patients with anorexia- or bulimia-like symptoms may deny their problematic behaviors in the hope of achieving unrealistic weight goals. They may justify these behaviors as common sequelae of surgery, including the need to limit the amounts and types of foods ingested, and may attribute the occurrence of vomiting and/or dumping to the surgery even if those behaviors are self-induced. In such cases, the patients' low level of commitment to change may be particularly challenging, and an empathic, nonjudgmental but firm approach will be needed to address the underlying motivation for these problematic behaviors. At all times, educating patients about the risks of certain eating behaviors or eating disorders and about how early detection of problematic symptoms may improve outcome of surgery and enhance psychological functioning will facilitate cooperation and openness.

Binge-eating disorder (BED), binge eating, and so-called loss-of-control eating are the most commonly reported eating disorder problems in patients before and after bariatric surgery. However, in bariatric surgery candidates, little is known about the prevalence of either full or subthreshold bulimia nervosa (BN), and anorexia nervosa (AN) is excluded because these patients do not meet the low-weight criteria. The development of classic eating disorders after bariatric surgery is now recognized, and although incidence rates are not well established, they appear to be very low. Nonetheless, in rare cases inpatient eating disorder treatment may be required (Conceição et al. 2013a). Presentations following surgery may be atypical because of age at onset (bariatric surgery patients are usually older), the difficulties in deciding what should be considered a normal or low body mass index (BMI), dissatisfaction with body image after massive weight loss, and some of the specific compensatory behaviors that are unique to this population.

Clinicians must distinguish between symptoms of an eating disorder and changes in behavior necessitated by alterations to the GI tract. After surgery, patients require a very restrictive diet and are instructed to limit meal size, to systematically follow an eating schedule, to weigh their food, and often to cut food into small pieces. They are also told to avoid certain foods that may be intolerable (e.g., red meat), to chew food extensively, and to monitor and control their weight. In fact, some level of patient self-responsibility and self-control regarding food intake is strongly encouraged by professionals caring for these patients to facilitate weight loss. These self-responsibility and self-control behaviors may resemble those expected in treatment of individuals with eating disorders. Thus, in evaluating such behaviors, the clinician needs to determine whether the patient's behaviors result from excessive concerns about weight and shape or from the desire to strictly adhere to recommendations to avoid complications following surgery.

Similarly, episodic vomiting is frequent among patients following bariatric surgery (de Zwaan et al. 2010) and usually occurs in response to the ingestion of intolerable foods (e.g., red meat), eating too quickly, or chewing food insufficiently. At times, vomiting is used to reduce physical discomfort from plugging symptoms (problems with the small opening of the stomach becoming plugged with food) or from having eaten too much at one time. However, a minority of patients (12% in the study by de Zwaan et al. [2010]) also utilize vomiting as a means to control their weight.

Atypical compensatory behaviors also may emerge in patients following bariatric surgery. Dumping syndrome–the rapid movement of undigested food into the small bowel, causing abdominal cramps, nausea, and diarrhea–is a common GI event after surgery. Dumping syndrome has typically been described as an involuntary event, but dumping also is induced purposefully with the ingestion of specific foods by some patients to compensate for overeating or to enhance weight loss.

Additional concerns emerge when assessing low weight in post–bariatric surgery patients. It has not yet been determined what constitutes a low BMI for patients who were formerly severely obese and have lost massive amounts of weight following surgery. A BMI of 25 kg/m^2 has been recommended as a useful line between overweight and so-called normal weight in the general population; however, there is little agreement on what should be regarded as a low or normal BMI in patients following bariatric surgery (Dixon et al. 2005). In reality, the majority of those who successfully lose weight postsurgery do not reach a BMI lower than 25 kg/m^2, which would be difficult to achieve outside of severely restricting their food intake and risking malnutrition (Dixon et al. 2005). Moreover, postsurgery BMI is also affected by patients' excess skin, which averages 4.8 kg but can account for up to 15 kg of weight following massive weight loss (Ortega et al. 2010). A detailed weight history and exploration of the patient's expectations regarding weight may facilitate the evaluation of BMI in this population.

Among patients being assessed after surgery, the clinician should also assess the age at onset and duration of obesity, past history of weight loss and weight loss attempts, the patient's view about his or her current weight, the patient's ideal weight and desired weight after surgery, weight loss since surgery, and recent weight fluctuations and their impact on self-esteem and mood. Patients' perspectives about their ideal weight, the weight they think they can achieve and maintain in a healthy way, fear of weight regain, coping strategies for weight stabilization, and behaviors to facilitate weight loss may help in deciding whether the weight goal is appropriate and whether it is being pursued or maintained with problematic or inappropriate eating behaviors.

Addressing weight or shape concerns in individuals who are undergoing massive changes in weight poses additional challenges. When addressing the role of body weight and body image in self-evaluation, the clinician should consider the fact that substantial weight loss facilitates many activities of daily living, improves perceived quality of life and social functioning, and is usually reinforced by others, which naturally results in weight being a salient aspect of self-evaluation (van Hout et al. 2006). Following surgery, individuals not only may have a realistic fear of weight regain, but excess loose skin, skin envelopes, and fat deposits also have a great impact on body image and may contribute to severe body dissatisfaction, as well as social embarrassment, despite weight loss (Odom et al. 2010). Weight concerns appear to peak when much of the expected weight loss has been achieved and patients reach a plateau in their rate of weight change (Conceição et al. 2013b). The slower weight loss rate at this time may trigger increased fears of weight regain (Conceição et al. 2013b) and greater efforts to control weight, resulting in overly restrictive eating behaviors that may result in malnutrition.

Special considerations and specific probe questions for the assessment eating disorder criteria in bariatric surgery patients are summarized in Table 5–1.

Binge Eating and Loss-of-Control Eating

An *objective binge-eating episode,* as defined by DSM-5, is determined by two characteristics: 1) a sense of loss of control over eating, or not being able to resist eating or stop eating once started, and 2) ingestion of an excessively large amount of food in a discrete period of time (see Chapter 10, "Use of the Eating Disorder Assessment for DSM-5"). Assessing binge eating prior to bariatric surgery poses challenges similar to those faced in the assessment of this behavior in any overweight individual (see Chapter 4, "Eating Problems in Individuals With Overweight and Obesity"). Considerations include 1) evaluating the presence of loss of control, which is often not as distinct among obese individuals as among individuals with BN, because feelings of loss of control may not be as intense and disorganizing for severely obese individuals and for BN patients and many of these patients may feel that they "gave up" trying to control or limit the amount of food they eat because of unsuccessful previous attempts; 2) deciding what constitutes a large amount of food in the context of eating episodes may be challenging because it may not be as distinctively different from other non-binge meals as it is in BN patients; and 3) the absence of inappropriate

TABLE 5–1. Summary of special considerations when assessing eating-disordered criteria after bariatric surgery and specific probe questions

Required for DSM-5 diagnosis	Criterion	Special considerations after surgery	Specific probe questions (to be used in addition to the questions concerning formal eating disorder diagnosis)
AN	Restriction of energy intake relative to requirements leading to a significantly low body weight in the context of age, sex, developmental trajectory, and physical health	A highly restrictive diet is prescribed in the initial months after surgery. The amount of food tolerated is limited. There are no clear rules for defining underweight in postoperative patients. Considering the weight loss trajectory and physical health are particularly important.	Could you describe your regular eating patterns for me? What is the prescribed nutritional plan for your follow-up? Do you avoid any foods, not because of the physical discomfort they may cause you but because you believe they will have an impact on your weight? Have you experienced any symptoms of starvation (e.g., cold intolerance, hypotension)? Do you have a problem with excess hanging skin?
	Intense fear of gaining weight or becoming fat and persistent behaviors to control weight	Fear of weight gain is to some extent realistic and based on past experience.	What strategies do you use to control your weight? Do you count calories? Do you avoid any food or nutritional supplements that were recommended to you? Do you limit the amount of food you eat at each meal? How often do you weigh yourself? How would you feel if you regained 5 pounds? 10 pounds?

TABLE 5–1. Summary of special considerations when assessing eating-disordered criteria after bariatric surgery and specific probe questions *(continued)*

Required for DSM-5 diagnosis	Criterion	Special considerations after surgery	Specific probe questions (to be used in addition to the questions concerning formal eating disorder diagnosis)
AN, BN, BED	Undue influence of body weight or shape on self-evaluation	Aesthetic alterations characterized by loose skin, skin envelopes, and fat deposits have important impacts on body image, causing dissatisfaction and social embarrassment.	What areas of your body are affected by extra hanging skin? What activities do you avoid because of excess skin? What types of clothing do you avoid?
BN, BED	Recurrent episodes of binge eating	Assessing the amount of food requires knowledge about the nutritional needs of each patient in their stage of treatment, the gastric capacity, and the type of surgery. Loss of control may be the only feature present in postoperative bariatric patients.	How is the amount of food eaten in a binge-eating episode different from the regular amount of food you eat in your typical meals? Do you often have the feeling of plugging from the food in your stomach? Do you experience dumping syndrome? Do you keep eating even though you know food will feel plugged, you will vomit, or you will experience dumping?

TABLE 5–1. Summary of special considerations when assessing eating-disordered criteria after bariatric surgery and specific probe questions *(continued)*

Required for DSM-5 diagnosis	Criterion	Special considerations after surgery	Specific probe questions (to be used in addition to the questions concerning formal eating disorder diagnosis)
BN	Recurrent inappropriate compensatory behaviors in order to prevent weight gain	Spontaneous or voluntary vomiting is commonly associated with the ingestion of intolerable foods or with eating too rapidly, or is secondary to physical discomfort after eating, and is not necessarily influenced by body weight or shape concerns. Atypical compensatory behaviors such as dumping may emerge.	What are your motives for vomiting and/or dumping? Does episodic vomiting happen because you feel plugged or physically uncomfortable with the food eaten? Did you overeat because you knew you would easily vomit or compensate through dumping?

Note. AN=anorexia nervosa; BED=binge-eating disorder; BN=bulimia nervosa.

compensatory behaviors, such as vomiting at the termination of an eating episode, as is seen in BN, possibly making occurrences more difficult to recognize as episodes of binge eating.

After surgery, physical restriction greatly limits the amount of food that can fit into a small gastric pouch/stomach created by bariatric surgery. However, it is still possible for individuals to report feeling a loss of control over eating, although the amount of food eaten is not objectively large (Colles et al. 2008). Therefore, the decision as to what constitutes a large amount of food eaten by individuals following bariatric surgery is not always straightforward, and emerging data suggest that this distinction may not be as important as the feature of loss of control over eating (Fitzsimmons-Craft et al. 2014; Niego et al. 1997). In fact, research with different patient samples showed that those presenting with *subjective binge eating* (loss of control over amounts of food not "large" but viewed by the individual as excessive) were similar to those reporting objective binge eating on eating disorder features, general psychopathology, and negative affect (Brownstone et al. 2013; Palavras et al. 2013). Additionally, subjective binge eating seems to be associated with depressive symptoms, anxiety, social avoidance, insecure attachment, and cognitive distortion (Brownstone et al. 2013; Fitzsimmons-Craft et al. 2014).

A number of studies have evaluated the presence of binge eating prior to bariatric surgery in an attempt to identify eating behaviors that might be predictive of attenuated weight loss after surgery, but research has failed to consistently demonstrate a significant relationship between preoperative binge eating and outcome. Some studies have found an association with poorer weight outcomes, whereas other studies have found no association or even greater weight loss (Livhits et al. 2012; Meany et al. 2014). However, the presence of binge eating prior to surgery can be associated with the risk of postsurgical binge eating or loss-of-control eating, both of which have been more consistently associated with less weight loss and/or increased weight regain over time (Meany et al. 2014; White et al. 2010). Binge eating prior to surgery has been related to increased psychological distress and other eating-disordered symptoms (Colles et al. 2008). Therefore, assessing binge eating prior to surgery plays an important role in screening for a subgroup of patients who may pose additional challenges following surgery.

Other problematic eating behaviors, such as grazing and emotional eating, have also been associated with loss-of-control eating (Allison et al. 2010; Conceição et al. 2014) and ultimately with risk of increased weight regain (Colles et al. 2008). See Table 5-1 for the special considerations that must be taken into account when assessing eating disorders in post–bariatric surgery patients.

Night Eating Syndrome

Night eating syndrome, listed in DSM-5 as one of the other specified feeding or eating disorders, is characterized by evening/nocturnal hyperphagia and associated emotional distress (Allison et al. 2010). With a wide range of prevalence rates reported, the prevalence of night eating syndrome is estimated to be as high as 55% among obese patients seeking surgical treatment (Colles and Dixon 2006). No consistent relationship has been observed between presurgery night eating syndrome and presurgery psychological distress or postsurgery weight loss, loss-of-control eating, grazing, or night eating syndrome (Colles and Dixon 2006). However, preoperative night eating syndrome has been associated with BED, lower cognitive restraint, increased social eating, eating when tired, and less consumption of protein, which can be highly problematic for patients following bariatric surgery (Colles and Dixon 2006; Colles et al. 2008). Thus, night eating syndrome seems to be part of a disorganized, high-risk eating pattern that may require treatment before or after bariatric surgery. Night eating syndrome should be distinguished from sleep-related eating disorder, a rare condition often related to the use of certain sedatives or hypnotics and associated with other sleep disorders such as restless legs syndrome (Colles and Dixon 2006). Sleep-related eating disorder is characterized by partial arousal from sleep, reduced levels of awareness, and impaired recall.

Grazing

Different definitions of the term grazing have been employed in the literature, which has led to some confusion. Recently, with our colleagues, we proposed that *grazing* be defined as the repetitive eating (more than twice in the same period of time without prolonged gaps between) of small or modest amounts of food in an unplanned manner and/or not in response to sensations of hunger or satiety (Conceição et al. 2014). Two subtypes were also suggested: 1) *compulsive grazing*—trying to resist but not being able to, returning repetitively to snack on food, and 2) *noncompulsive grazing*—repetitively eating in a distracted and mindless way (Conceição et al. 2014). Constructs similar to grazing that have been described in the literature include picking, nibbling, and repetitive snack eating; however, there is little research regarding the extent to which these behaviors overlap.

After surgery, owing to reduced gastric capacity, most patients must eat multiple small meals in order to consume a sufficient amount of food. This behavior should not be considered grazing, because this eating pattern demonstrates appropriate control. Grazing should also be distin-

TABLE 5–2. Summary of and differentiation between different eating behaviors found in postoperative bariatric patients and their associated level of control over eating

Episode	Sense of control	Description
Normal	0	Eating behavior that is planned, controlled, and mindful of hunger and satiety. Repetitive eating of small amounts of food in order to accommodate the required daily amounts.
Deliberate overeating	0	Plan to fractionate and repeatedly eat small amounts to intentionally overeat and accommodate the amount of food desired (e.g., dessert). No sense of loss of control.
Grazing, noncompulsive subtype	1	"Mindless" and distracted eating of whatever is available. Not planned.
Grazing, compulsive subtype	2	Attempting to resist but returning repeatedly to eat small/modest portions of tempting foods; associated with cravings for food.
Binge eating; loss of control	3	Eating in a circumscribed period of time with a sense that one cannot resist eating or stop eating.

Source. Adapted from Conceição et al. 2014.

guished from intentional overeating, a behavior in which individuals fractionate and eat smaller portions of a large amount over an extended time in order to purposefully overeat. The planned nature of intentional overeating distinguishes it from grazing. Grazing should also be differentiated from binge eating with moderate amounts of food (subjective binge eating), because grazing does not involve the sense that one cannot stop or resist eating in a circumscribed period of time.

Grazing may be characterized by some level of lack of control that is clinically different from the loss of control experienced in binge-eating episodes and that might be captured with a more flexible rating scheme. Some have advocated the use of a continuous rating scale for loss of control (see example in Table 5–2) instead of the more typical dichotomous (present/absent) nomenclature (Conceição et al. 2014; Mitchell et al. 2012).

Little is known about the clinical importance or prevalence of grazing prior to surgery, but the emergence of grazing postoperatively has been the focus of some research. Postoperative grazing has been suggested to serve the same function as presurgery binge eating, which is no longer possible because of the anatomical changes (Saunders 2004). Also, the unplanned, repetitive nature of the behavior may result in excessive caloric intake and ultimately less weight loss and/or greater weight regain. Grazing behavior after bariatric surgery may also be associated with binge eating and/or loss-of-control eating, and the overall combined pattern may lead to increased weight regain (Conceição et al. 2014). Although inconsistent, initial evidence points to an association between grazing and depressive symptoms, emotional eating, mindless eating, and poorer mental health and quality of life (Colles et al. 2008; Kofman et al. 2010). Although there is no clear evidence to argue that grazing is necessarily a psychopathological eating behavior in the general population, it does seem that grazing may compromise weight outcomes after bariatric surgery.

Emotional Eating

Although a standardized definition of *emotional eating* is lacking, the phenomenon has been described as "the tendency to eat in response to emotional distress and during stressful life situations" (Canetti et al. 2009, p. 109). Before surgery, emotional eating has been associated with higher levels of depression and binge eating and with more frequent eating in response to external cues (Fischer et al. 2007). Emotional eating is thought to be common among bariatric surgery candidates and postoperative patients and has been associated with binge eating (Pinaquy et al. 2003), grazing, uncontrolled eating, and snack eating (Chesler 2012). Additionally, some authors have considered emotional eating to be a risk factor for poorer outcomes after surgery, although data addressing this issue are quite limited (e.g., Canetti et al. 2009; Chesler 2012). Although emotional eating has been suggested to play a mediating role in treatment outcomes, including weight loss and quality of life (Canetti et al. 2009), contradictory results have been reported about the impact of emotional eating on weight outcomes after surgery (Fischer et al. 2007).

Dumping Syndrome

Dumping syndrome refers to a constellation of GI and vasomotor symptoms associated with the consumption of foods containing high concentrations of carbohydrates or sugar and/or with eating excessively following bariatric surgery (Deitel 2008). Dumping syndrome is estimated to occur in about three-quarters of patients undergoing malabsorptive bariatric procedures (Mechanick et al. 2013), typically develops 10–30 minutes postprandially, and has been referred to as early dumping by some authors. The syndrome occurs following rapid gastric emptying, leading to a hyperosmolar load in the intestine and subsequent fluid shifts (Deitel 2008), which are accompanied by an autonomic vasomotor response.

Dumping usually involves diarrhea, and there are anecdotal reports of patients using dumping as a compensatory behavior, relying on this GI consequence to compensate for overeating or binge eating. Thus, clinicians need to be aware that dumping is not only a frequent problem in the initial months after surgery, particularly until patients learn to eat slowly and to avoid foods that trigger these symptoms, but also an inappropriate method to compensate for eating and to regulate weight. Uncontrolled severe dumping can also result in a fear of certain foods or of eating, resulting in accentuated weight loss and even malnutrition (Lin and Hasler 1995).

Some patients have reported another condition similar to dumping that has been termed by some authors late dumping, as opposed to the early dumping that corresponds to dumping syndrome. Despite the similarity of symptoms reported by patients (dizziness, fatigue, diaphoresis, and weakness), the physiological mechanism underlying these conditions is not the same, and they should be considered distinct conditions. Late dumping occurs about 1–3 hours after a meal because of an exaggerated insulin response to hyperglycemia, resulting in subsequent reactive hypoglycemia (Ceppa et al. 2012; Deitel 2008); when intense and recurrent, this may result in blackouts, seizures, and other severe complications, including death as a rare outcome (Ceppa et al. 2012). Whereas early dumping usually develops shortly after surgery, late dumping typically develops a year to several years later. Clinicians should assess for dumping syndromes and educate patients about common triggers and consequences. Patients who experience late dumping may require dietary modifications to reduce carbohydrate intake, may need to take medications, or, in rare treatment-resistant cases, may require pancreatic resection.

Assessment of Current Eating Behaviors

To perform a comprehensive evaluation of a patient's current eating behaviors, the clinician should inquire about the frequency and content of meals and snacks, problematic eating behaviors, and GI problems. Important concerns include the following:

1. Level of *restriction and avoidance* of certain foods. The amount of food ingested by patients following bariatric surgery is naturally limited, and

some foods (e.g., meat and pasta) are best avoided because of intolerance and physical discomfort. The motives underlying restrictive behaviors should be probed, along with expectations about the influence of restriction on weight. Recurrent thinking about calories; establishment or maintenance of a very low calorie plan; and frequent weighing, body pinching, or body checking may be of concern.

2. Presence, frequency, and duration of *binge-eating* and/or *loss-of-control episodes,* including the amounts and the types of food ingested during these episodes.
3. Presence, frequency and duration of any *purging behaviors.* Besides those behaviors typically reported by individuals with AN and BN, the occurrence of dumping should be assessed. Clinicians should differentiate vomiting related to the ingestion of intolerable foods or to excessively rapid eating from vomiting related to weight or shape concerns.
4. Frequency and intensity of *exercise.*
5. Presence, frequency, and duration of *grazing* (Conceição et al. 2014).
6. Presence and frequency of *overeating* by intentionally fractionating large amounts of food into smaller portions to be eaten over an extended time.
7. *Emotional eating,* which has two subtypes (Chesler 2012): 1) a conscious behavior to cope with emotional distress and 2) an automatic/reflexive reaction to misidentified feelings and emotions or alexithymia, which is common among bariatric surgery candidates and postoperative patients (Noli et al. 2010).
8. Presence, frequency, and duration of *night eating symptoms* (Allison et al. 2010).

Assessment of Prior Eating Disturbances

In addition to assessing current eating behaviors and related symptoms, the clinician needs to assess whether a patient has had prior clinically significant eating problems. For example, a history of intensive dietary restriction and low weight because of AN may indicate that a patient is more likely to subscribe to rigid, inflexible attitudes regarding eating and weight and to have these attitudes reinforced by the extreme weight loss and the facilitation of control over eating that surgery permits. A past history of BN, BED, or night eating may be informative regarding the potential for loss-of-control eating and the prior use of compensatory behaviors (e.g., vomiting, dumping) that may reemerge because they are facilitated by the surgery. Finally, information about past treatments and responses to them may be useful in anticipating what may be most helpful in the future.

Structured Clinical Interviews and Self-Report Measures

Providers may use the general guidelines provided in this chapter in conducting clinical interviews but may also consider the use of structured diagnostic assessment instruments. Table 5–3 provides a brief summary of clinical interviews and self-report measures to assess disordered eating behavior among individuals following bariatric surgery (see also Part 3, "Assessment Tools," in this volume).

Clinical Interview: Additional Considerations

As part of the clinical interview, in addition to soliciting the information relevant to eating disorders, providers should also assess other past and co-occurring psychiatric conditions of particular relevance for bariatric surgery patients.

Mood and Anxiety Disorders

Among bariatric surgery candidates, the presence of BED has been associated with current or past history of both mood and anxiety disorders. Although significant improvement often occurs after surgery, postoperative BED or loss of control has also been associated with continued anxiety and depression and ultimately poorer outcomes (de Zwaan et al. 2011).

Impulse-Control Disorders

Impulse-control disorders such as skin-picking disorder, compulsive buying, or intermittent explosive disorder have been estimated to occur in up to 19% of bariatric surgery candidates (Schmidt et al. 2012).

Alcohol Use Disorder

Although presurgery binge eating has not been found to be a significant predictor of postsurgery alcohol abuse (King et al. 2012), individuals with eating disorders are at increased risk of alcohol abuse (Ferriter and Ray 2011). Extant evidence suggests that bariatric surgery patients have a greater sensitivity to the intoxicating effects of alcohol after surgery and are vulnerable to the development of alcohol use disorder, particularly following gastric bypass (King et al. 2012).

TABLE 5–3. Clinical interviews and self-report measures for eating-disordered behaviors and associated features in bariatric surgery patients

	Measure (authors)	Type of measure	Description	Examples of studies on bariatric surgery patients
Eating disorders	EDQ (Mitchell 2005)	Self-report	Designed to collect comprehensive data about disordered eating symptoms (current and lifetime); psychosocial, medical, and psychiatric history; and weight history.	NA
	EDE–Bariatric Surgery Version (Fairburn et al. 2008; modified by de Zwaan et al. 2010)	Semistructured interview	45- to 75-minute interview. Assesses eating-disordered behaviors and symptomatology and gastrointestinal problems. Generates global score and four subscores: Restraint, Eating Concerns, Shape Concern, and Weight Concern. Also addresses behaviors specific to bariatric surgery patients.	Kalarchian et al. 2000
	EDE-Q (Fairburn and Beglin 2008)	Self-report	Self-report version of EDE. Assesses eating-disordered behaviors and symptomatology. Generates global score and four subscores: Restraint, Eating Concern, Shape Concern, and Weight Concern.	Grilo et al. 2013; Kalarchian et al. 2000
	BES (Gormally et al. 1982)	Self-report	16-item questionnaire with a total score reflecting severity of binge-eating behaviors.	Grupski et al. 2013; Hood et al. 2013
	DEBQ (van Strien et al. 1986)	Self-report	33-item questionnaire assessing three patterns of eating, resulting in three subscores: Restrained Eating, Emotional Eating, and External Eating.	van Hout et al. 2007

TABLE 5–3. Clinical interviews and self-report measures for eating-disordered behaviors and associated features in bariatric surgery patients *(continued)*

	Measure (authors)	Type of measure	Description	Examples of studies on bariatric surgery patients
Grazing	Rep(eat) (Conceição et al. 2014)	Semistructured interview	15- to 45-minute interview. Assesses eating behaviors including grazing and allows decision on the presence/absence and characterization of grazing behavior.	(Conceição et al., work in progress)
	Rep(eat)-Q (Conceição et al. 2014)	Self-report	15-item questionnaire. Assesses grazing and generates a total score reflecting levels of associated symptomatology.	(Conceição et al., work in progress)
Night eating syndrome	NEQ (Allison et al. 2008)	Self -report	14-item questionnaire. Assesses behavioral and psychological symptoms of night eating syndrome. Generates a total score reflecting levels of associated symptomatology.	Rand et al. 1997
Emotional eating	EES (Arnow et al. 1995)	Self-report	25-item scale. Assesses tendency to eat in response to emotional triggers. Generates three subscores: Depression, Anxiety, and Anger.	Castellini et al. 2014
Dumping	Sigstad's Clinical Diagnostic Index (Sigstad 1970)	Self-report	Generates an index score based on the weight of 16 symptoms of dumping. A score of 7 or more points is suggestive of dumping.	Kalarchian et al. 2014

Note. BES=Binge-Eating Scale; DEBQ=Dutch Eating Behavior Questionnaire; EDE–Bariatric Surgery Version=Eating Disorder Examination–Bariatric Surgery Version; EDE-Q=Eating Disorder Examination Questionnaire; EDQ=Eating Disorder Questionnaire; EES=Emotional Eating Scale; NA=none available; NEQ=Night Eating Questionnaire; Rep(eat)=Repetitive Eating Interview; Rep(eat)-Q=Repetitive Eating Questionnaire.

Medical Complications and Physical Assessment

Disordered eating behaviors in patients who have undergone bariatric surgery may have physical consequences that require medical attention. Disordered eating behaviors may be associated with compromised intake of vitamins and minerals, such as vitamin B_{12}, calcium, vitamin D, thiamine, folic acid, iron, zinc, and magnesium (Malone 2008). Deficiency secondary to surgery and/or due to lack of compliance with replacement regimens should be addressed, as should dumping syndrome and recurrent vomiting.

Conclusion

Assessment of eating disorders and problematic eating behaviors in bariatric candidates poses challenges to both clinicians and researchers attempting to improve the support provided to these patients and to enhance weight outcomes. Particularly in the postoperative period, the subsyndromal presentations of eating disorders and the fact that some compensatory behaviors may be facilitated by the surgical procedures make the line between normative and problematic behaviors difficult to establish. Further, problematic eating behaviors that do not constitute DSM diagnoses should also be assessed as they may compromise weight maintenance in the long term.

Research has been proliferating in the development and validation of assessment instruments, and there are a variety of semistructured interviews and self-report measures validated to assess eating behaviors and problematic eating in both preoperative and postoperative bariatric surgery patients. However, despite the growing evidence that eating behaviors are predictors of outcomes, it seems that it is the long-term presentation of problematic eating that best predicts poor weight loss or weight regain, shedding light on the importance of longitudinal assessment of these patients.

Key Clinical Points

- The presence of problematic eating behaviors and subsyndromal presentations of eating disorders are common in bariatric surgery patients, but no diagnostic terms have been specifically developed for these patients.

- Restriction of energy intake in patients following bariatric surgery must be assessed in light of the highly restrictive diet initially prescribed for these patients and the limitations on the amount of food that can be physically tolerated following surgery.
- There is no clear definition of what constitutes being underweight among patients following bariatric surgery.
- On the basis of previous experience, patients' fear of weight gain following bariatric surgery is, at least to some extent, realistic.
- Excessive loose skin, skin envelopes, and fat deposits following surgery can have a major negative impact on body image, causing body dissatisfaction and social embarrassment.
- The experience of loss of control may be the only feature of binge eating following surgery.
- Spontaneous, involuntary vomiting is commonly associated with physical discomfort and may not be related to excessive concern about body weight or shape. Atypical compensatory behaviors such as dumping may emerge following surgery.
- Grazing, night eating, and emotional eating have been related to loss-of-control eating, increased psychopathology, and adverse bariatric surgery weight outcomes.

References

Allison KC, Lundgren JD, O'Reardon JP, et al: The Night Eating Questionnaire (NEQ): psychometric properties of a measure of severity of the night eating syndrome. Eat Behav 9(1):62–72, 2008 18167324

Allison KC, Lundgren JD, O'Reardon JP, et al: Proposed diagnostic criteria for night eating syndrome. Int J Eat Disord 43(3):241–247, 2010 19378289

American Psychiatric Association: Diagnostic and Statistical Manual of Mental Disorders, 5th Edition. Arlington, VA, American Psychiatric Association, 2013

Arnow B, Kenardy J, Agras WS: The Emotional Eating Scale: the development of a measure to assess coping with negative affect by eating. Int J Eat Disord 18(1):79–90, 1995 7670446

Brownstone LM, Bardone-Cone AM, Fitzsimmons-Craft EE, et al: Subjective and objective binge eating in relation to eating disorder symptomatology, negative affect, and personality dimensions. Int J Eat Disord 46(1):66–76, 2013 23109272

Canetti L, Berry EM, Elizur Y: Psychosocial predictors of weight loss and psychological adjustment following bariatric surgery and a weight-loss program: the mediating role of emotional eating. Int J Eat Disord 42(2):109–117, 2009 18949765

Castellini G, Godini L, Amedei SG, et al: Psychological effects and outcome predictors of three bariatric surgery interventions: a 1-year follow-up study. Eat Weight Disord 19(2):217–224, 2014 24737175

Ceppa EP, Ceppa DP, Omotosho PA, et al: Algorithm to diagnose etiology of hypoglycemia after Roux-en-Y gastric bypass for morbid obesity: case series and review of the literature. Surg Obes Relat Dis 8(5):641–647, 2012 21982939

Chesler BE: Emotional eating: a virtually untreated risk factor for outcome following bariatric surgery. ScientificWorldJournal 2012:365961, 2012 22566765

Colles SL, Dixon JB: Night eating syndrome: impact on bariatric surgery. Obes Surg 16(7):811–820, 2006 16839476

Colles SL, Dixon JB, O'Brien PE: Grazing and loss of control related to eating: two high-risk factors following bariatric surgery. Obesity (Silver Spring) 16(3):615–622, 2008 18239603

Conceição E, Orcutt M, Mitchell J, et al: Eating disorders after bariatric surgery: a case series. Int J Eat Disord 46(3):274–279, 2013a 23192683

Conceição E, Vaz A, Bastos AP, et al: The development of eating disorders after bariatric surgery. Eat Disord 21(3):275–282, 2013b 23600557

Conceição EM, Mitchell JE, Engel SG, et al: What is "grazing"? Reviewing its definition, frequency, clinical characteristics, and impact on bariatric surgery outcomes, and proposing a standardized definition. Surg Obes Relat Dis 10(5):973–982, 2014 25312671

Deitel M: The change in the dumping syndrome concept. Obes Surg 18(12):1622–1624, 2008 18941845

de Zwaan M, Hilbert A, Swan-Kremeier L, et al: Comprehensive interview assessment of eating behavior 18–35 months after gastric bypass surgery for morbid obesity. Surg Obes Relat Dis 6(1):79–85, 2010 19837012

de Zwaan M, Enderle J, Wagner S, et al: Anxiety and depression in bariatric surgery patients: a prospective, follow-up study using structured clinical interviews. J Affect Disord 133(1–2):61–68, 2011 21501874

Dixon JB, McPhail T, O'Brien PE: Minimal reporting requirements for weight loss: current methods not ideal. Obes Surg 15(7):1034–1039, 2005 16105403

Fairburn CG, Beglin SJ: Eating Disorder Examination Questionnaire (EDE-Q 6.0), in Cognitive Behavior Therapy and Eating Disorders. Edited by Fairburn CG. New York, Guilford, 2008, pp 309–314

Fairburn CG, Cooper Z, O'Connor M: Eating Disorder Examination (16.0D), in Cognitive Behavior Therapy and Eating Disorders. Edited by Fairburn CG. New York, Guilford, 2008, pp 265–308

Ferriter C, Ray LA: Binge eating and binge drinking: an integrative review. Eat Behav 12(2):99–107, 2011 21385638

Fischer S, Chen E, Katterman S, et al: Emotional eating in a morbidly obese bariatric surgery-seeking population. Obes Surg 17(6):778–784, 2007 17879578

Fitzsimmons-Craft EE, Ciao AC, Accurso EC, et al: Subjective and objective binge eating in relation to eating disorder symptomatology, depressive symptoms, and self-esteem among treatment-seeking adolescents with bulimia nervosa. Eur Eat Disord Rev 22(4):230–236, 2014 24852114

Gormally J, Black S, Daston S, et al: The assessment of binge eating severity among obese persons. Addict Behav 7(1):47–55, 1982 7080884

Grilo CM, Henderson KE, Bell RL, et al: Eating Disorder Examination-Questionnaire factor structure and construct validity in bariatric surgery candidates. Obes Surg 23(5):657–662, 2013 23229951

Grupski AE, Hood MM, Hall BJ, et al: Examining the Binge Eating Scale in screening for binge eating disorder in bariatric surgery candidates. Obes Surg 23(1):1–6, 2013 23104387

Hood MM, Grupski AE, Hall BJ, et al: Factor structure and predictive utility of the Binge Eating Scale in bariatric surgery candidates. Surg Obes Relat Dis 9(6):942–948, 2013 22963818

Kalarchian MA, Wilson GT, Brolin RE, et al: Assessment of eating disorders in bariatric surgery candidates: self-report questionnaire versus interview. Int J Eat Disord 28(4):465–469, 2000 11054796

Kalarchian MA, Marcus MD, Courcoulas AP, et al: Self-report of gastrointestinal side effects after bariatric surgery. Surg Obes Relat Dis 10(6):1202–1207, 2014 25443069

King WC, Chen J-Y, Mitchell JE, et al: Prevalence of alcohol use disorders before and after bariatric surgery. JAMA 307(23):2516–2525, 2012 22710289

Kofman MD, Lent MR, Swencionis C: Maladaptive eating patterns, quality of life, and weight outcomes following gastric bypass: results of an Internet survey. Obesity (Silver Spring) 18(10):1938–1943, 2010 20168309

Lin H, Hasler W: Disorders of gastric emptying, in Textbook of Gastroenterology. Edited by Yamada T, Alpers D, Owyang C. Philadelphia, PA, JB Lippincott, 1995, pp 1318–1346

Livhits M, Mercado C, Yermilov I, et al: Preoperative predictors of weight loss following bariatric surgery: systematic review. Obes Surg 22(1):70–89, 2012 21833817

Magro DO, Geloneze B, Delfini R, et al: Long-term weight regain after gastric bypass: a 5-year prospective study. Obes Surg 18(6):648–651, 2008 18392907

Malone M: Recommended nutritional supplements for bariatric surgery patients. Ann Pharmacother 42(12):1851–1858, 2008 19017827

Meany G, Conceição E, Mitchell JE: Binge eating, binge eating disorder and loss of control eating: effects on weight outcomes after bariatric surgery. Eur Eat Disord Rev 22(2):87–91, 2014 24347539

Mechanick JI, Youdim A, Jones DB, et al; American Association of Clinical Endocrinologists; Obesity Society; American Society for Metabolic and Bariatric Surgery: Clinical practice guidelines for the perioperative nutritional, metabolic, and nonsurgical support of the bariatric surgery patient–2013 update: cosponsored by American Association of Clinical Endocrinologists, The Obesity Society, and American Society for Metabolic and Bariatric Surgery. Obesity (Silver Spring) 21 (suppl 1):S1–S27, 2013 23529939

Mitchell J: A standardized database, in Assessment of Eating Disorders. Edited by Mitchell JE, Peterson CB. New York, Guilford, 2005, pp 57–78

Mitchell JE, Karr TM, Peat C, et al: A fine-grained analysis of eating behavior in women with bulimia nervosa. Int J Eat Disord 45(3):400–406, 2012 21956763

Niego SH, Pratt EM, Agras WS: Subjective or objective binge: is the distinction valid? Int J Eat Disord 22(3):291–298, 1997 9285266

Noli G, Cornicelli M, Marinari GM, et al: Alexithymia and eating behaviour in severely obese patients. J Hum Nutr Diet 23(6):616–619, 2010 20487173

Odom J, Zalesin KC, Washington TL, et al: Behavioral predictors of weight regain after bariatric surgery. Obes Surg 20(3):349–356, 2010 19554382

Ortega J, Navarro V, Cassinello N, et al: Requirement and postoperative outcomes of abdominal panniculectomy alone or in combination with other procedures in a bariatric surgery unit. Am J Surg 200(2):235–240, 2010 20591405

Palavras MA, Morgan CM, Borges FMB, et al: An investigation of objective and subjective types of binge eating episodes in a clinical sample of people with co-morbid obesity. J Eat Disord 1:26, 2013 24999405

Pinaquy S, Chabrol H, Simon C, et al: Emotional eating, alexithymia, and binge-eating disorder in obese women. Obes Res 11(2):195–201, 2003 12582214

Rand CS, Macgregor AM, Stunkard AJ: The night eating syndrome in the general population and among postoperative obesity surgery patients. Int J Eat Disord 22(1):65–69, 1997 9140737

Saunders R: "Grazing": a high-risk behavior. Obes Surg 14(1):98–102, 2004 14980042

Schmidt F, Körber S, de Zwaan M, et al: Impulse control disorders in obese patients. Eur Eat Disord Rev 20(3):e144–e147, 2012 22367789

Sigstad H: A clinical diagnostic index in the diagnosis of the dumping syndrome: changes in plasma volume and blood sugar after a test meal. Acta Med Scand 188(6):479–486, 1970 5507449

van Hout GC, Boekestein P, Fortuin FA, et al: Psychosocial functioning following bariatric surgery. Obes Surg 16(6):787–794, 2006 16756745

van Hout GC, Jakimowicz JJ, Fortuin FA, et al: Weight loss and eating behavior following vertical banded gastroplasty. Obes Surg 17(9):1226–1234, 2007 18074499

van Strien T, Frijters J, Bergers G, et al: The Dutch Eating Behavior Questionnaire (DEBQ) for assessment of restrained, emotional, and external eating behavior. Int J Eat Disord 5(2):295–315, 1986

White MA, Kalarchian MA, Masheb RM, et al: Loss of control over eating predicts outcomes in bariatric surgery patients: a prospective, 24-month follow-up study. J Clin Psychiatry 71(2):175–184, 2010 19852902

6 Eating-Related Pathology in Men and Boys

Thomas Hildebrandt, Psy.D.
Katherine Craigen, Ph.D.

The clinical assessment of males with eating problems requires several important conceptual considerations. First, such problems have a very diverse presentation among men and boys. Second, the motivations that drive such problems may differ from those typically cited among females. Finally, male body image disturbances often differ in their quality and content from female equivalents. These conceptual distinctions may assist with the assessment and diagnosis of men and boys with eating disorders, particularly when uncertainty exists about whether an eating disorder is even present. This guidance, however, should not replace existing validated methods, because men and boys can also present with classic syndromes identical to those of women and girls. Video 4, "Assessing eating problems in men," addresses specific issues related to assessment and treatment of male patients.

Conceptual Overview of Assessing Men and Boys With Eating-Related Pathology

A number of diffuse conditions (e.g., reverse anorexia, bigorexia, muscle dysmorphia, anabolic-androgenic steroid use) with links to traditional eating disorders potentially have a higher prevalence among males than females (Grieve et al. 2009; Hildebrandt et al. 2011a). Several studies have demonstrated superficial overlap of clinical features between traditionally recognized eating disorders and these other presentations. The most notable symptom cluster in males is a subtype of body dysmorphic disorder termed muscle dysmorphia (Pope et al. 1997). *Muscle dysmorphia* is characterized by obsessional and compulsive behaviors intended to achieve a lean and muscular physique. Men with anorexia nervosa (AN) and men with muscle dysmorphia display similar severity levels of compulsive exercise, body image disturbance, and disordered eating (Murray et al. 2012). Core psychological constructs associated with eating disorders (perfectionism, difficulty tolerating negative moods, and low self-esteem) also correlate with muscle dysmorphia symptoms (Murray et al. 2013) and act as antecedents to symptom onset (McFarland and Kaminski 2009).

Empirical classification studies suggest that symptoms of obsessive-compulsive disorder and bulimia nervosa (BN) cluster with symptoms of muscle dysmorphia (Hildebrandt et al. 2006), leading to the suggestion that muscle dysmorphia should be considered an eating disorder in the *Diagnostic and Statistical Manual of Mental Disorders* (Murray et al. 2010). Despite these suggestions, as well as the superficial overlap in symptoms, a core distinction between muscle dysmorphia and AN remains: the primary importance of eating pathology. Although patients with muscle dysmorphia report engaging in a number of weight-regulating behaviors, including some forms of disordered eating (Contesini et al. 2013), their primary disturbance relates to body image, whereas AN and other eating disorders are primarily defined by a core disturbance in eating. Consequently, any clinical assessment of men and boys may require differentiating distress and impairment related primarily to eating from that related to concerns about body image. Should the latter be primary, we recommend following clinical guidelines for men and boys with body dysmorphic disorder (see Hartmann et al. 2013).

The core motivations for men and boys to control or influence their appearance through eating and weight control often differ from those of their female counterparts. One approach to understanding this potential divergence is to consider how shape and appearance serve different functions for each sex. For instance, the functional (as contrasted to appearance) demands of the male body are often the primary source of evaluation, meaning that men or boys will have greater investment in how fast they run or how well they fight. Consequently, male body dissatisfaction may more likely be triggered by some actual or perceived failure to perform physically in an athletic or similar setting where physical performance rather than appearance is the primary focus of evaluation (Edman et al. 2014). This difference yields a qualitatively distinct experience for many men and boys and contributes to the clinical heterogeneity found in treatment-seeking populations. For instance, a boy who idealizes an Olympic swimmer may express a desire for leanness and endurance, choosing a range of behaviors designed to keep weight and body fat down while maintaining a high level of fitness. Alternatively, a boy who idealizes an American professional football player may express a desire for muscularity, choosing weight-control methods that favor muscle development and raw strength.

Body image disturbances among males can be conceptually defined along two orthogonal dimensions of muscularity and body fat. Depending on an individual's current placement along these dimensions (e.g., high muscularity and low body fat) and the desired change (e.g., larger or smaller), the types of weight- and shape-controlling behavior can be predicted (Hildebrandt et al. 2010). Men and boys who desire leanness but have little concern for muscularity may be more likely to present with classic eating disorder concerns about thinness. Conversely, men and boys who present with greater desire for muscularity but little concern for leanness may be more likely to present with symptoms of muscle dysmorphia. Males who have a high degree of concern about both leanness and muscularity may have elements of both muscle dysmorphia and an eating disorder and may engage in distinct behaviors linked to these motivations. Notably, it is also the latter group that is most likely to abuse performance-enhancing drugs (Pope et al. 2012).

Illicit substances used to control one's outward appearance or level of physical fitness are termed *appearance- and performance-enhancing drugs* (APEDs). These drugs encompass an evolving market of synthetic chemicals designed to target and enhance the natural breakdown and repair of energy stores and muscle (Hildebrandt et al. 2007). Not surprisingly, men who use these substances are generally at risk for eating or body image pathology and tend to evaluate the functional aspects of their bodies and traditionally masculine body parts (e.g., shoulders, biceps) (Walker et al. 2009). These males are also more likely to be concerned with aspects of body hair, head hair, physical height, and penis size (Tiggemann et al. 2008), each of which is associated with its own set of behavioral checking and avoidance strategies.

In summary, assessing men and boys for eating disorder symptoms requires an understanding of what symptoms (eating, body image, or drug use) drive the primary distress and impairment. To make such distinctions, the assessment strategy used by clinicians working with men and boys requires an understanding of the unique motivations for the weight- and shape-controlling behaviors. These motivations may involve traditional investment in thinness but also may involve scrutiny of specific functional components of body image (e.g., strength, speed). In addition, the assessment strategy requires a thorough evaluation of APED use, because this may be a more common approach to dealing with body image disturbances in men and boys than in women and girls.

Challenges in the Assessment of Eating-Related Pathology in Men and Boys

The role of gender in the assessment and diagnosis of eating disorders should not be underestimated. Increasing knowledge of the unique clinical presentations of men and boys with disordered eating behaviors and attitudes has increased understanding of important considerations for clinical assessment.

Video 4 demonstrates special issues that may arise in the assessment and treatment of male patients.

Video Illustration 4: Assessing eating problems in men (5:32)

Table 6–1 describes the key areas of assessment for men and boys who present for treatment with likely eating and related psychopathology. Generally, querying about these domains should involve a professional nonjudgmental style. The questions should be direct and reflect some knowledge of the domain. This approach is particularly important for questions pertaining to APED use, because the patient may assume that the clinician is ignorant about the nature of these drugs, their effects, and the relative risks associated with their use. The interviewer's demonstration of some understanding of street use (e.g., how drugs are sourced or used) or brands of these substances will increase the likelihood of the patient's disclosure. Similarly, questions about body image or disturbances in eating should be direct and begin with the goal of generating a general understanding of how a patient experiences his body (appearance and function) as well as what approach(es) he takes to influencing his body (appearance and function) and in what context. Many body image–controlling behaviors can be healthy or normative in the appropriate context (e.g., heavy exercising or weight change for athletic competition). The interviewer, however, must determine whether these behaviors are functionally impairing given the specific context provided by the patient.

The following is a review of additional common challenges and important features that the clinician should consider for the successful assessment of males struggling with eating and body image issues.

TABLE 6–1. Relevant questions in the assessment of eating-related problems in men and boys

Topic	Information relevant to eating disorder	Sample inquiries
Weight history	Recent weight change	What is your current weight? What has been your highest and lowest weight? Have you experienced any recent weight loss or weight gain?
Body checking	Excessive in quantity or compulsive/ritualistic	How do you evaluate your outward appearance? How do you evaluate yourself physically?
Exercise patterns	Compulsive and compensatory in nature	Do you feel compelled to exercise? How bad do you feel if you miss or have to limit your amount or intensity of exercise?
Eating habits	Evidence of restriction, dietary rules	How would you describe a typical day's eating? What influences your day-to-day decisions about eating?
Binge eating	Overeating with loss of control	Have you ever consumed what others might consider an unusually large amount of food?
Supplement/ illicit drug use	Steroids, muscle-building supplements, fat-burning supplements, hormones	Have you ever taken a fitness supplement, weight-control drug, or synthetic hormone such as an anabolic steroid? How would you describe your pattern of fitness supplement use?

Diagnosis Bias

Males suffering from body image and eating issues have a significant stigma to overcome, because U.S. culture typically considers eating disorders and obsession with appearance to be "women's issues." Although AN and BN continue to be more common among women than men, the gap is narrowing. Prevalence rates suggest that binge-eating disorder is about as common in men as in women (Lewinsohn et al. 2002; Mond and Hay

2007; Striegel-Moore et al. 2009). Recent data suggest that for both AN and BN, the ratio of women to men is approximately 3:1 (Hudson et al. 2007). It is difficult to determine whether the rising prevalence rates of males with AN and BN represent an increasing number of actual cases, a greater awareness of this problem in men and boys, or an improvement in diagnostic criteria that are less gender biased. For example, the amenorrhea criterion for AN in DSM-IV (American Psychiatric Association 1994) may have primed clinicians to be more likely to consider girls and women for that diagnosis. Clinicians should be sensitive to their own gender biases regarding eating disorder diagnoses. Men may be more likely to be misdiagnosed and less likely to receive treatment or be referred to specialized eating disorder programs (Currin et al. 2007).

Shame and Gender Roles

Cultural stereotypes about women and eating disorders may also present challenges for male patients seeking help for their eating-disordered behaviors and attitudes. Men often experience shame about their eating-disordered behaviors and about reporting those behaviors, which can lead to total avoidance of help seeking for these issues or underreporting of symptom severity (Robinson et al. 2013). Adherence to traditional gender role norms that encourage men to exercise emotional control may interfere with help-seeking behavior (Good et al. 2005; Mahalik et al. 2003). It is therefore important for clinicians to consider the experience of shame within the context of cultural gender role norms for men and boys.

Data on the relationship between body and muscle dissatisfaction and gender roles among men are mixed. Research suggests that only certain aspects of masculinity are associated with dissatisfaction. Specifically, placing an emphasis on winning, emotional control, risk taking, violence, dominance, power over women, and pursuit of status seems to place men at risk for higher levels of dissatisfaction with their muscularity and muscularity-oriented disordered eating (Blashill 2011; Griffiths et al. 2015).

Sexual Orientation

Research has demonstrated that sexual orientation is a risk factor for disordered eating and that bisexual and gay men, compared with heterosexual men, report significantly greater disordered eating and higher body dissatisfaction (Carlat et al. 1997; Feldman and Meyer 2007; Jones and Morgan 2010; Russell and Keel 2002). Although the reason for this remains uncertain, it has been suggested that gay culture places a heightened emphasis on physical appearance and that certain subcultures may therefore be at greater risk when trying to attract other men as romantic partners (Siever 1994). Supporting this theory, several studies have found that both heterosexual and gay men tend to place more emphasis on appearance when looking for a romantic partner than do heterosexual and gay women (Legenbauer et al. 2009; Tiggemann et al. 2007; Yelland and Tiggemann 2003). Cultural pressures and aesthetic ideals therefore appear to be more salient for gay and bisexual men.

Eating Disorder Measures in the Assessment of Males

Eating disorder research has begun to recognize that it may be inappropriate to draw conclusions about males with eating disorders based on their responses to questionnaires designed for females. Such measures have demonstrated lower rates of reliability for men than for women (Boerner et al. 2004), which may be due to the intention for these instruments to assess symptoms that are more relevant to the presentation of eating disorders in women than in men. The following measures are recommended for the assessment of eating-disordered behaviors and attitudes in men and boys because they have been specifically designed for or normed with males.

Eating Disorder Examination Questionnaire

The Eating Disorder Examination Questionnaire (EDE-Q; Fairburn and Beglin 1994, 2008) is a self-report version of the Eating Disorder Examination (EDE) interview (Cooper and Fairburn 1987) (for details, see Chapter 9, "Self-Report Assessments of Eating Pathology"). The EDE-Q is used for both research and clinical purposes, and normative data are now available for adolescent boys (Mond et al. 2014) and undergraduate men (Lavender et al. 2010).

Eating Disorder Inventory

The Eating Disorder Inventory (EDI; Garner et al. 1983) is a six-point, forced-choice, self-report measure. The three subscales (Drive for Thinness, Bulimia, and Body Dissatisfaction) assess levels of eating-disordered behaviors and attitudes (for details, see Chapter 9). The EDI is a commonly used measure; however, studies have found that men and boys score lower on the three core subscales and that the scale is somewhat less reliable for males than females.

Male Body Checking Questionnaire

The Male Body Checking Questionnaire (MBCQ; Hildebrandt et al. 2010) is a 19-item measure that assesses the frequency of body checking behaviors and results in scores on four subscales: Global Muscle Checking, Chest and Shoulder Checking, Other Comparative Body Checking, and Body Testing. The questionnaire has demonstrated good reliability and discriminant validity with a young adult male population.

Muscle Dysmorphia Disorder Inventory

The Muscle Dysmorphia Disorder Inventory (MDDI; Hildebrandt et al. 2004) is a 13-item self-report measure of muscle dysmorphia symptomatology with three subscales (Drive for Size, Appearance Impairment, and Functional Impairment) that map onto the DSM-5 (American Psychiatric Association 2013) criteria for body dysmorphic disorder with muscle dysmorphia specifier. Higher scores represent greater likelihood of having muscle dysmorphia, with the Functional Impairment subscale having the greatest discriminative validity.

Body Change Inventory

The Body Change Inventory (BCI; Ricciardelli and McCabe 2002) is an 18-item self-report tool designed for adolescent boys and girls that evaluates three body change strategies: Strategies to Decrease Body Size, Strategies to Increase Body Size, and Strategies to Increase Muscle Size. This scale has demonstrated good internal consistency and discriminant validity (Ricciardelli and McCabe 2002) for adolescents up to age 17.

Male Eating Behavior and Body Image Evaluation

The Male Eating Behavior and Body Image Evaluation (MEBBIE; Kaminski et al. 2002; P.L. Kaminski and J. Caster, The Male Eating Behaviors and Body Image Evaluation, unpublished test, 1994, available from P.L. Kaminski [kaminski@unt.edu]) is a 57-item self-report scale designed to assess men's attitudes and behaviors regarding eating, exercise, and body image. The MEBBIE yields scores on seven subscales: Body Dissatisfaction, Drive for Muscularity, Emotional Eating, Drive for Thinness, Overexercise, Fear of Fatness, and Distorted Cognitions.

Drive for Muscularity Scale

The Drive for Muscularity Scale (DMS; McCreary and Sasse 2000) is a 14-item self-report measure of muscularity-oriented attitudes and behaviors.

Each item is scored on a six-point scale, ranging from "always" to "never." The internal reliability has been shown to be 0.84 for adolescent boys and 0.87 in a combined high school and college male sample. This measure has been widely used to examine body image issues in gay men.

Appearance and Performance Enhancing Drug Use Schedule

The Appearance and Performance Enhancing Drug Use Schedule (APEDUS; Hildebrandt et al. 2011b) is a semistructured interview that assesses the use of substances (e.g., anabolic-androgenic steroids) to effect change in appearance, as well as assessing associated behaviors such as intense exercise and dietary control. For the assessment of eating-disordered behaviors in men, the clinician would use only the sections pertaining to subscales addressing the associated features (Compulsive Exercise, Dietary Control, and Body Image Disturbance). This measure has demonstrated interrater agreement and reliability as well as convergent validity with adult men.

Physical Assessment

Chapter 2, "Eating Problems in Adults," and Chapter 3, "Eating Problems in Children and Adolescents," provide comprehensive descriptions of the types of physical assessments needed for the evaluation of eating disorders. There are no data to suggest that specific gender-appropriate modifications are needed other than ensuring assessment of male gonadal hormone function. The assessment of physical signs and complications related to APED use is beyond the scope of this chapter; see Langenbucher et al. 2008 for a comprehensive discussion of the physical complications of this type of drug use.

Conclusion

The assessment of men and boys with eating problems reflects diagnostic heterogeneity associated with body image disturbance. Special attention to the differential diagnosis of muscle dysmorphia, eating disorders, and substance use disorders is required, and the symptom assessments suggested in this chapter may assist in the evaluation. It is also essential to recognize challenges (e.g., diagnosis bias, impact of shame and gender roles, sexual orientation) related to help seeking in this population. A well-informed clinician should adapt his or her assessment approach to incorporate these issues effectively.

Key Clinical Points

- Men and boys who desire leanness but have little concern for muscularity may be more likely to present with classic eating disorder concerns about thinness.
- Conversely, men and boys who present with greater desire for muscularity or both leanness and muscularity may be more likely to present with symptoms of muscle dysmorphia.
- The assessment strategy for clinicians working with men and boys requires an understanding of the unique motivations for the weight- and shape-controlling behaviors.
- Men who use appearance- and performance-enhancing drugs are generally at risk for eating or body image pathology and tend to evaluate the functional aspects of their bodies and traditionally masculine body parts.
- Gender biases in the diagnosis of eating disorders are important to understand. Although anorexia nervosa and bulimia nervosa continue to be more common among women than men, the gap is smaller in the general population than in clinical populations, and binge-eating disorder is about as common in men as women.
- Shame related to gender role biases in help-seeking behavior may lead to underreporting of severity.
- Sexual orientation is a risk factor for disordered eating; bisexual and gay men report significantly greater disordered eating and higher body dissatisfaction than heterosexual men.

References

American Psychiatric Association: Diagnostic and Statistical Manual of Mental Disorders, 4th Edition. Washington, DC, American Psychiatric Association, 1994

American Psychiatric Association: Diagnostic and Statistical Manual of Mental Disorders, 5th Edition. Arlington, VA, American Psychiatric Association, 2013

Blashill AJ: Gender roles, eating pathology, and body dissatisfaction in men: a meta-analysis. Body Image 8(1):1–11, 2011 20952263

Boerner LM, Spillane NS, Anderson KG, et al: Similarities and differences between women and men on eating disorder risk factors and symptom measures. Eat Behav 5(3):209–222, 2004 15135333

Carlat DJ, Camargo CA Jr, Herzog DB: Eating disorders in males: a report on 135 patients. Am J Psychiatry 154(8):1127–1132, 1997 9247400

Contesini N, Adami F, Blake MD, et al: Nutritional strategies of physically active subjects with muscle dysmorphia. Int Arch Med 6(1):25, 2013 23706013

Cooper Z, Fairburn C: The Eating Disorder Examination: A semi-structured interview for the assessment of the specific psychopathology of eating disorders. Int J Eat Disord 6:1–8, 1987

Currin L, Schmidt U, Waller G: Variables that influence diagnosis and treatment of the eating disorders within primary care settings: a vignette study. Int J Eat Disord 40(3):257–262, 2007 17167756

Edman JL, Lynch WC, Yates A: The impact of exercise performance dissatisfaction and physical exercise on symptoms of depression among college students: a gender comparison. J Psychol 148(1):23–35, 2014 24617269

Fairburn CG, Beglin SJ: Assessment of eating disorders: Interview or self-report questionnaire? Int J Eat Disord 16:363–370, 1994

Fairburn CG, Beglin SJ: Eating Disorder Examination Questionnaire (EDE-Q 6.0), in Cognitive Behavior Therapy and Eating Disorders. Edited by Fairburn CG. New York, Guilford, 2008, 309–314

Feldman MB, Meyer IH: Eating disorders in diverse lesbian, gay, and bisexual populations. Int J Eat Disord 40(3):218–226, 2007 17262818

Garner DM, Olmstead MP, Polivy J: Development and validation of a multidimensional eating disorder inventory for anorexia nervosa and bulimia. Int J Eat Disord 2:15–34, 1983

Good GE, Thomson DA, Braithwaite AD: Men and therapy: critical concepts, theoretical frameworks, and research recommendations. J Clin Psychol 61(6):699–711, 2005 15732084

Grieve FG, Truba N, Bowersox S: Etiology, assessment, and treatment of muscle dysmorphia. J Cogn Psychother 23(4):306–314, 2009 17167756

Griffiths S, Murray SB, Touyz S: Extending the masculinity hypothesis: an investigation of gender role conformity, body dissatisfaction, and disordered eating in young heterosexual men. Psychology of Men and Masculinity 16(1):108–114, 2015

Hartmann AS, Greenberg JL, Wilhelm S: The relationship between anorexia nervosa and body dysmorphic disorder (Research Support, Non-U.S. Gov't Review). Clin Psychol Rev 33(5):675–685, 2013 23685673

Hildebrandt T, Langenbucher J, Schlundt DG: Muscularity concerns among men: development of attitudinal and perceptual measures. Body Image 1(2):169–181, 2004 18089149

Hildebrandt T, Schlundt D, Langenbucher J, et al: Presence of muscle dysmorphia symptomology among male weightlifters. Compr Psychiatry 47(2):127–135, 2006 16490571

Hildebrandt T, Langenbucher JW, Carr SJ, et al: Modeling population heterogeneity in appearance- and performance-enhancing drug (APED) use: applications of mixture modeling in 400 regular APED users. J Abnorm Psychol 116(4):717–733, 2007 18020718

Hildebrandt T, Walker DC, Alfano L, et al: Development and validation of a male specific body checking questionnaire. Int J Eat Disord 43(1):77–87, 2010 19247988

Hildebrandt T, Lai JK, Langenbucher JW, et al: The diagnostic dilemma of pathological appearance and performance enhancing drug use. Drug Alcohol Depend 114(1):1–11, 2011a 21115306

Hildebrandt T, Langenbucher JW, Lai JK, et al: Development and validation of the Appearance and Performance Enhancing Drug Use Schedule. Addict Behav 36(10):949–958, 2011b 21640487

Hudson JI, Hiripi E, Pope HG Jr, et al: The prevalence and correlates of eating disorders in the National Comorbidity Survey Replication. Biol Psychiatry 61(3):348–358, 2007 16815322

Jones WR, Morgan JF: Eating disorders in men: a review of the literature. J Public Ment Health 9:23–31, 2010

Kaminski PL, Slaton SR, Caster J, et al: The Male Eating Behavior and Body Image Evaluation (MEBBIE): a scale to measure eating, exercise, and body image concerns in men. Poster presented at the annual convention of the Texas Psychological Association, San Antonio, 2002

Langenbucher J, Hildebrandt T, Carr S: Medical consequences of anabolic steroids, in Handbook of Medical Consequences of Drug Abuse. Edited by Brick J. Binghamton, NY, Hawthorn Press, 2008, pp 385–422

Lavender JM, De Young KP, Anderson DA: Eating Disorder Examination Questionnaire (EDE-Q): Norms for undergraduate men. Eat Behav 11(2):119–121, 2010 20188296

Legenbauer T, Vocks S, Schäfer C, et al: Preference for attractiveness and thinness in a partner: influence of internalization of the thin ideal and shape/weight dissatisfaction in heterosexual women, heterosexual men, lesbians, and gay men. Body Image 6(3):228–234, 2009 19443281

Lewinsohn PM, Seeley JR, Moerk KC, et al: Gender differences in eating disorder symptoms in young adults. Int J Eat Disord 32(4):426–440, 2002 12386907

Mahalik JR, Good GE, Englar-Carlson M: Masculinity scripts, presenting concerns, and help seeking: implications for practice and training. Prof Psychol Res Pr 34:123–131, 2003

McCreary DR, Sasse DK: An exploration of the drive for muscularity in adolescent boys and girls. J Am Cell Health 48(6):297–304, 2000 10863873

McFarland MB, Kaminski PL: Men, muscles, and mood: the relationship between self-concept, dysphoria, and body image disturbances. Eat Behav 10(1):68–70, 2009 19171324

Mond JM, Hay PJ: Functional impairment associated with bulimic behaviors in a community sample of men and women. Int J Eat Disord 40(5):391–398, 2007 17497705

Mond J, Hall A, Bentley C, et al: Eating-disordered behavior in adolescent boys: eating disorder examination questionnaire norms. Int J Eat Disord 47(4):335–341, 2014 24338639

Murray SB, Rieger E, Touyz SW, et al: Muscle dysmorphia and the DSM-V conundrum: where does it belong? A review paper. Int J Eat Disord 43(6):483–491, 2010 20862769

Murray SB, Rieger E, Hildebrandt T, et al: A comparison of eating, exercise, shape, and weight related symptomatology in males with muscle dysmorphia and anorexia nervosa. Body Image 9(2):193–200, 2012 22391410

Murray SB, Rieger E, Karlov L, et al: An investigation of the transdiagnostic model of eating disorders in the context of muscle dysmorphia. Eur Eat Disord Rev 21(2):160–164, 2013 22865715

Pope HG Jr, Gruber AJ, Choi P, et al: Muscle dysmorphia: an underrecognized form of body dysmorphic disorder. Psychosomatics 38(6):548–557, 1997 9427852

Pope HG Jr, Kanayama G, Hudson JI: Risk factors for illicit anabolic-androgenic steroid use in male weightlifters: a cross-sectional cohort study. Biol Psychiatry 71(3):254–261, 2012 21839424

Ricciardelli LA, McCabe MP: Psychometric evaluation of the Body Change Inventory: an assessment instrument for adolescent boys and girls. Eat Behav 3(1):45–59, 2002 15001019

Robinson KJ, Mountford VA, Sperlinger DJ: Being men with eating disorders: perspectives of male eating disorder service-users. J Health Psychol 18(2):176–186, 2013 22453166

Russell CJ, Keel PK: Homosexuality as a specific risk factor for eating disorders in men. Int J Eat Disord 31(3):300–306, 2002 11920991

Siever MD: Sexual orientation and gender as factors in socioculturally acquired vulnerability to body dissatisfaction and eating disorders. J Consult Clin Psychol 62(2):252–260, 1994 8201061

Striegel-Moore RH, Rosselli F, Perrin N, et al: Gender difference in the prevalence of eating disorder symptoms. Int J Eat Disord 42(5):471–474, 2009 19107833

Tiggemann M, Martins Y, Kirkbride A: Oh to be lean and muscular: body image ideals in gay and heterosexual men. Psychol Men Masc 8:15–24, 2007

Tiggemann M, Martins Y, Churchett L: Beyond muscles: unexplored parts of men's body image. J Health Psychol 13(8):1163–1172, 2008 18987089

Walker DC, Anderson DA, Hildebrandt T: Body checking behaviors in men. Body Image 6(3):164–170, 2009 19482568

Yelland C, Tiggemann M: Muscularity and the gay ideal: body dissatisfaction and disordered eating in homosexual men. Eat Behav 4(2):107–116, 2003 15000974

7 Eating Problems in Special Populations

Cultural Considerations

Anne E. Becker, M.D., Ph.D., S.M.

Clinical effectiveness in multicultural and cross-cultural settings in general warrants sensitivity to variations in illness experience and symptom reporting as well as expectations, values, and preferences that drive risk, presentation, help seeking, and therapeutic engagement in health care delivery. Attunement to culturally and socially patterned characteristics of clinical presentation is essential to an informed and accurate mental health assessment, given the importance of the psychiatric interview and patient report of experiential symptoms to the diagnostic formulation. Understanding cultural variation is especially germane to identifying, evaluating, and managing feeding and eating disorders, given the dimensional nature of many core symptoms, the salience of cultural contextual factors in ascertaining diagnostic criteria, and the critical importance of decisions to seek help and disclose symptoms. Video 5, "Cultural considerations in the assessment of eating problems," highlights cultural factors.

Epidemiology of Eating Disorders Across Social Contexts

Historical and cross-cultural data support that anorexia nervosa (AN) and bulimia nervosa (BN) are mental disorders associated with the sociocultural contexts of modernization. After sentinel case reports of AN in the nineteenth century, aesthetic ideals and valuation of thinness emerged in the United States and other historically Western cultural regions in the twentieth century, and the documented prevalence of AN rose concomitantly (Brumberg 1988). By the late twentieth century, the presence of AN and BN was recognized in North America, Europe, Australia, and New Zealand, whereas eating disorders were viewed as relatively rare outside postindustrialized, Westernized societies. In this respect, the argument that eating disorders are "culture bound" to the West or to Western cultures has been made (e.g., Keel and Klump 2003; Swartz 1985).

The Global Burden of Disease Study demonstrates, however, that the health burdens associated with eating disorders, as measured both in disability-adjusted life years and in years lived with disability, have shown steep percentage increases globally over the past two decades (Murray et al. 2012; Vos et al. 2012). Given that the prevalence of AN and BN does not appear have increased in Europe, the United States, and other high-income regions over the past few decades (Smink et al. 2012), these data support the possibility that eating disorders may be increasingly prevalent in low- and middle-income countries. Transnational migration and widespread participation in the global economy have resulted in similarly widespread exposure to ideas, values, and products originating in historically Western societies. Cross-cultural epidemiological data, moreover, support the association of eating disorders with some of these Western cultural exposures, even across socially diverse populations. These exposures occur, for example, through acculturation associated with both migration and in-country rapid social and economic development (e.g., Becker 2004; Becker et al. 2002, 2010a; Nasser et al. 2001). Furthermore, emerging communication platforms–including televised and other media–that enable the rapid and broad global distribution of ideas, images, and products may foster accelerated distribution of cultural exposures that elevate risk for disordered eating (Becker et al. 2011; Gerbasi et al. 2014; Grabe et al. 2008; Levine and Murnen 2009).

Within the United States, eating disorders are also more broadly distributed across sociodemographic strata than previously understood. Epidemiological data collected in representative community-based samples of the U.S. population indicate that eating disorders occur across each major census group residing in the United States (Alegria et al. 2007; Nicdao et al. 2007; Striegel-Moore et al. 2011; Taylor et al. 2013). Although clinicians should be aware of sociodemographic variation in patterns of eating disorder presentation, they should also understand that it is neither possible nor advisable to summarize clinical features that "typify" eating disorders within a particular ethnic, racial, or social group. For example, there is substantial heterogeneity within any one of the major census groups, relating to country of origin and postmigration generation. In addition, cultural exposures arise not only from the family's country or ethnic heritage of origin but also from the so-called host or dominant culture, global culture (accessed through the media and Internet), and other immigrant communities.

It may be that the only valid assumption relating ethnicity to eating disorders for clinical assessment is that any individual could be at risk, regardless of ethnic, racial, or social background. Clinicians should be aware that although eating disorders may present in conventional ways across diverse populations (Shaw et al. 2004), disclosure and presentation of symptoms may vary across sociodemographic groups. For this reason, implementation of the DSM-5 Cultural Formulation Interview (American Psychiatric Association 2013a) and its additional supplementary modules (American Psychiatric Association 2013b) can be especially helpful in eliciting the patient's understanding and experience of symptoms as well as his or her preferences and expectations about treatment. Because of lay and clinical stereotyping of AN as a disease associated with affluence and white ethnicity, ethnic minority patients are at risk of a double stigma attached to having an eating disorder (Becker et al. 2010b). Stigma, moreover, may have different kinds of impact for different health care consumers. For example, in China, Tong et al. (2014) reported a 39% refusal rate for an interview among study participants who were likely to meet diagnostic criteria on the basis of screening; they suggested that this may have been driven by concerns about stigma and shame (Tong et al. 2014).

Cultural Patterning and Other Contextual Influences on Diagnostic Assessment

Evidence of culture-specific phenotypes and patterning of symptoms (Franko et al. 2007; Lee et al. 2010; Pike and Mizushima 2005; Striegel-Moore et al. 2011; Thomas et al. 2011) suggests that cultural factors may have more of a dimensional than categorical role in influencing the kind and presentation of symptoms. For example, in Fiji, the use of traditional herbal purgatives has been identified as a weight management behavior among adolescent girls. Individuals with this behavior–along with those reporting more familiar and conventional purging behaviors–have greater eating psychopathology than individuals who do not engage in purging; in addition, and perhaps more unexpectedly, the use of traditional herbal purgatives appears to be associated with greater distress and impairment than is the more familiar and conventional bulimia-like purging behavior (Thomas et al. 2011).

Lee and colleagues have extensively documented another example of a culture-specific phenotype of AN. They described a variant of AN among the Hong Kong Chinese distinguished by an absence of "fear of fatness," a characteristic that has been regarded as a core diagnostic feature of AN. This presentation, termed *non-fat-phobic AN,* characterized a sizable proportion of individuals presenting to a tertiary psychiatric clinic in this Hong Kong setting in the mid-1980s (Lee et al. 2010). Notably, these patients provided a different–but culturally salient–rationale for their dietary restriction and failure to gain weight (Lee 1995, 1996; Lee et al. 2001). Additional studies identified non-fat-phobic AN in other Asian study populations, including in Japan, Singapore, and China (e.g., Pike and Borovoy 2004). Non-fat-phobic AN has also been documented in the United States (Becker et al. 2009b).

The phenomenological diversity of feeding and eating disorders is reflected in the substantial proportion of cases that are assigned to the residual category even after the publication of revised criteria in DSM-5 (Machado et al. 2013; Nakai et al. 2013). Wide cultural variability in dietary patterns and variability in body size and weight ideals and their salience across the life course (Becker 1995) amplify this diversity further and may contribute to the absence of clinical detection of an eating disorder, which is frequent in primary care settings. Other major challenges in the diagnostic assessment of feeding and eating disorders include the dimensionality of key symptoms that lie on a continuum with socially normative dietary patterns and weight concerns. Intrinsic to several of these criteria is their relativity to cultural context. For instance, ascertainment of Criterion D for BN requires a judgment about whether the influence of shape and weight on an individual's self-evaluation is "undue." Likewise, Criterion A for both BN and binge-eating disorder operationalizes a binge episode in relation to an amount that most individuals "would eat in a similar period of time under similar circumstances" (American Psychiatric Association 2013a, pp. 345, 350). As a result, clinical assessment requires understanding of the prevailing social norms within the patient's cultural milieu. In the absence of observable behaviors or collateral history that can inform ascertainment of cognitive symptoms intrinsic to the feeding and eating disorders, their assessment relies on patient report, which can be affected by maturity, insight, and willingness to disclose (Becker et al. 2005, 2009a). Furthermore, whether a patient is able or willing to formulate or provide information about the departure from these norms may also be governed by cultural style. Additional related symptoms such as "marked distress" or "feeling uncomfortably full" (American Psychiatric

Association 2013a, p. 350) also require interpretation of subjective experience, which may be informed by socialization to culturally grounded standards and expectations. Collateral information from other sources is also likely filtered through a cultural lens.

A Clinical Approach to Eating Problems Across Culturally and Socially Diverse Patient Populations

DSM-5 has replaced the older term "culture-bound syndrome" with several new terms that better frame and capture the multiple cultural dimensions that influence experience, presentation, and help seeking (American Psychiatric Association 2013a, p. 758). Definitions are summarized in Table 7–1 with some corresponding examples. A culturally informed approach to assessment of feeding and eating disorders in multicultural clinical settings will benefit from referencing relevant cultural syndromes, idioms of distress, and cultural explanations with regard to the disordered eating and comorbid psychiatric symptoms and disorders, including anxiety and depressive disorders. However, because these cultural influences are neither temporally fixed nor uniform within any particular social group, a process-based approach to cross-cultural diagnostic formulation–such as is set forth in the Cultural Formulation Interview (CFI) in DSM-5–has optimal clinical utility. The CFI can also be accessed at www.psychiatry.org/practice/dsm/dsm5/online-assessment-measures#Cultural.

Video 5 demonstrates cultural factors in the assessment of individuals with eating problems.

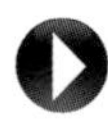

Video Illustration 5: Cultural considerations in the assessment of eating problems (6:10)

Overcoming Social and Cultural Barriers to Treatment

Eating disorders are serious mental disorders, yet nearly half of individuals with an eating disorder in the United States do not receive specialty care for this problem (Hudson et al. 2007). Available evidence, moreover, points to ethnic disparities in care access for an eating disorder in the United States (Marques et al. 2011). Factors associated with both clinicians and health consumers likely contribute to suboptimal care access. For ex-

TABLE 7–1. Cultural dimensions of illness experience, expression, and expectations relevant to mental health assessment

Cultural concept	DSM-5 definition	Examples relevant to disordered eating
Cultural syndromes	"[C]lusters of symptoms and attributions that tend to co-occur among individuals in specific cultural groups, communities, or contexts and that are recognized locally as coherent patterns of experience"	*Macake* (Fijian)–a loss of appetite associated with rhinorrhea, fever, oral candidiasis, which can cause dangerous weight loss (Becker 1995)
Cultural idioms of distress	"[W]ays of expressing distress that may not involve specific symptoms or syndromes, but that provide collective, shared ways of experiencing and talking about personal or social concerns"	Non-fat-phobic anorexia nervosa among Hong Kong Chinese–in lieu of concerns about fatness or weight gain, patients provide an alternative rationale for dietary restriction, such as fullness or other gastrointestinal symptoms, which is culturally salient (Lee et al. 2001)
Cultural explanations or perceived causes	"[L]abels, attributions, or features of an explanatory model that indicate culturally recognized meaning or etiology for symptoms, illness, or distress"	*Macake* (Fijian)–often perceived to be caused by social neglect that leads to a diet that is of poor quality or otherwise inadequate (Becker 1995)

Note. Definitions are excerpted from American Psychiatric Association 2013a, p. 758. Used with permission.

ample, consumer demand for care may be low in certain ethnic groups, and clinician recognition of and response to patients with a feeding or eating disorder may also vary across patient ethnicity. Community-based epidemiological survey data demonstrate that service utilization for an eating disorder is significantly lower among African Americans, Latinos, and Asian Americans than among non-Hispanic white populations in the United States (Marques et al. 2011). One study, controlling for severity of symptoms, found that clinicians in a college-based screening program were less likely to refer Latino participants than non-Latino white participants, when controlling for severity of symptoms (Becker et al. 2003). A qualitative study showed that some health consumers experience ethnicity-based stereotyping by clinicians specific to their eating or weight complaints (Becker et al. 2010b). Clinician bias related to other psychiatric diagnoses has also been reported (Good 1992–1993). Unfortunately, these clinician and health consumer factors can both reinforce reluctance to seek care and reify the impression that feeding and eating disorders are uncommon among ethnic minorities. It is advisable, therefore, for clinicians to consider whether patient distrust may adversely affect a patient's willingness to engage in care. The CFI includes a probe question (question 16) that clinicians can use to address this sensitive issue in a respectful way along with other social and cultural barriers to help seeking. The CFI Supplementary Module 8 ("Patient-Clinician Relationship") provides additional guidance for addressing factors in the patient-clinician relationship that might undermine care. This module can be accessed in its entirety online (see American Psychiatric Association 2013b). Table 7–2 excerpts five relevant questions that clinicians can ask a patient to expand on CFI question 16.

A variety of additional cultural and social factors influence patterns of help seeking for mental disorders. For example, the stigma frequently associated with mental disorders may present a barrier to care if there are perceived intolerable social costs to the patient or family. Likewise, patients and their caregivers may experience the therapeutic benefits of care in nonclinical settings as superior or preferable. Family and social factors that either enable or undermine adherence can be elicited using the CFI Supplementary Module 3 ("Social Network"). Example questions from this module are included in Table 7–2, and the module can be accessed in its entirety online (see American Psychiatric Association 2013b).

Many individuals with an eating disorder are initially reluctant to disclose their symptoms to a clinician but may be willing to admit to symptoms when asked directly (Becker et al. 2005). Self-report assessments, such as the Eating Disorder Examination Questionnaire (EDE-Q; Fairburn and Beglin 1994) and the SCOFF questionnaire (Morgan et al. 1999), which have demonstrated validity in several languages and study populations, may be useful in promoting case identification when used alongside clinician-based assessment. For example, they can augment a clinical interview or prime a conversation about disordered eating symptoms. Because the item content in these measures may not tap all relevant domains in all cultural settings, clinicians working with populations in multiethnic settings or regions outside of Europe, North America, Australia, and New Zealand should consider supplementing these screeners–as well as clinical interviews–with questions assessing local dietary and weight management behaviors. In addition to inquiring about conventional symptoms, clinicians should consider asking patients about use of complementary and al-

TABLE 7–2. Excerpted questions from Cultural Formulation Interview (CFI) supplementary modules addressing the patient-clinician relationship and the patient's social network

Patient-Clinician Relationship (related to CFI question 16)

QUESTIONS FOR THE PATIENT:

1. What kind of experiences have you had with clinicians in the past? What was most helpful to you?
2. Have you had difficulties with clinicians in the past? What did you find difficult or unhelpful?
3. Now let's talk about the help that you would like to get here. Some people prefer clinicians of a similar background (for example, age, race, religion, or some other characteristic) because they think it may be easier to understand each other. Do you have any preference or ideas about what kind of clinician might understand you best?
4. Sometimes differences among patients and clinicians make it difficult for them to understand each other. Do you have any concerns about this? If so, in what way? [RELATED TO CFI Q#16.]
5. What patients expect from their clinicians is important. As we move forward in your care, how can we best work together?

Social Network (related to CFI questions 5, 6, 12, 15)

INTRODUCTION FOR THE INDIVIDUAL BEING INTERVIEWED: I would like to know more about how your family, friends, colleagues, co-workers, and other important people in your life have had an impact on your [PROBLEM].

Composition of the individual's social network

2. Is there anyone in particular whom you trust and can talk with about your [PROBLEM]? Who? Anyone else?

Social network understanding of problem

4. What ideas do your family and friends have about the nature of your [PROBLEM]? How do they understand your [PROBLEM]?

Social network response to problem

6. What advice have family members and friends given you about your [PROBLEM]?

Social network as a stress/buffer

9. What have your family, friends, and other people in your life done to make your [PROBLEM] better or easier for you to deal with? (IF UNCLEAR: How has that made your [PROBLEM] better?)

11. What have your family, friends, and other people in your life done to make your [PROBLEM] worse or harder for you to deal with? (IF UNCLEAR: How has that made your [PROBLEM] worse?)

Social network in treatment

15. How would involving family or friends make a difference in your treatment?

Source. Excerpted from American Psychiatric Association 2013b. Used with permission.

ternative medicines and products, including over-the-counter natural supplements. Because use of natural supplements and traditional purgatives varies across ethnicities (Kelly et al. 2006) and may be regarded as normative in some social milieus, and may also be common among individuals with BN (Roerig et al. 2003), clinicians should inquire directly about usage and probe further for misuse that reflects eating disorder psychopathology.

Although little is known about the global epidemiology of the feeding and eating disorders, avoidant/restrictive food intake disorder and rumination disorder, there are numerous prevalence studies of pica eating. For example, in some African regions, geophagia is prevalent among schoolchildren (e.g., near or exceeding 75% in Zambia [Nchito et al. 2004] and Western Kenya [Geissler et al. 1998a]) as well as among women attending antenatal clinics (e.g., approximately half of women sampled in Kenya [Geissler et al. 1998b]). Pica eating in these regions often falls within local social norms (e.g., in Western Kenya, Zambia, and Dar es Salaam [Geissler et al. 1999; Kawai et al. 2009; Nchito et al. 2004]). For example, in some regions, local vendors sometimes sell earth for consumption. Consequently, clinicians not only should consider assessing for pica eating in migrant populations in which pica eating is prevalent but also should evaluate whether or not it is socially normative if intervention is indicated.

In assessing AN, clinicians should probe for persistent dietary restriction or compensatory behaviors that prevent weight gain even if the presence of intense fear of weight gain or fatness is not apparent. When these behaviors are present, the patient's rationale should be evaluated. If present, unconventional rationales for dietary restriction, such as gastrointestinal (GI) discomfort, which are commonly seen in Chinese patients (Lee et al. 2012) and which persist in undermining weight gain despite appropriate intervention, should be considered and assessed.

Clinicians should be aware that social structural barriers, such as poverty or limited knowledge of English, may impede access to treatment settings and also influence clinical presentation. The differential diagnosis for AN should encompass nutritional deficits due to food insecurity. The U.S. Department of Agriculture reports that 14.5% of U.S. households were food insecure in 2012. In addition, 7 million American households (5.7%) experienced very low food security (operationalized by disruption of eating patterns and reduction of food intake by at least one household member because of poverty). Nearly half of these households with very low food security reported weight loss due to inadequate money for food (Coleman-Jensen et al. 2013). Clinicians may find the questions used to assess household food security as part of the Current Population Survey (item content available at www.ers.usda.gov/media/1183208/err-155.pdf; Coleman-Jensen et al. 2013) to be a useful guide for assessing food insecurity; they should also ask about the specific impact of food insecurity, if any, on the identified patient. Household characteristics associated with food insecurity in the United States include those with children and headed by a single adult, those at or below the poverty line, and those with identified as black or Hispanic (Coleman-Jensen et al. 2013). Although the relationship between food insecurity and disordered eating is not yet well understood, neither poverty nor presence of hunger excludes the possibility of an eating disorder, because both can be simultaneously present.

Physical Assessment

Physical examination is crucial to excluding medical causes of signs and symptoms and planning nutritional, medical, pharmacological, and psychosocial management. Psychoeducation for the patient and his or her family, when appropriate, about the physical health impacts of disordered eating may be especially helpful if they are unfamiliar with eating disorders and their associated risks. In addition to a comprehensive physical and laboratory examination to evaluate general health, clinicians should consider and evaluate additional possible health and psychosocial exposures among patients who have recently emigrated from or traveled to their country of origin. A patient's weight and height should be measured and assessed against international standards for body mass index (BMI) and BMI centiles, as well as in the context of population-specific benchmarks, growth history, and family history. For example, clinicians should be aware that the relationship among BMI, adiposity, and health risk varies across some Asian, white, and Pacific Islander populations (Duncan et al. 2009; Rush et al. 2009; WHO Expert Consultation 2004).

Although GI symptoms are common complaints among patients with feeding or eating disorders, these symptoms may have no discernible physiological correlate. Moreover, if a GI symptom or another somatic complaint is a culturally preferred idiom for distress, then some patient populations may present with these complaints with greater frequency than others. In addition to considering and ruling out GI disorders and conditions (Becker and Baker 2010), clinicians should consider and exclude helminthic and other parasitic infections that can affect appetite and weight (Stephenson 1994) and that differentially affect certain populations in the United States (Hotez 2008).

Conclusion

Eating disorders have broad global distribution and occur across diverse social and cultural contexts. Given sociocultural variation in help seeking for, and the presentation and experience of, mental disorders, it is important for clinicians to consider the potential influence of the cultural and social contexts in which symptoms have developed in the diagnostic assessment of an eating disorder. Clinicians, moreover, should be mindful of social barriers to treatment in framing recommendations and formulating a care management plan. The DSM-5 Cultural Formulation Interview can be a helpful supplemental tool in evaluating social and cultural factors germane to the diagnosis and treatment of an eating disorder.

Key Clinical Points

- Eating disorders occur across all of the major U.S. census groups as well as around the world. The measurable global health burdens associated with eating disorders increased substantially over the past few decades.
- Service utilization for eating disorders varies substantially across major ethnic groups, and thus certain ethnic groups are at higher risk for lack of access to care; social barriers to care for an eating disorder include clinician stereotyping and stigma. Ethnic variation in service utilization for feeding disorders is unknown.
- Cultural variation has been observed in eating disorder symptom presentation. However, cultural influences on prevalence and phenomenology of disordered eating are fluid and dynamic and therefore cannot be generalized for application in any particular ethnically or culturally defined population.
- Clinicians should include food insecurity in their differential diagnosis of anorexia nervosa, particularly among high-risk households.
- Clinicians should inquire about use of herbal, indigenous, or traditional supplements that affect appetite, weight, or gastrointestinal function.
- Clinicians should reference dietary behaviors against local social norms, using collateral history from the patient's family, when appropriate.
- Clinicians should consider conducting a patient-centered interview, using the DSM-5 Cultural Formulation Interview and supplementary modules, to elicit symptoms or terms with salience for the patient that might not otherwise emerge when using questions with conventional medical or psychiatric ideas or terms.

References

Alegria M, Woo M, Cao Z, et al: Prevalence and correlates of eating disorders in Latinos in the United States. Int J Eat Disord 40(suppl):S15–S21, 2007 17584870

American Psychiatric Association: Diagnostic and Statistical Manual of Mental Disorders, 5th Edition. Arlington, VA, American Psychiatric Association, 2013a

American Psychiatric Association: Supplementary Modules to the Core Cultural Formulation Interview. 2013b. Available at: http://www.psychiatry.org/practice/dsm/dsm5/online-assessment-measures#Cultural. Accessed March 16, 2015.

Becker AE: Body, Self, and Society: The View From Fiji. Philadelphia, PA, University of Pennsylvania Press, 1995

Becker AE: Television, disordered eating, and young women in Fiji: negotiating body image and identity during rapid social change. Cult Med Psychiatry 28(4):533–559, 2004 15847053

Becker AE, Baker CW: Eating disorders, in Sleisenger and Fordtran's Gastrointestinal and Liver Disease, 9th Edition. Edited by Feldman M, Friedman LS, Brandt LJ. Philadelphia, PA, Elsevier, 2010 pp 121–138

Becker AE, Burwell RA, Gilman SE, et al: Eating behaviours and attitudes following prolonged exposure to television among ethnic Fijian adolescent girls. Br J Psychiatry 180:509–514, 2002 12042229

Becker AE, Franko DL, Speck A, et al: Ethnicity and differential access to care for eating disorder symptoms. Int J Eat Disord 33(2):205–212, 2003 12616587

Becker AE, Thomas JJ, Franko DL, et al: Disclosure patterns of eating and weight concerns to clinicians, educational professionals, family, and peers. Int J Eat Disord 38(1):18–23, 2005 15971235

Becker AE, Eddy KT, Perloe A: Clarifying criteria for cognitive signs and symptoms for eating disorders in DSM-V. Int J Eat Disord 42(7):611–619, 2009a 19650082

Becker AE, Thomas JJ, Pike KM: Should non-fat-phobic anorexia nervosa be included in DSM-V? Int J Eat Disord 42(7):620–635, 2009b 19655370

Becker AE, Fay K, Agnew-Blais J, et al: Development of a measure of "acculturation" for ethnic Fijians: methodologic and conceptual considerations for application to eating disorders research. Transcult Psychiatry 47(5):754–788, 2010a 21088103

Becker AE, Hadley Arrindell A, Perloe A, et al: A qualitative study of perceived social barriers to care for eating disorders: perspectives from ethnically diverse health care consumers. Int J Eat Disord 43(7):633–647, 2010b 19806607

Becker AE, Fay KE, Agnew-Blais J, et al: Social network media exposure and adolescent eating pathology in Fiji. Br J Psychiatry 198(1):43–50, 2011 21200076

Brumberg JJ: Fasting Girls: The History of Anorexia Nervosa. Cambridge, MA, Harvard University Press, 1988

Coleman-Jensen A, Nord M, Singh A: Household Food Security in the United States in 2012. Economic Research Service, U.S. Department of Agriculture. September 2013. Available at: http://www.ers.usda.gov/media/1183208/err-155.pdf. Accessed March 16, 2015.

Duncan JS, Duncan EK, Schofield G: Accuracy of body mass index (BMI) thresholds for predicting excess body fat in girls from five ethnicities. Asia Pac J Clin Nutr 18(3):404–411, 2009 19786389

Fairburn CG, Beglin SJ: Assessment of eating disorders: interview or self-report questionnaire? Int J Eat Disord 16(4):363–370, 1994 7866415
Franko DL, Becker AE, Thomas JJ, et al: Cross-ethnic differences in eating disorder symptoms and related distress. Int J Eat Disord 40(2):156–164, 2007 17080449
Geissler PW, Mwaniki DL, Thiong'o F, et al: Geophagy, iron status and anaemia among primary school children in Western Kenya. Trop Med Int Health 3(7):529–534, 1998a 9705186
Geissler PW, Shulman CE, Prince RJ, et al: Geophagy, iron status and anaemia among pregnant women on the coast of Kenya. Trans R Soc Trop Med Hyg 92(5):549–553, 1998b 9861377
Geissler PW, Prince RJ, Levene M, et al: Perceptions of soil-eating and anaemia among pregnant women on the Kenyan coast. Soc Sci Med 48(8):1069–1079, 1999 10390045
Gerbasi ME, Richards LK, Thomas JJ, et al: Globalization and eating disorder risk: peer influence, perceived social norms, and adolescent disordered eating in Fiji. Int J Eat Disord 47(7):727–737, 2014 25139374
Good BJ: Culture, diagnosis and comorbidity. Cult Med Psychiatry 16(4):427–446, 1992–1993 1305525
Grabe S, Ward LM, Hyde JS: The role of the media in body image concerns among women: a meta-analysis of experimental and correlational studies. Psychol Bull 134(3):460–476, 2008 18444705
Hotez PJ: Neglected infections of poverty in the United States of America. PLoS Negl Trop Dis 2(6):e256, 2008 18575621
Hudson JI, Hiripi E, Pope HG Jr, et al: The prevalence and correlates of eating disorders in the National Comorbidity Survey Replication. Biol Psychiatry 61(3):348–358, 2007 16815322
Kawai K, Saathoff E, Antelman G, et al: Geophagy (soil-eating) in relation to anemia and helminth infection among HIV-infected pregnant women in Tanzania. Am J Trop Med Hyg 80(1):36–43, 2009 19141837
Keel PK, Klump KL: Are eating disorders culture-bound syndromes? Implications for conceptualizing their etiology. Psychol Bull 129(5):747–769, 2003 12956542
Kelly JP, Kaufman DW, Kelley K, et al: Use of herbal/natural supplements according to racial/ethnic group. J Altern Complement Med 12(6):555–561, 2006 16884347
Lee S: Self-starvation in context: towards a culturally sensitive understanding of anorexia nervosa. Soc Sci Med 41(1):25–36, 1995 7667670
Lee S: Reconsidering the status of anorexia nervosa as a Western culture-bound syndrome. Soc Sci Med 42(1):21–34, 1996 8745105
Lee S, Lee AM, Ngai E, et al: Rationales for food refusal in Chinese patients with anorexia nervosa. Int J Eat Disord 29(2):224–229, 2001 11429985
Lee S, Ng KL, Kwok K, et al: The changing profile of eating disorders at a tertiary psychiatric clinic in Hong Kong (1987–2007). Int J Eat Disord 43(4):307–314, 2010 19350649
Lee S, Ng KL, Kwok KP, et al: Gastrointestinal dysfunction in Chinese patients with fat-phobic and nonfat-phobic anorexia nervosa. Transcult Psychiatry 49(5):678–695, 2012 23002113

Levine MP, Murnen SK: "Everybody knows that mass media are/are not [pick one] a cause of eating disorders": a critical review of evidence for a causal link between media, negative body image, and disordered eating in females. J Soc Clin Psychol 28:9–42, 2009

Machado PP, Gonçalves S, Hoek HW: DSM-5 reduces the proportion of EDNOS cases: evidence from community samples. Int J Eat Disord 46(1):60–65, 2013 22815201

Marques L, Alegria M, Becker AE, et al: Comparative prevalence, correlates of impairment, and service utilization for eating disorders across U.S. ethnic groups: implications for reducing ethnic disparities in health care access for eating disorders. Int J Eat Disord 44(5):412–420, 2011 20665700

Morgan JF, Reid F, Lacey JH: The SCOFF questionnaire: assessment of a new screening tool for eating disorders. BMJ 319(7223):1467–1468, 1999 10582927

Murray CJL, Vos T, Lozano R, et al: Disability-adjusted life years (DALYs) for 291 diseases and injuries in 21 regions, 1990–2010: a systematic analysis for the Global Burden of Disease Study 2010. Lancet 380(9859):2197–2223, 2012 23245608

Nakai Y, Fukushima M, Taniguchi A, et al: Comparison of DSM-IV versus proposed DSM-5 diagnostic criteria for eating disorders in a Japanese sample. Eur Eat Disord Rev 21(1):8–14, 2013 23059695

Nasser M, Katzman MA, Gordon RA (eds): Eating Disorders and Cultures in Transition. Hove, UK, Brunner-Routledge, 2001

Nchito M, Geissler PW, Mubila L, et al: Effects of iron and multimicronutrient supplementation on geophagy: a two-by-two factorial study among Zambian schoolchildren in Lusaka. Trans R Soc Trop Med Hyg 98(4):218–227, 2004 15049460

Nicdao EG, Hong S, Takeuchi DT: Prevalence and correlates of eating disorders among Asian Americans: results from the National Latino and Asian American Study. Int J Eat Disord 40(suppl):S22–S26, 2007 17879986

Pike KM, Borovoy A: The rise of eating disorders in Japan: issues of culture and limitations of the model of "Westernization." Cult Med Psychiatry 28(4):493–531, 2004 15847052

Pike KM, Mizushima H: The clinical presentation of Japanese women with anorexia nervosa and bulimia nervosa: a study of the Eating Disorders Inventory-2. Int J Eat Disord 37(1):26–31, 2005 15690462

Roerig JL, Mitchell JE, de Zwaan M, et al: The eating disorders medicine cabinet revisited: a clinician's guide to appetite suppressants and diuretics. Int J Eat Disord 33(4):443–457, 2003 12658674

Rush EC, Freitas I, Plank LD: Body size, body composition and fat distribution: comparative analysis of European, Maori, Pacific Island and Asian Indian adults. Br J Nutr 102(4):632–641, 2009 19203416

Shaw H, Ramirez L, Trost A, et al: Body image and eating disturbances across ethnic groups: more similarities than differences. Psychol Addict Behav 18(1):12–18, 2004 15008681

Smink FRE, van Hoeken D, Hoek HW: Epidemiology of eating disorders: incidence, prevalence and mortality rates. Curr Psychiatry Rep 14(4):406–414, 2012 22644309

Stephenson LS: Helminth parasites, a major factor in malnutrition. World Health Forum 15(2):169–172, 1994 8018283

Striegel-Moore RH, Rosselli F, Holtzman N, et al: Behavioral symptoms of eating disorders in Native Americans: results from the ADD Health Survey Wave III. Int J Eat Disord 44(6):561–566, 2011 21823140

Swartz L: Anorexia nervosa as a culture-bound syndrome. Soc Sci Med 20(7):725–730, 1985 4012359

Taylor JY, Caldwell CH, Baser RE, et al: Classification and correlates of eating disorders among blacks: findings from the National Survey of American Life. J Health Care Poor Underserved 24(1):289–310, 2013 23377735

Thomas JJ, Crosby RD, Wonderlich SA, et al: A latent profile analysis of the typology of bulimic symptoms in an indigenous Pacific population: evidence of cross-cultural variation in phenomenology. Psychol Med 41(1):195–206, 2011 20346191

Tong J, Miao S, Wang J, et al: A two-stage epidemiologic study on prevalence of eating disorders in female university students in Wuhan, China. Soc Psychiatry Psychiatr Epidemiol 49(3):499–505, 2014 23744441

Vos T, Flaxman AD, Naghavi M, et al: Years lived with disability (YLDs) for 1160 sequelae of 289 diseases and injuries 1990–2010: a systematic analysis for the Global Burden of Disease Study 2010. Lancet 380(9859):2163–2196, 2012 23245607

WHO Expert Consultation: Appropriate body-mass index for Asian populations and its implications for policy and intervention strategies. Lancet 363(9403):157–163, 2004 14726171

PART III

Assessment Tools

8 Assessment Measures, Then and Now

A Look Back at Seminal Measures and a Look Forward to the Brave New World

Jennifer J. Thomas, Ph.D.
Christina A. Roberto, Ph.D.
Kelly C. Berg, Ph.D., LP

Assessment is perceived by some people to be pedantic and boring. One may envision a group of research assistants sitting around a conference table quibbling over whether a sleeve of crackers counts as a "binge." However, accurate and reliable diagnostic evaluation is the foundation for everything we do as clinicians and researchers. The way data are captured and recorded informs diagnoses, treatment plans, insurance requests, research results, and public policy.

Eating disorder assessment has come a long way over the last quarter century. Just over 25 years ago, no structured interviews for assessing eating psychopathology existed, and eating disorders were rarely evaluated in large-scale epidemiological studies. Since then, a plethora of interview measures have emerged, each with its own advantages and disadvantages. Seminal measures, most notably the Eating Disorder Examination (EDE; Cooper and Fairburn 1987), have irrevocably shaped understanding of the core psychopathology of eating disorders. Newer measures, such as the Eating Disorder Assessment for DSM-5 (EDA-5; Sysko et al. 2015), have pioneered the assessment of novel constructs of feeding psychopathology. Recently, synergistic factors, including the publication of DSM-5 (American Psychiatric Association 2013) criteria that incorporate feeding disorders into a combined diagnostic scheme with eating disorders, improvements in the understanding of psychometrics, and advances in mobile technology, have converged to create a brave new world of feeding and eating disorder assessment that will shape the next quarter century of research and clinical care. Video 1, "Diagnostic issues in the age of DSM-5," presents a discussion of the changes in DSM-5.

A Look Back at Seminal Measures

Eating disorders have historically been assessed with either eating disorder–specific or general psychiatric interviews. Both types of measures have strengths and weaknesses. In general, these measures were not designed to incorporate the measurement of feeding disorders; however, exceptions are noted in the descriptions of the interviews in this chapter. The currently available instruments are summarized in Table 8–1.

Eating Disorder–Specific Interviews

The first and most widely used eating disorder–specific interview has undoubtedly been the EDE (Cooper and Fairburn 1987). Other specialty interviews that help in diagnosing eating disorders include the Structured Interview for Anorexic and Bulimic Disorders (SIAB; Fichter et al. 1990), the Interview for the Diagnosis of Eating Disorders (IDED; Williamson 1990), and an eating disorder–focused adaptation of the Longitudinal Interval Follow-up Evaluation (LIFE-EAT-3; K.T. Eddy, H.B. Murray, J.J. Thomas, unpublished work, July 2015).[1] These measures differ with respect to the specific diagnoses derived, the constructs assessed, the generation of dimensional severity ratings, and the assessment of current versus lifetime symptoms.

Eating Disorder Examination

The EDE was the first structured interview to assess current eating disorder psychopathology. This widely used instrument has long been consid-

[1] Other eating disorder–specific interviews, such as the Yale-Brown-Cornell Eating Disorder Scale (Sunday et al. 1995) and the Clinical Eating Disorder Rating Instrument (Palmer et al. 1987), can also be used to assess the severity of eating disorder psychopathology and associated features. However, they are not discussed in this chapter because neither can be used to make eating disorder diagnoses.

TABLE 8–1. Characteristics of currently available structured interviews for eating disorder diagnosis

Measure	Clinical expertise required	Age range (years)	Administration time	Feeding and eating disorder diagnoses assessed	Current or lifetime diagnoses	Updated for DSM-5
Eating disorder–specific interviews						
EDE-17.0D (Fairburn et al. 2014)	Yes	14 and up	1 hour	AN, BN, BED, OSFED	Current	Yes
Child EDE (Bryant-Waugh et al. 1996)	Yes	8–14	1 hour	AN, BN, OSFED	Current	No
SIAB-EX (Fichter et al. 1998)	Yes	12–65	30–60 minutes	AN, BN, BED	Both	No
IDED (Williamson 1990)	Yes	Adolescents and adults	30 minutes	AN, BN, BED	Current	No
LIFE-EAT-3 (K.T. Eddy, H.B. Murray, J.J. Thomas, unpublished work, July 2015)	Yes	10 and up	15–20 minutes	AN, BN, BED, ARFID, pica, rumination disorder, OSFED	Both	Yes
EDA-5 (Sysko et al. 2015)	Some	Adult	15 minutes	AN, BN, BED, ARFID, pica, rumination disorder, OSFED	Current	Yes
General psychiatric interviews						
SCID-5 (First et al. 2015)	Yes	Adult	1–2 hours[a]	AN, BN, BED, OSFED (ARFID optional)	Both	Yes

TABLE 8–1. Characteristics of currently available structured interviews for eating disorder diagnosis *(continued)*

Measure	Clinical expertise required	Age range (years)	Administration time	Feeding and eating disorder diagnoses assessed	Current or lifetime diagnoses	Updated for DSM-5
KSADS-PL (J. Kaufman, B. Birmaher, D. Axelson, F. Perepletchikova, D. Brent, Neal Ryan, working draft, 2013)	Yes	6–18	1.25 hours[a]	AN, BN, BED	Both	Yes
CIDI (Robins et al. 1988)	No	Adult	1.5 hours[a]	AN, BN, BED	Both	No
DISC-IV (Shaffer et al. 2000)	No	6–17	1.5 hours[a]	AN, BN, pica	Both	No

Note. AN=anorexia nervosa; ARFID=avoidant/restrictive food intake disorder; BED=binge-eating disorder; BN=bulimia nervosa; CIDI=Composite International Diagnostic Interview; DISC-IV=Diagnostic Interview Schedule for Children Version IV; EDA-5=Eating Disorder Assessment for DSM-5; EDE-17.0D=Eating Disorder Examination Version 17; IDED=Interview for the Diagnosis of Eating Disorders; KSADS-PL=Schedule for Affective Disorders and Schizophrenia for School-Age Children–Present and Lifetime version; LIFE-EAT-3=Longitudinal Interval Follow-up Evaluation eating disorder adaptation; OSFED=other specified feeding or eating disorder; SCID-5=Structured Clinical Interview for DSM-5; SIAB=Structured Interview for Anorexic and Bulimic Disorders.

[a]Reflects administration time for full interview, not just eating disorder section.

ered the gold standard for eating disorder assessment (for review, see Thomas et al. 2014). The EDE was created primarily as a research tool for studies of psychopathology and treatment response; it requires specialized training to administer. To minimize recall bias (e.g., Teasdale and Fogarty 1979), the interview begins by orienting the respondent to the 28-day time frame that is the focus of most of the interview, with the exception of diagnostic questions, which assess the frequency of behaviors over the past 3 months. Respondents are provided at the outset with a calendar and asked to describe any events (e.g., holidays, days off work) that would help them remember the time period; the calendar is then referenced throughout the interview. This type of timeline follow-back procedure, which was originally developed for the retrospective recall of alcohol consumption (Sobell et al. 1979), helps orient respondents to the time period for the assessment and provides contextual information during the interview. Each interview item includes a mandatory probe and optional additional questions designed to elicit the necessary information for the assessor to make a rating. The EDE generates scores for four subscales: Restraint, Eating Concern, Weight Concern, and Shape Concern. These scores are averaged to produce a global score. Constructs originally introduced in the EDE (e.g., overvaluation of shape and weight) later became central to revised diagnostic criteria for bulimia nervosa (BN). Items are coded based on either the frequency of a behavior or cognition (e.g., present every day) or the severity (e.g., to an extreme amount) using a seven-point Likert scale with unequal spacing and an absolute zero point (Fairburn et al. 2008). The EDE also assesses key behavioral features of eating disorders, including three forms of overeating (objective overeating, objective bulimic episodes, and subjective bulimic episodes) based on the amount of food consumed and the degree of loss of control over eating. The frequency scores generated from these questions (e.g., number of objective bulimic episodes in the past 28 days) can be analyzed dimensionally or used categorically to derive a diagnosis of anorexia nervosa (AN), BN, or binge-eating disorder (BED). The EDE has recently been updated to version 17 (i.e., EDE-17.0D; Fairburn et al. 2014; available for free from www.credo-oxford.com/6.2.html) to better reflect diagnostic algorithms for DSM-5 criteria; however, the interview itself was not altered from the prior version (EDE-16.0D). To facilitate the assessment of youths, both parent (Couturier et al. 2007) and child (Bryant-Waugh et al. 1996) versions of the EDE are available.

The EDE-17.0D has several strengths, including 1) the lack of skip logic (i.e., every respondent answers every question, regardless of previous responses), which ensures that subthreshold eating disorder symptoms are captured rather than overlooked (e.g., Swanson et al. 2011); 2) empirical support for aspects of its reliability and validity (for review, see Berg et al. 2012); 3) free availability; and 4) inclusion of items that enable the assessment of some–but not all–other specified feeding or eating disorder (OSFED) example presentations (i.e., subthreshold BN, subthreshold BED, and purging disorder). In addition, as the most widely used interview assessment of eating disorders, it has provided a consistent measure of clinical response across treatment outcome studies (Fairburn et al. 2009; le Grange et al. 2007) and is ideal for capturing clinically significant change, even over brief time periods (e.g., 4 weeks).

The EDE also has a number of limitations. Perhaps the most important are theoretical in nature and include 1) a bias toward assessing the psychopathology of BN; 2) a focus on concepts most relevant to cognitive-behavioral therapy; and 3) a lack of empirical support for the proposed factor structure (Thomas et al. 2014). There are also a number of logistical and functional limitations, including 1) the lack of empirical support for the clinical or research value of specific items (e.g., picking and nibbling, concern over body composition); 2) unnecessary item redundancy throughout the interview (Berg 2010) and some overly complex questions; 3) limited accessibility of the specialized training needed to administer the interview; 4) rating scales with unequal intervals that limit the statistical utility of certain items; 5) a diagnostic algorithm that does not fully represent DSM-5 criteria; 6) a lack of items assessing feeding disorders or concepts relevant to avoidant/restrictive food intake disorder (ARFID), pica, and rumination disorder; and 7) the length of time required to conduct the interview (usually an hour or more).

Structured Interview for Anorexic and Bulimic Disorders

The SIAB (Fichter et al. 1990) was originally developed as both a self-report questionnaire (SIAB-S) and a semistructured interview or expert rating scale (SIAB-EX). The SIAB-EX (Fichter et al. 1998) was subsequently revised to be compatible with DSM-IV (American Psychiatric Association 1994) and the International Classification of Diseases (ICD-10; World Health Organization 1992) and can be used to derive eating disorder diagnoses.[2] Additionally, the SIAB-EX includes subscales that provide dimensional measures of eating disorder–specific psychopathology as well as additional symptoms and characteristics that are commonly as-

[2] The SIAB-EX is freely available online for research purposes (www.klinikum.uni-muenchen.de/Klinik-und-Poliklinik-fuer-Psychiatrie-und-Psychotherapie/en/forschung/epidemiologie). Alternatively, it can be obtained by contacting the primary author, Manfred Fichter, at MFichter@schoen-kliniken.de or at the Department of Psychiatry, University of Munich, Nussbaumstrasse 7, 80336 Munich, Germany.

sociated with eating disorder diagnoses (Body Image and Slimness Ideal, General Psychopathology, Sexuality and Social Integration, Bulimic Symptoms, Measures to Counteract Weight Gain, Fasting, Substance Abuse, and Atypical Binges). The strengths of the SIAB-EX include the following: 1) it is the only eating disorder–specific interview that was designed to measure both current and lifetime symptoms, making it ideal for use in genetic studies (e.g., the Price Foundation Collaborative Group [2001] used the SIAB to evaluate lifetime eating disorder phenotypes in a large multisite genetics collaboration); 2) it is currently the only eating disorder interview that can be used to derive both DSM and ICD diagnoses; 3) it was designed to be used both dimensionally and categorically, a feature that broadens the utility of the instrument; and 4) the manual and coding forms include detailed descriptions of each construct being assessed as well as additional probes, which may enhance the validity with which these constructs are assessed as well as the reliability of ratings between assessors. Limitations of the SIAB-EX include the following: 1) although there are plans to update the instrument,[3] it has not yet been modified to reflect changes in DSM-5 criteria for AN, BN, and BED[4]; 2) it does not assess symptoms associated with ARFID, pica, or rumination disorder; 3) it is a long interview (87 items), which may be prohibitive in terms of time and cost; 4) it is meant to be administered by someone who has expertise in the field of eating disorders, and untrained clinicians require substantial training prior to administering the interview; and 5) some of the items assess constructs that may not be a priority in some settings (e.g., internal achievement motivation, grazing, substance use).

Interview for the Diagnosis of Eating Disorders

The IDED (Williamson 1990) was originally developed to derive descriptive and diagnostic information about AN, BN, compulsive overeating, and obesity. The interview begins with general assessment and history to elicit descriptive information about the onset and course of eating- and weight-related problems, weight history, and associated medical problems. Three additional sections are devoted to the psychopathology of AN, BN, and compulsive overeating, with a focus on questions related to diagnostic criteria. The IDED has been subsequently revised, most re-

---

[3] There are plans to update the SIAB-EX for both ICD-11 and DSM-5 once ICD-11 is finalized and released (M. Fichter, personal communication, September 2014).

[4] The current version of SIAB-EX is incompatible with DSM-5 because frequencies of binge eating and compensatory behaviors are measured on a Likert scale that does not include a frequency anchor for one episode per week.

cently to ensure compatibility with DSM-IV criteria for AN, BN, and BED (IDED-IV; Kutlesic et al. 1998).[5] Strengths of the IDED-IV include the following: 1) it can be used either categorically to derive diagnoses or dimensionally to describe eating disorder psychopathology; 2) diagnostic coding is relatively straightforward; and 3) research has demonstrated preliminary support for interrater reliability and for the content, concurrent, and discriminant validity of the instrument to assess and derive diagnostic data on eating disorders (Kutlesic et al. 1998). Limitations of the IDED-IV include the following: 1) there are no plans to update the instrument for DSM-5 (e.g., changes to the diagnostic criteria for AN, BN, and BED will not be reflected; V. Kutlesic, personal communication, September 2014); 2) it does not assess ARFID, pica, and rumination disorder; 3) it does not assess specific symptom frequencies (e.g., binge eating, vomiting), which decreases its utility for certain types of analyses and increases the likelihood of ceiling and/or floor effects; and 4) its focus on the diagnostic criteria necessarily precludes a rich and detailed assessment of specific facets of eating disorder psychopathology (e.g., weight/shape concern, cognitive restraint) or the assessment of constructs relevant to eating disorders that are not reflected in diagnostic criteria. Owing in part to these limitations, the IDED has been used much less frequently in eating disorder research than the EDE or the SIAB.

Longitudinal Interval Follow-up Evaluation

The LIFE (Keller et al. 1987) was developed for use in longitudinal studies, and the eating disorder adaptation (LIFE-EAT) was created for one of the longest-running longitudinal studies of eating disorders, ongoing since 1987 (Eddy et al. 2008). LIFE-EAT-3 was recently updated to reflect DSM-5 criteria (K. Eddy, personal communication, June 2015). The LIFE-EAT-3 assesses the relative severity of diagnostic features of AN, BN, BED, ARFID, pica, rumination disorder, and OSFED over a prespecified length of time determined by the study purpose. The assessor uses a calendar to collect detailed weekly data to track longitudinal fluctuations in eating disorder symptoms. On the basis of these findings, the assessor confers a transdiagnostic psychiatric status rating (PSR) on a six-point severity scale, ranging from "definite criteria severe" to "complete recovery."

---

[5] The IDED-IV can be obtained by contacting the primary author, Vesna Kutlesic, at vesna.kutlesic@nih.gov or at 6100 Executive Boulevard, Room 2A01B, MSC 7510, Bethesda, MD 20892-7510.

Strengths include 1) the free availability of the measure[6]; 2) the collection of weekly symptom data that can be used to ascertain clinically significant change, persistence, recurrence, time to recovery, or diagnostic crossover over time; and 3) the recent update to reflect DSM-5 criteria. The primary limitation of the LIFE-EAT-3 is the lack of reliability and validity data for the most recent version.

General Psychiatric Interviews

Because eating disorder–specific interviews are typically time-consuming and require specialized training to administer, general psychiatric interviews provide a viable alternative that allows eating disorders to be assessed alongside other potentially comorbid disorders. The clear standard in patient-oriented research is the semistructured assessment that requires some degree of clinical expertise to administer. These instruments include the Structured Clinical Interview for DSM Axis I disorders (SCID; First et al. 2002b), which is used to assess adults, and the Schedule for Affective Disorders and Schizophrenia for School-Age Children (KSADS; Ambrosini 2000), which is used to assess both children and adolescents. In contrast, epidemiological studies typically employ highly structured interviews that can be delivered by nonclinicians. These interviews include the Composite International Diagnostic Interview (CIDI; Robins et al. 1988), used with adults, and the Diagnostic Interview Schedule for Children Version IV (DISC-IV; Shaffer et al. 2000), used with children and adolescents.

Structured Clinical Interview for DSM Axis I Disorders

The SCID is a widely used semistructured interview designed to assess DSM diagnostic criteria for psychiatric disorders. It includes modules that cover a range of psychiatric diagnoses, including eating disorders. The SCID is published by the American Psychiatric Association, which also publishes DSM. Prior to the 2013 publication of DSM-5, the SCID-IV, based on DSM-IV criteria, was most widely used, with different versions for researchers (First et al. 2002b), for clinicians (First et al. 1996), and for use with community samples (First et al. 2002a). (A version for children, called the KID-SCID [Matzner et al. 1997], is freely available but does not

---

[6] To obtain a copy of LIFE-EAT-3, please contact Kamryn T. Eddy at keddy@mgh.harvard.edu or at the Massachusetts General Hospital Eating Disorders Clinical and Research Program, 2 Longfellow Place, Suite 200, Boston, MA 02114.

have published reliability and validity data and, more importantly, does not have a module for eating disorders.) The recently available SCID-5 (First et al. 2015) assesses the DSM-5 diagnostic criteria for AN, BN, and BED and also covers some OSFED presentations and contains an optional module to assess ARFID.

To conduct the SCID, assessors read mandatory probe questions that include suggested follow-up items designed to evaluate a specific diagnostic criterion. The SCID uses extensive skip logic that prompts the assessor to skip subsequent questions when sufficient diagnostic criteria are not met to warrant further questioning. The SCID assesses both current and lifetime diagnoses, with criteria for partial or full remission, and prompts the assessor to capture age at illness onset and to rate current illness severity. Scoring the SCID for an eating disorder diagnosis can be done in a few minutes by the assessor after administration of the module. Ideally, the SCID is completed by an assessor who has enough clinical knowledge that he or she could conduct a diagnostic interview in the absence of a structured interview (First et al. 2008), but those with less knowledge or experience can administer the SCID provided they receive appropriate training and have been observed by an experienced assessor. The SCID and training DVDs can be ordered online (www.scid4.org). In a major multisite study of SCID-III-R test-retest reliability, good to excellent reliability was obtained for AN and BN diagnoses in patient samples (Williams et al. 1992). Another study found substantial interrater reliability for eating disorder diagnoses ascertained through an unstructured clinical interview versus the SCID-IV (Thomas et al. 2010).

The SCID-5 has several strengths, including 1) generating diagnoses based on DSM-5 criteria, although probes remain largely consistent with DSM-IV queries; 2) empirical support for the reliability and validity of prior versions, although additional data will be needed to support the SCID-5 itself; and 3) an eating disorder module that can be administered and scored relatively quickly. There are also two key improvements from the SCID-IV, including the addition of specific questions (under OSFED) to establish impairment, helping the assessor to distinguish between an eating disorder or non–eating disorder diagnosis, and specific guidance on assigning severity categories for AN (based on a table of adult heights and weights for each severity category) and BN (based on frequency of compensatory behaviors). The SCID-5 also has several limitations: 1) pica and rumination disorder are excluded; 2) the ARFID module is *optional,* which likely means that limited data will be collected to further the understanding of this new diagnostic category; 3) the extensive use of skip logic creates missed opportunities to capture useful diagnostic information that might be of interest to researchers or clinicians; 4) options for assigning

OSFED diagnoses include a list of OSFED presentations but no interview prompts to guide their identification; and 5) it must be purchased.

Schedule for Affective Disorders and Schizophrenia for School-Age Children

The KSADS is a semistructured interview that generates psychiatric diagnoses for youths ages 6–18 (Ambrosini 2000). The KSADS was adapted from the Schedule for Affective Disorders and Schizophrenia (SADS) for adults (Endicott and Spitzer 1978), with the "K" standing for kiddie. Parallel versions of the KSADS include options to interview the child alone and/or both the child and parent separately and subsequently to create a summary score from the child and all collateral sources (e.g., parent, child, teacher, medical record). The KSADS–Present and Lifetime (PL) version 2013 Working Draft (J. Kaufman, B. Birmaher, D. Axelson, F. Pereplet-chikova, D. Brent, Neal Ryan) has been updated to reflect DSM-5 criteria, including both severity and remission specifiers. The KSADS eating disorder screen begins with 2–3 minutes of open-ended questions to gather information about typical eating habits and feelings about shape and weight, followed by items keyed to specific DSM-5 diagnostic criteria, which can be assessed as present, subthreshold, or threshold. If the respondent meets any key criteria, the assessor then asks additional diagnostic questions from the eating disorder supplement. The KSADS produces current and lifetime diagnoses of AN, BN, and BED.

Strengths of the KSADS include 1) the flexibility of the semistructured style that allows assessors to ask additional unscripted questions and apply their own clinical judgment; 2) the lengthy screen with queries about a variety of eating disorder symptoms (e.g., fear of weight gain, low weight, binge eating, purging), which trigger application of the supplement if answered affirmatively, thereby reducing the probability of missing clinically significant presentations; 3) a recent update to reflect DSM-5 criteria; and 4) free availability.[7] In contrast, the weaknesses include 1) the lack of ARFID, pica, and rumination disorder items; 2) the necessity for a trained clinician to administer the interview, thus reducing ease of dissemination; and 3) the length of time required for assessment (approximately 1.25 hours) (Ambrosini 2000).

---

[7] To obtain a copy of the KSADS-PL, please contact the primary author, Joan Kaufman, at joan.kaufman@yale.edu or at the Department of Psychiatry, Yale School of Medicine, Congress Place, 301 Cedar Street, P.O. Box 208098, New Haven, CT 06520.

Composite International Diagnostic Interview

The CIDI was developed by the World Health Organization to be relevant cross-culturally and reflective of both DSM and ICD criteria (Robins et al. 1988). A unique feature of the CIDI is its cross-cultural applicability (e.g., items assessing the criteria for alcohol use disorders query not just about absenteeism from salaried employment but also about failure to complete chores, which may be more relevant to rural subsistence farmers in developing countries). The CIDI assesses both current and lifetime AN, BN, and BED. Of special note for the eating disorders field, the CIDI was the instrument used to establish the widely cited eating disorder prevalence rates from the United States–based National Comorbidity Survey Replication (Hudson et al. 2007). Because administration is fully computerized and questions are close-ended, trained lay assessors can administer the interview without a formal clinical degree.

Strengths of the CIDI include 1) enhanced cross-cultural validity in comparison to other interviews; 2) ease of use by lay assessors after brief training; and 3) free accessibility online (www.hcp.med.harvard.edu/wmhcidi). Weaknesses include the following: 1) because eating disorders are considered "non-core" disorders, they are not assessed on the abridged "core" version of the measure; 2) OSFED, ARFID, pica, and rumination disorder are not assessed; 3) skip logic requires that respondents who do not endorse twice-weekly binge eating will *not* be asked about purging, meaning that clinically significant presentations (e.g., purging disorder) may be missed; and 4) it has not yet been updated to reflect DSM-5, likely because the update will need to wait until the publication of ICD-11, anticipated in 2017.

Diagnostic Interview Schedule for Children Version IV

The DISC-IV (Shaffer et al. 2000) is a highly structured psychiatric interview, originally based on the adult Diagnostic Interview Schedule (Robins et al. 1981) and developed by the National Institute of Mental Health (NIMH). The DISC-IV features options for direct administration to youths ages 9–17 and parallel administration versions for parents/caretakers and youths ages 6–17. The youth (DISC-IV-Y) and parent (DISC-IV-P) versions are nearly identical except for pronoun usage (i.e., "you" vs. "him" or "her"). Now in its fourth revision, the DISC-IV generates current and optional lifetime diagnoses adhering very strictly to DSM-IV and ICD-10 criteria. In addition to assessing AN and BN, the DISC-IV is one of the few currently available psychiatric interviews–either general or eating disorder–specific–that assesses the diagnostic criteria for pica (i.e., "eating things that aren't food, like peeling paint...or ashes...or dirt...or pebbles" for at least 4 weeks with associated impairment).

The DISC-IV has many pros: 1) it can be administered by lay assessors after brief training, thereby making it an ideal measure for large-scale epidemiological studies; 2) questions are read verbatim and are never open-ended, so administration is extremely straightforward; 3) assessors are encouraged to use the computer-assisted version, which standardizes administration, reduces data entry burden, and identifies positive diagnoses based on a computer algorithm; and 4) it assesses pica.[8] Cons include the following: 1) it does not assess BED, ARFID, rumination disorder, or OSFED; 2) it employs a very strict skip-out structure and scoring algorithm that may miss clinically significant diagnoses, especially atypical presentations; and 3) it has not yet been updated for DSM-5.

A Look Forward to the Brave New World

Despite their seminal role in defining the field, existing measures–both eating disorder–specific and general psychiatric–have limitations, particularly in the assessment of DSM-5 constructs, most notably feeding disorders. A newly published interview, the EDA-5 (Sysko et al. 2015), overcomes many of these limitations, although it is not without its own drawbacks. The combination of feeding and eating disorders into a single DSM-5 chapter introduces new challenges but ultimately presents a unique opportunity to shape the field by developing new assessments that will better define these emerging phenotypes.

See Video 1, which features a roundtable discussion with B. Timothy Walsh, M.D., and colleagues involved in changes to feeding and eating disorder diagnoses in DSM-5.

 **Video Illustration 1:** Diagnostic issues in the age of DSM-5 (8:11)

Eating Disorder Assessment for DSM-5

The EDA-5 (Sysko et al. 2015) is a brief, semistructured interview specifically developed to derive feeding and eating disorder diagnoses using DSM-5 criteria (see Chapter 10, "Use of the Eating Disorder Assessment for DSM-5"). Originally developed as a paper-and-pencil instrument, it has been modified for use as a Web-based application ("app") for comput-

---

[8] To obtain a copy of the DISC-IV, please e-mail disc@childpsych.columbia.edu or write to DISC Development Group, Columbia University, 1051 Riverside Drive, Unit 78, New York, NY 10032.

ers and mobile devices (freely available at www.eda5.org). The app allows the assessor to enter information provided by the respondent directly into the app's answer fields. The app then moves the assessor through the interview (and diagnostic criteria) based on the information being provided by the respondent. At the end of the interview, the app provides the diagnosis that best fits the respondent's reported symptoms as well as key symptoms associated with the diagnostic criteria (e.g., current body mass index [BMI], frequency of binge eating, frequency of compensatory behaviors). The EDA-5 is relatively brief to administer (i.e., approximately 15 minutes; Sysko et al. 2015), which can be attributed to its primary focus on feeding and eating disorder diagnostic criteria and its use of skip rules. Research comparing the EDA-5 to the diagnostic items of the EDE and unstructured clinical interviews has demonstrated preliminary evidence of the validity of the EDA-5 to determine diagnoses and the test-retest reliability of derived diagnoses (Sysko et al. 2015).

There are several advantages of the EDA-5, particularly in comparison with other currently available interviews. First, the EDA-5 is the first–and currently the only–comprehensive interview that assesses *all* symptoms of feeding and eating disorders described in DSM-5, which, at least conceptually, would enhance one's ability to derive accurate diagnoses. Second, it can be administered by individuals with limited training, is available as a Web-based application, and is compatible with mobile devices, which enhances its portability and ease of use (e.g., it automatically follows skip rules, calculates BMI, and runs diagnostic algorithms that derive diagnoses). Finally, it is a brief instrument, which minimizes the burden on both the respondent and the assessor. Minimizing assessment burden can enhance the validity of the information gathered during an assessment, reduce costs associated with the assessment (e.g., salary/wages for assessor, payment for research participation), and allow time for the assessment of other relevant symptoms or constructs.

Although the instrument's specificity as a diagnostic measure of DSM-5 feeding and eating disorders has inherent strengths, it also has limitations. For example, symptoms or features that are often associated with eating disorders but are not included in the DSM-5 criteria (e.g., perfectionism, impulsivity) are not assessed by the EDA-5. Additionally, because the EDA-5 was developed as a diagnostic tool, the data provided are primarily categorical; the tool provides only minimal dimensional data. These features of the EDA-5 mean that if assessors are interested in gathering information above and beyond diagnosis and frequency of disordered behaviors, the inclusion of other assessment instruments (e.g., a dimensional self-report measure of eating psychopathology) is likely to be necessary. In the age of the NIMH Research Domain Criteria (Insel et al.

2010), which are based on dimensional assessment, the focus on categorical diagnoses could negate the strengths of the EDA-5 as a brief measure for use in research settings.

Additionally, although the use of skip rules does minimize the time needed to complete the instrument, skip rules can result in failure to capture clinically significant symptoms. Indeed, prior research on skip rules suggests that this loss of information can lead to an underestimation of the prevalence and severity of symptoms (Swanson et al. 2014). For example, the first three items of the EDA-5, which function to determine whether a feeding or eating disorder might be present, are skip-out items. Unless the respondent endorses at least two of these items,[9] the interview ends without an assigned diagnosis. Given that inadvertent or deliberate minimization of symptoms is common among individuals with eating disorders (Becker et al. 2009), the use of skip rules so early in the interview may be problematic. Another consideration is that data entered into the app version of the EDA-5 are not saved and must later be entered by hand. Finally, the EDA-5 is relatively new and its psychometric properties have not been thoroughly tested or replicated.

Feeding Disorder Assessment

Few currently available interviews assess the specific psychopathology of feeding disorders. ARFID is assessed only on the EDA-5 and in an optional SCID module, pica is assessed only on the EDA-5 and DISC-IV, and rumination disorder is assessed only on the EDA-5. Importantly, all existing interviews that assess feeding disorders are purely diagnostic, and none of them feature dimensional measures of feeding disorder severity. Current knowledge of feeding disorders is scattered across disciplines, including not only psychiatry but also speech pathology, occupational therapy, and gastroenterology. Indeed, apart from the EDA-5, the only other structured interview to assess rumination behavior is the Rome-III Diag-

[9] A curiosity of the EDA-5 is that of the first three items, the only one that respondents must endorse to move forward in the interview is the item that assesses impairment/distress, a symptom that is not required for DSM-5 diagnoses of AN, BN, BED, pica, rumination disorder, and ARFID. Even if the respondent answers affirmatively to the other two items, the interview will end and the respondent will receive a diagnosis of no feeding or eating disorder if the respondent does not endorse impairment/distress. The EDA-5 does specify that the assessor can use additional sources of information such as clinical observation, treatment providers, and family members to help determine whether impairment/distress is present. However, these sources of information may not always be available.

nostic Questionnaire for Functional Gastrointestinal Disorders (Walker et al. 2006). The Rome-III items may be instructive to feeding disorder researchers because they differentiate "adolescent rumination syndrome" from gastroesophageal reflux disease, in part by querying about pain and nausea associated with regurgitation.

Just as the development of structured interviews played a major role in refining eating disorder phenotypes over the last quarter century, so too could the development of structured assessments for feeding disorders over the next 25 years. Owing to the overlapping nature of feeding and eating symptoms, the two will likely need to be evaluated side by side. Indeed, rumination can be challenging to separate from frank purging in the context of shape and weight concerns (Delaney et al. 2015), and the consumption of nonfood items to suppress appetite (sometimes observed in patients with AN; Delaney et al. 2015) would not meet DSM-5 criteria for pica. Thus, there is currently a critical need for specialized interviews and self-report questionnaires on feeding pathology; we cannot study what we do not measure.

Conclusion

The last quarter century of eating disorder assessment has demonstrated that the development of structured interviews was vital to the advancement of the field. However, these historical measures, including the gold standard EDE, are not without limitations. The newly published EDA-5 is currently the only measure that captures all DSM-5 feeding and eating disorder diagnoses, but it may not be suitable for all clinical and research applications. The addition of feeding disorders in a joint DSM-5 category with eating disorders poses a diagnostic challenge but will ultimately present an opportunity for further refining phenotypes over the next quarter century.

Key Clinical Points

- Accurate and reliable assessment is the foundation for clinical and research efforts. The way in which data are captured and recorded informs diagnoses, treatment plans, insurance requests, research results, and public policy. Structured interviews fall into two categories: eating disorder–specific and general psychiatric.
- The Eating Disorder Examination (EDE-17) is the most widely used eating disorder–specific interview, and its seminal value to the field is reflected in the current understanding of the core psychopathol-

ogy of anorexia nervosa and bulimia nervosa. This instrument has a number of strengths, including comprehensive assessment of eating disorder psychopathology, empirical support for aspects of its reliability and validity, and free availability. However, it is limited by a bias toward assessing bulimia nervosa, a focus on concepts specific to cognitive-behavioral therapy, a lack of feeding disorder coverage, and minimal support for the proposed factor structure.
- The Structured Clinical Interview for DSM (SCID) disorders is the most widely used general psychiatric interview applicable for eating disorders, and the SCID-5 is the most recent version. It captures DSM-5 diagnostic criteria, and it can be scored easily and quickly. Prior versions have shown good to excellent reliability. However, the SCID-5 is limited by the use of skip rules, minimal coverage of feeding disorders, and a lack of prompts to help assessors assign specific examples of other specified feeding or eating disorders.
- The Eating Disorder Assessment for DSM-5 (EDA-5) is a promising new diagnostic interview for eating disorders. Benefits include its brevity, compatibility with DSM-5 criteria, and use of technology (i.e., a mobile app). However, limitations include its specificity, use of skip rules, minimal dimensional assessment, and limited psychometric data.
- Few currently available interviews assess the specific psychopathology of feeding disorders. This poses a challenge for establishing prevalence, severity, and treatment response but also presents a unique opportunity to shape the field by creating new assessments that more clearly define feeding disorder phenotypes.

References

Ambrosini PJ: Historical development and present status of the Schedule for Affective Disorders and Schizophrenia for School-Age Children (K-SADS). J Am Acad Child Adolesc Psychiatry 39(1):49–58, 2000 10638067

American Psychiatric Association: Diagnostic and Statistical Manual of Mental Disorders, 4th Edition. Washington, DC, American Psychiatric Association, 1994

American Psychiatric Association: Diagnostic and Statistical Manual of Mental Disorders, 5th Edition. Arlington, VA, American Psychiatric Association, 2013

Becker AE, Eddy KT, Perloe A: Clarifying criteria for cognitive signs and symptoms for eating disorders in DSM-V. Int J Eat Disord 42(7):611–619, 2009 19650082

Berg KC: A study of the validity of the Eating Disorder Examination. Unpublished doctoral dissertation, University of Minnesota, Minneapolis, MN, 2010

Berg KC, Peterson CB, Frazier P, et al: Psychometric evaluation of the Eating Disorder Examination and Eating Disorder Examination-Questionnaire: a systematic review of the literature. Int J Eat Disord 45(3):428–438, 2012 21744375

Bryant-Waugh RJ, Cooper PJ, Taylor CL, et al: The use of the Eating Disorder Examination with children: a pilot study. Int J Eat Disord 19(4):391–397, 1996 8859397

Cooper Z, Fairburn C: The Eating Disorder Examination: a semi-structured interview for the assessment of the specific psychopathology of eating disorders. Int J Eat Disord 6:1–8, 1987

Couturier J, Lock J, Forsberg S, et al: The addition of a parent and clinician component to the Eating Disorder Examination for children and adolescents. Int J Eat Disord 40(5):472–475, 2007 17726771

Delaney CB, Eddy KT, Hartmann AS, et al: Pica and rumination behavior among individuals seeking treatment for eating disorders or obesity. Int J Eat Disord 48(2):238–248, 2015 24729045

Eddy KT, Dorer DJ, Franko DL, et al: Diagnostic crossover in anorexia nervosa and bulimia nervosa: implications for DSM-V. Am J Psychiatry 165(2):245–250, 2008 18198267

Endicott J, Spitzer RL: A diagnostic interview: the Schedule for Affective Disorders and Schizophrenia. Arch Gen Psychiatry 35(7):837–844, 1978 678037

Fairburn CG, Cooper Z, O'Connor M: Eating Disorder Examination, Edition 16.0D, in Cognitive Behavior Therapy and Eating Disorders. Edited by Fairburn CG. New York, Guilford, 2008, pp 265–308

Fairburn CG, Cooper Z, Doll HA, et al: Transdiagnostic cognitive-behavioral therapy for patients with eating disorders: a two-site trial with 60-week follow-up. Am J Psychiatry 166(3):311–319, 2009 19074978

Fairburn CG, Cooper Z, O'Connor M: Eating Disorder Examination, Edition 17.0D. The Center for Research on Dissemination at Oxford. April 2014. Available at: http://www.credo-oxford.com/6.2.html. Accessed March 17, 2015.

Fichter MM, Elton M, Engel K, et al: The Structured Interview for Anorexia and Bulimia Nervosa (SIAB): development and characteristics of a (semi-)standardized instrument, in Bulimia Nervosa: Basic Research, Diagnoses, and Therapy. Edited by Fichter MM. Chichester, UK, Wiley, 1990, pp 55–70

Fichter MM, Herpertz S, Quadflieg N, et al: Structured Interview for Anorexic and Bulimic Disorders for DSM-IV and ICD-10: updated (third) revision. Int J Eat Disord 24(3):227–249, 1998 9741034

First MB, Spitzer RL, Gibbon M, et al: Structured Clinical Interview for DSM-IV Axis I Disorders, Clinician Version (SCID-CV). Washington, DC, American Psychiatric Press, 1996

First MB, Spitzer RL, Gibbon M, et al: Structured Clinical Interview for DSM-IV-TR Axis I Disorders, Research Version, Non-patient Edition (SCID-I/NP). New York, Biometrics Research, New York State Psychiatric Institute, 2002a

First MB, Spitzer RL, Gibbon M, et al: Structured Clinical Interview for DSM-IV-TR Axis I Disorders, Research Version, Patient Edition (SCID-I/P). New York, Biometrics Research, New York State Psychiatric Institute, 2002b

First MB, Spitzer RL, Gibbon M, et al: Structured Clinical Interview for DSM-IV Axis I Disorders (SCID-I), in Handbook of Psychiatric Measures, 2nd Edition. Edited by Rush AJ, First MB, Blacker D. Washington, DC, American Psychiatric Publishing, 2008, pp 40–43

First MB, Williams JB, Karg RS, Spitzer RL: Structured Clinical Interview for DSM-5 Disorders, Clinician Version (SCID-5-CV). Washington, DC, American Psychiatric Publishing, 2015

Hudson JI, Hiripi E, Pope HG Jr, et al: The prevalence and correlates of eating disorders in the National Comorbidity Survey Replication. Biol Psychiatry 61(3):348–358, 2007 16815322

Insel T, Cuthbert B, Garvey M, et al: Research domain criteria (RDoC): toward a new classification framework for research on mental disorders. Am J Psychiatry 167(7):478–451, 2010 20595427

Keller MB, Lavori PW, Friedman B, et al: The Longitudinal Interval Follow-up Evaluation: a comprehensive method for assessing outcome in prospective longitudinal studies. Arch Gen Psychiatry 44(6):540–548, 1987 3579500

Kutlesic V, Williamson DA, Gleaves DH, et al: The Interview for the Diagnosis of Eating Disorders-IV: application to DSM-IV diagnostic criteria. Psychol Assess 10:41–48, 1998

le Grange D, Crosby RD, Rathouz PJ, et al: A randomized controlled comparison of family based treatment and supportive psychotherapy for adolescent bulimia nervosa. Arch Gen Psychiatry 64(9):1049–1056, 2007 17768270

Matzner F, Silva R, Silvan M, et al: Preliminary test-retest reliability of the KID-SCID. Paper presented at the annual meeting of the American Psychiatric Association, San Diego, CA, May 17–22, 1997

Palmer R, Christie M, Cordle C, et al: The Clinical Eating Disorder Rating Instrument (CEDRI): a preliminary description. Int J Eat Disord 6:9–16, 1987

Price Foundation Collaborative Group: Deriving behavioural phenotypes in an international, multi-centre study of eating disorders. Psychol Med 31(4):635–645, 2001 11352366

Robins LN, Helzer JE, Croughan J, et al: National Institute of Mental Health Diagnostic Interview Schedule: its history, characteristics, and validity. Arch Gen Psychiatry 38(4):381–389, 1981 6260053

Robins LN, Wing J, Wittchen HU, et al: The Composite International Diagnostic Interview: an epidemiologic instrument suitable for use in conjunction with different diagnostic systems and in different cultures. Arch Gen Psychiatry 45(12):1069–1077, 1988 2848472

Shaffer D, Fisher P, Lucas CP, et al: NIMH Diagnostic Interview Schedule for Children Version IV (NIMH DISC-IV): description, differences from previous versions, and reliability of some common diagnoses. J Am Acad Child Adolesc Psychiatry 39(1):28–38, 2000 10638065

Sobell LC, Maisto SA, Sobell MB, et al: Reliability of alcohol abusers' self-reports of drinking behavior. Behav Res Ther 17(2):157–160, 1979 426744

Sunday SR, Halmi KA, Einhorn A: The Yale-Brown-Cornell Eating Disorder Scale: a new scale to assess eating disorder symptomatology. Int J Eat Disord 18(3):237–245, 1995 8556019

Swanson SA, Crow SJ, Le Grange D, et al: Prevalence and correlates of eating disorders in adolescents: results from the National Comorbidity Survey Replication Adolescent Supplement. Arch Gen Psychiatry 68(7):714–723, 2011 21383252

Swanson SA, Brown TA, Crosby RD, et al: What are we missing? The costs versus benefits of skip rule designs. Int J Methods Psychiatr Res 23:474–485, 2014 24030679

Sysko R, Glasofer DR, Hildebrandt T, et al: The Eating Disorder Assessment for DSM-5 (EDA-5): development and validation of a structured interview for feeding and eating disorders. Int J Eat Disord Jan 30, 2015 [Epub ahead of print] 25639562

Teasdale JD, Fogarty SJ: Differential effects of induced mood on retrieval of pleasant and unpleasant events from episodic memory. J Abnorm Psychol 88(3):248–257, 1979 500952

Thomas JJ, Delinsky SS, St Germain SA, et al: How do eating disorder specialist clinicians apply DSM-IV diagnostic criteria in routine clinical practice? Implications for enhancing clinical utility in DSM-5. Psychiatry Res 178(3):511–517, 2010 20591498

Thomas JJ, Roberto CA, Berg KC: The Eating Disorder Examination: a semi-structured interview for the assessment of the specific psychopathology of eating disorders. Advances in Eating Disorders: Theory, Research, and Practice 2:190–203, 2014

Walker LS, Caplan A, Rasquin A III: Rome III diagnostic questionnaire for the pediatric functional GI disorders, in Rome III: The Functional Gastrointestinal Disorders, 3rd Edition. Edited by Drossman, DA. McLean, VA, Degnon Associates, 2006, pp 961–990

Williams JBW, Gibbon M, First MB, et al: The Structured Clinical Interview for DSM-III-R (SCID), II: multisite test-retest reliability. Arch Gen Psychiatry 49(8):630–636, 1992 1637253

Williamson DA: Assessment of Eating Disorders: Obesity, Anorexia, and Bulimia Nervosa. New York, Pergamon, 1990

World Health Organization: The ICD-10 Classification of Mental and Behavioural Disorders: Clinical Descriptions and Diagnostic Guidelines. Geneva, World Health Organization, 1992

9 Self-Report Assessments of Eating Pathology

Kelsie T. Forbush, Ph.D., LP
Kelly C. Berg, Ph.D., LP

Self-report measures of eating psychopathology are important tools for understanding disordered eating behaviors across a wide variety of contexts, ranging from routine clinical care to large-scale epidemiological research studies. In the era of managed health care, the selection of self-report measures with evidence to support their reliability and validity has become increasingly important within clinical settings. Indeed, managers of mental health organizations face pressures to reduce or eliminate unnecessary costs, while maintaining strong quality of care, which has led to an increased emphasis on the need for tracking of clinical outcomes (Burlingame et al. 1995).

Tracking clinical outcomes is important not only from the perspective of managed care but also because results from randomized studies have shown that when therapists are provided with objective feedback from assessments of clients' progress, a variety of improved client outcomes, including increased therapy attendance, greater achievement of clinically significant or reliable change, and reduced deterioration of therapeutic gains after treatment termination, occur (Hatfield et al. 2010; Lambert and Shimokawa 2011; Lambert et al. 2002; Reese et al. 2010). For patients who were predicted to have a good prognosis at the beginning of therapy, assessment feedback has been shown to result in a reduced number of therapy sessions without reducing positive therapeutic outcomes (Lambert et al. 2002).

Although the assessment of eating disorder behaviors provides an important foundation for empirical research studies and is a crucial component of clinical care, few resources summarize the psychometric properties and clinical utility of available self-report measures. The current chapter aims to offer a useful resource for clinicians and researchers alike. We provide information on the development, reliability, and validity of commonly used self-report measures of eating pathology. We also mention issues in the assessment of disordered eating behaviors and cognitions among specific demographic populations, such as men, overweight or obese persons, and individuals in ethnic or racial minorities, as a complement to the descriptions in other chapters of the book (e.g., Chapter 6, "Eating-Related Pathology in Men and Boys," and Chapter 7, "Eating Problems in Special Populations"). Given the large number of available eating disorder measures, we limit the chapter to popular "all-in-one" self-report assessments of eating pathology that assess multiple dimensions of eating disorder psychopathology within a single measure. The measures we have chosen have strong psychometric properties, are easily available to clinicians, and/or have a substantial research base. Another reason we focus on multidimensional measures is because they represent an efficient way for busy clinicians to assess their clients for eating psychopathology (i.e., the all-in-one measures can be used instead of a battery of several self-report measures to assess the same thoughts and behaviors). We conclude with a discussion of the strengths and limitations of self-report assessments of eating disorders and suggestions for future research.

Scale Development Methods

Although the initial development and validation of eating disorder self-report measures are crucial considerations in instrument selection, the busy eating disorder professional may overlook their importance. Many of the issues with reliability and validity subsequently discussed in this chapter stem from outdated scale development and testing, and we are not aware of any published articles or chapters in the field of eating disorders that describe optimal methods for scale construction. Given that tracking client outcomes and interpreting research findings often hinge on the psychometric properties of the selected test battery, it is important to have at least a cursory knowledge of scale development procedures.

Rationally and Empirically Based Methods

At one end of the scale development spectrum are rationally based methods, which are based primarily (or exclusively) on theory and in which empirical (statistical) methods are not used to eliminate questions from the initial item pool (although statistics may be used after the measure is finalized to test the reliability and validity of the measure). At the extreme other end are purely empirically based methods, which use statistical approaches in the absence of theory to identify a set of questionnaire items that best distinguish among criterion groups (e.g., items may be selected that best distinguish individuals with anorexia nervosa [AN] from those with bulimia nervosa [BN]). Each of these approaches has a serious problem: rational measures tend to have a large number of psychometric issues that hamper their reliability and validity; empirical measures are limited to the samples in which they were developed (Clark and Watson 1995; Comrey 1988). As an example of the latter, if an eating disorder measure was designed to distinguish patients with AN from those with BN, it would not be appropriate to use that measure with persons with binge-eating disorder (BED) without additional validation. The need to validate an empirically based measure to each population in which it could be used (e.g., diagnostic group, age group, racial/ethnic group) has the potential to significantly limit the usefulness of these types of measures.

Hybrid-Based Methods

Modern scale development recommendations highlight the importance of hybrid-based methods (Clark and Watson 1995; Comrey 1988). These approaches incorporate both a heavy emphasis on using theory to develop the initial item pool and the use of empirical analyses to remove poorly performing items from the scale by employing exploratory and confirmatory factor analyses. These factor analytic techniques are designed to identify latent unobserved dimensions (or "factors") based on the pattern of correlations among items in the item pool. Myriad data in other areas of psychopathology suggest that hybrid-based approaches are more likely to result in the development of measures with strong psychometric properties, such as good convergent validity (the measure or scale is correlated moderately to strongly with other measures or scales of the same construct) and discriminant validity (the measure or scale is *not* correlated substantially with measures or scales assessing different constructs). We direct the interested reader to classic papers by Clark and Watson (1995), Loevinger (1957), and Smith et al. (2000) for additional information on best practices for scale development and testing.

Overview of Multidimensional Eating Disorder Self-Report Assessments

Eating Disorder Inventory

The Eating Disorder Inventory (EDI; Garner et al. 1983), now in its third edition (EDI-3; Garner 2004), is a widely used measure designed to assess cognitive and behavioral features that underlie AN and BN. Expert clinicians who were familiar with the research literature on AN and had treated patients with eating disorders developed the initial item pool. The items were administered to independent samples of individuals (males and females) with AN (n=113) and female control subjects without AN (n=577). The authors retained items only if they were able to significantly differentiate between individuals with AN and control subjects without AN and only if they were more highly correlated with the scale to which they were hypothesized to belong than with other scales.

In the second phase of development, additional items were written; the scale was administered to independent samples of individuals with AN and female control subjects; and criterion validity (the ability of a measure or scale to predict a criterion, such as psychiatric diagnosis, either concurrently or in the future) was tested in a variety of samples that included men (n=166) and participants with BN (n=195), obesity (n=44), past history of obesity (n=52), or past history of AN (n=17). The results of these analyses led to the development of eight scales: Drive for Thinness (excessive concern with dieting, weight preoccupation, and the pursuit of thinness), Bulimia ("uncontrollable" overeating episodes and the desire to engage in self-induced vomiting), Body Dissatisfaction (the belief that body parts that are generally associated with shape change or weight gain during puberty are too large), Ineffectiveness (feelings of inadequacy, insecurity, and lack of control over one's life), Perfectionism (excessively high personal and achievement standards), Interpersonal Distrust (disinclination to form close relationships and feelings of alienation), Interoceptive Awareness (lack of ability to identify emotions, satiety, and hunger), and Maturity Fears (desire to retreat to the security of preadolescence because of the stressors and demands of adulthood). Scores from the three eating disorder–specific scales (Drive for Thinness, Bulimia, and Body Dissatisfaction) can be summed to create the Eating Disorder Risk Composite score.

In 1991, a second version of the EDI was developed (EDI-2; Garner 1991), which retains the original EDI format and adds 27 new items in three additional subscales: Asceticism, Impulse Regulation, and Social Insecurity. The EDI was revised again in 2004 (EDI-3; Garner 2004) to provide a new 0- to 4-point scoring system and the calculation of age- and diagnosis-adjusted *T* scores. Although new scales were introduced, including Low Self-Esteem, Personal Alienation, Interpersonal Insecurity, Interpersonal Alienation, and Emotion Dysregulation, the eating disorder–specific scale content was not changed from the EDI-2 to the EDI-3.

Eating Disorder Examination Questionnaire

The Eating Disorder Examination Questionnaire (EDE-Q; Fairburn and Beglin 1994) is a self-report version of the Eating Disorder Examination

(EDE) interview (Cooper and Fairburn 1987), which is considered by many in the field to represent the gold standard of eating disorder psychopathology assessment (see Chapter 8, "Assessment Measures, Then and Now"). The EDE was developed based on 1) comprehensive literature reviews, in which the authors identified key elements of eating disorder psychopathology, and 2) unstructured interviews with patients with AN or BN to elicit detailed descriptions of their behaviors and attitudes. Items were written to assess the hypothesized key elements of eating disorders, and the interview was administered to patients with eating disorders and matched control subjects (sample sizes not published) to test the EDE's interrater reliability. From published articles (Cooper and Fairburn 1987; Fairburn and Beglin 1994), it appears that no statistical analyses were conducted to remove items from the EDE during the initial scale development and validation process, suggesting that the EDE and EDE-Q were developed using rational methods.

The EDE and EDE-Q contain four rationally derived subscales: Restraint, Eating Concern, Shape Concern, and Weight Concern. The most recent version of the EDE interview (Fairburn 2008) contains an item assessing night eating, but this content is not included in the EDE-Q. Although the EDE interview is able to generate diagnoses for AN, BN, BED, and a variety of other specified feeding or eating disorders, such as purging disorder (Keel et al. 2005), the questionnaire is intended to obtain information regarding dimensions of eating disorder psychopathology and was not developed as a self-report diagnostic measure. In addition to scores for the four subscales listed above, the EDE-Q provides a global score that represents the composite (sum) of scores from the four subscales and includes specific items that assess binge eating, driven exercise, and purging behaviors. (For information on the child version of the EDE-Q, please refer to Chapter 11, "Diagnosis of Feeding and Eating Disorders in Children and Adolescents.")

Eating Pathology Symptoms Inventory

The Eating Pathology Symptoms Inventory (EPSI; Forbush et al. 2013) was developed using a hybrid scale development approach in an effort to comprehensively assess a broad range of eating disorder dimensions. The initial item pool, developed on the basis of theoretical and empirical models of eating disorders, included 160 items designed to assess 20 potential dimensions of eating pathology and included items to assess all of the DSM-IV-TR (American Psychiatric Association 2000) criteria for eating disorders. The initial item pool was administered to large independent samples of college students (N=433) and community adults (N=407). Exploratory, confirmatory, and multiple-group factor analyses (which test to determine whether the structure of the measure is different across different groups of people) were used to eliminate poorly performing items from the pool. An 88-item revised measure was then administered to additional independent samples of patients with eating disorders (N=158) and general psychiatric outpatients (N=303). On the basis of the results of additional multivariate statistical analyses, the measure was revised a second time, which resulted in the final 45-item measure.

The EPSI contains eight scales: Body Dissatisfaction (dissatisfaction with body weight and/or shape), Binge Eating (ingestion of large amounts of food and accompanying cognitive symptoms), Cognitive Restraint (cognitive efforts to limit or avoid eating, whether or not such attempts are successful), Purging (self-induced vomiting, laxative use, diuretic use, and diet pill use), Muscle Building (desire for increased muscularity and muscle building supplement use), Restricting (concrete efforts to avoid or reduce food consumption), Excessive Exercise (physical exercise that is intense and/or compulsive), and Negative Attitudes Toward Obesity (negative attitudes toward individuals who are overweight or obese).

Reliability and Stability

Reliability refers to the consistency or precision of a measure. The critical question when evaluating reliability is whether test scores are sufficiently consistent and free from error to be useful.

Test-retest reliability measures the consistency of scores on an assessment over relatively short time intervals (e.g., several days to a month), during which time it would be highly unlikely that true change would have occurred. Correlations among test scores that are below 1.00 (indicating perfect agreement) are assumed to indicate the presence of time sampling error. Scores of at least 0.70 typically indicate evidence for good retest reliability (Joiner et al. 2005).

A related concept is *stability,* which is defined as the consistency of test scores over more extended time periods (e.g., months to years between assessments). Stability estimates are expected to be lower than test-retest reliability estimates because in addition to time sampling error, true change may have occurred (e.g., the patient may have experienced symptom improvement [Watson 2004]).

Finally, *internal consistency* refers to error in scores that results from fluctuations in items across a test scale. Low internal consistency manifests as low correlations among test items and is typically measured by coefficient α or the average inter-item correlation (Urbina 2011). In general, coefficient α values of at least 0.80 and average inter-item correlation values between 0.20 and 0.50 represent strong evidence for internal consistency (Clark and Watson 1995).

Eating Disorder Inventory

Coefficient α for the EDI-2 and EDI-3 appears to be good to excellent, with values generally exceeding 0.80. Nevertheless, in a large, well-conducted study by Clausen et al. (2011), Perfectionism, Asceticism, and several of the newer nonspecific EDI-3 scales (Personal Alienation, Interpersonal Alienation, and Emotion Dysregulation) had low coefficient α values in a sample of 561 patients with eating disorders. The coefficient α for the EDI-3 Asceticism scale was also very low (r=0.59) among control participants without eating disorders. Tasca et al. (2003) evaluated average inter-item correlation values for the EDI in a large sample of individuals seeking treatment for BED or BN. The results of their study indicated that except for the Asceticism scale, all scales had average inter-item correlation values within the 0.15–0.50 range, suggesting that high coefficient values for the EDI-3 do not appear to be due to redundant item content.

As indicated in Table 9–1, studies evaluating the retest reliability of the EDI suggest that this measure is highly reliable over short time intervals, and these findings have been replicated across both patients with eating disorders and general psychiatric patients who did not have an eating disorder diagnosis, as well as in nonclinical samples of college students. Stability estimates for the EDI are generally good across nonclinical samples of college females and in clinical eating disorder samples (Crowther et al. 1992; Tasca et al. 2003); however, very low stability was observed for the Bulimia scale (r=0.22) and Maturity Fears scale (r=0.26) among a subsample of college females at risk for an eating disorder (Crowther et al. 1992). Overall, the EDI has strong test-retest reliability over short time periods and good stability (with the exception of the Bulimia and Maturity Fears scales), and the eating disorder–specific EDI-3 scales demonstrate evidence for high internal consistency.

Eating Disorder Examination Questionnaire

Table 9-1 presents reliability and stability data for the EDE-Q. Internal consistency for the EDE-Q is generally good, with correlations close to or above 0.80 among female college undergraduates and community women (Luce and Crowther 1999; Mond et al. 2004a). However, other research has found that the Restraint, Eating Concern, and Weight Concern scales have lower internal consistency among individuals with bulimic syndromes (r ranged from 0.70 to 0.73 [Peterson et al. 2007]). We are not aware of published studies reporting average inter-item correlation values for the

TABLE 9–1. Reliability for multidimensional eating disorder self-report measures

Measure	Study sample	Test-retest reliability	Stability
EDI			
Crowther et al. 1992	282 female undergraduate students (31 participants were deemed at risk for the development of an eating disorder)	–	0.41–0.75 (total sample); 0.26–0.81 (at-risk sample)
Tasca et al. 2003	40 women seeking treatment for binge-eating disorder	–	0.67–0.82
Thiel and Paul 2006	327 female inpatients with eating disorders and 209 general psychiatric patients (without eating disorders)	0.81–0.89 (eating disorder patients); 0.75–0.94 (general psychiatric patients)	–
Wear and Pratz 1987	70 undergraduates (75.7% female)	0.90–0.97	–
EDE-Q			
Luce and Crowther 1999	139 female undergraduate students	0.81–0.92 (subscales[a]); 0.54–0.92 (behavioral items[b])	–
Mond et al. 2004a	802 community adult females	–	0.57–0.77 (subscales)
Reas et al. 2006	86 adults with binge-eating disorder (79.1% female)	0.66–0.77 (subscales)	–
EPSI			
Forbush et al. 2013	233 undergraduate students (58.15% female)	0.61–0.85	–

Note. Dash indicates that data are not available for the specific type of reliability that is listed in the column headings. EDE-Q=Eating Disorder Examination Questionnaire; EDI=Eating Disorder Inventory; EPSI=Eating Pathology Symptoms Inventory.

[a]The subscales on the EDE-Q are Weight Concern, Shape Concern, Eating Concern, and Dietary Restraint.

[b]Behavioral items on the EDE-Q include self-induced vomiting, binge eating, excessive exercise, diuretic misuse, and laxative misuse.

EDE-Q, so it is unclear whether high internal consistency was achieved, in part, because of item redundancy within scales.

Apart from self-induced vomiting, the behavioral features of the EDE-Q (i.e., binge eating, laxative misuse, diuretic misuse, excessive exercise) have lower than desirable test-retest reliability, ranging from 0.54 to 0.68 in female undergraduate students (Luce and Crowther 1999). Reas et al. (2006) found that the retest reliability for objective binge episodes in the EDE-Q was excellent; however, retest reliabilities were low for subjective binge episodes (r=0.51) and objective overeating episodes (r=0.39) in a sample of adults with BED. Finally, Mond et al. (2004a) conducted a stability study of the EDE-Q in a nationally representative sample of community women from Australia. Results indicated that subscale scores showed evidence of reasonable stability over an 11-month period, yet objective binge eating (r=0.44), subjective binge eating (r=0.24), and excessive exercise (r=0.31) had quite poor stability over time. Taken together, EDE-Q scores show evidence for high internal consistency among female college students and community women, and several scales possess good test-retest reliability and stability. However, concerns related to the reliability and stability of the EDE-Q behavioral items (e.g., self-induced vomiting, binge eating) have been documented in previous research studies.

Eating Pathology Symptoms Inventory

The EPSI has been shown to have good to excellent internal consistency across a range of samples, including men, women, obese participants, and psychiatric patients with and without eating disorders (Forbush et al. 2013, 2014). The majority of EPSI scales, except Negative Attitudes Toward Obesity (which showed some evidence of redundant item content), had average inter-item correlation values within the recommended range. Together, these findings indicate that the majority of EPSI scales are highly internally reliable across multiple populations.

Only one published study has evaluated the test-retest reliability of the EPSI (see Table 9–1). Most scales had excellent retest reliability, exceeding the recommended benchmark of 0.70. However, the retest reliability of the Cognitive Restraint scale was 0.61, indicating that this scale may not be as reliable or stable over time. These findings may reflect difficulties in measuring cognitive restraint using self-report measures, given that Forbush et al. (2013) found that the EDE-Q Restraint scale had an identical retest reliability of 0.61 in the same sample. Rigorous studies that have sought to evaluate the predictive validity of cognitive restraint (vs. more concrete efforts to restrict dietary intake) imply that the lowered reliability for restraint may also translate into poor validity for assessing dietary intake (Stice et al. 2004, 2007).

Comparison of Measures

Taken together, the results from reliability studies of multidimensional self-report assessments of eating disorders indicate evidence for good internal consistency and acceptable to excellent test-retest reliability and stability. Some caveats to this statement include the following: 1) certain EDI-3 scales that measure more general psychopathology (i.e., Maturity Fears, Perfectionism, Asceticism, Personal Alienation, Interpersonal Alienation, Emotion Dysregulation) show evidence for poor internal consistency and/or test-retest reliability; 2) EDE-Q behavioral items have lower test-retest reliability compared with scale scores; and 3) few data exist to describe the reliability of the EPSI. Despite these limitations, it is important to note that in many ways, the reduced reliability of EDE-Q behavioral items is to be expected because the majority of these EDE-Q behavioral items are assessed with only one or two items (compared with the EDE-Q subscales, which have several items). As a result of having fewer items, the EDE-Q behavioral items are inherently more susceptible to time sampling error. The EPSI includes scales that assess much of the behavioral content of the EDE-Q, but with more items, and these scales appear to be more reliable over time. Finally, despite the clear need for additional research to support the reliability of the EPSI, it is notable that Forbush et al. (2013) included men in the test-retest reliability sample, given that few reliability studies of eating disorder measures have included males (see Chapter 6, "Eating-Related Pathology in Men and Boys," for more information about self-report measures developed for males).

Validity

Eating Disorder Inventory

Comprehensive validity data for the first and second versions of the EDI are available; however, far less information is available about the validity of the EDI-3 as a multifactorial measure of eating disorder symptomatology. Although the EDI-3 includes the same item content as the EDI-2, changes to the factor structure, response indicators, and scoring necessitated a reexamination of the validity of the instrument. Independent investigations (Clausen et al. 2011; Stanford and Lemberg 2012) found that in both female and male samples, the EDI-3 successfully differentiated between eating disorder and control groups, with the eating disorder group scoring significantly higher on all subscales (thus providing evidence for criterion validity). The theorized factor structure of the EDI-3, which includes 12 subscales and 2 higher-order subscales representing eating disorder–specific pathology and general psychological disturbance, has also been replicated (Clausen et al. 2011). However, the authors noted that the model fit was minimally acceptable and suggested that this might be due to poor psychometric properties of several individual items on the EDI-3. In sum, early psychometric data on the EDI-3 are consistent with the psychometric data on the EDI-2; however, these conclusions must be tempered in light of the relative lack of information.

Eating Disorder Examination Questionnaire

The validity of the EDE-Q for the assessment of eating pathology has been investigated in several ways. First, research has consistently demonstrated that compared with control samples, individuals with eating disorders score higher on the EDE-Q (Aardoom et al. 2012; Engelsen and Laberg 2001; Mond et al. 2004b; Wilson et al. 1993), findings that support the criterion validity of the EDE-Q to distinguish between individuals with and without eating disorders. Second, with regard to convergent and discriminant validity, research has demonstrated that scores on the EDE-Q subscales are significantly and positively correlated with scores on the corresponding EDE subscales (for review, see Berg et al. 2012). The Restraint subscale, specifically, has been found to correlate more strongly with measures of similar constructs than with measures of dissimilar constructs (Bardone-Cone and Boyd 2007; Grilo et al. 2013). Finally, two studies have demonstrated that the frequencies of objective bulimic episodes reported on the EDE-Q were significantly correlated with the frequencies of these eating episodes recorded in daily food intake records (Grilo et al. 2001a, 2001b).

The factor structure of the EDE-Q has also been examined to determine the structural validity of the four EDE-Q subscales. Numerous factor analytic studies have failed to replicate the original, rationally derived subscales (Aardoom et al. 2012; Friborg et al. 2013; Grilo et al. 2013; Hrabosky et al. 2008; Peterson et al. 2007); interestingly, all of the analyses derived different factor structures. Two of the more recent factor analyses have suggested that there may be one general underlying dimension (Aardoom et al. 2012) or a nested general factor (Friborg et al. 2013), which could explain the inconsistent findings in previous studies.

Finally, given that the EDE-Q can also be used as a diagnostic measure, the validity of diagnoses derived from the EDE-Q has been investigated. When eating disorder diagnoses derived from the EDE-Q were compared with those derived from another self-report questionnaire, there was low diagnostic agreement between the two measures (Elder et al.

2006). However, moderate diagnostic agreement and similar latent structures have been found when comparing the EDE-Q with the EDE (Berg et al. 2012, 2013). In sum, there is support for the validity of the EDE-Q as a measure of eating disorder pathology; however, there is no empirical support for the original four subscales of the EDE-Q. Furthermore, additional data are needed on the validity of the EDE-Q as a diagnostic instrument.

Eating Pathology Symptoms Inventory

The EPSI subscale scores have been shown to successfully discriminate between eating disorder and general psychiatric outpatient samples (Forbush et al. 2013), between eating disorder and college student samples (Forbush et al. 2013, 2014), and between individuals with AN and individuals with BN (Forbush et al. 2013). Interestingly, the EPSI differentiated between nonpatient college males and females but not between male and female eating disorder patients (with the exception that males with eating disorders scored significantly higher on the EPSI Muscle Building subscale [Forbush et al. 2014]). Additionally, analyses in college samples have demonstrated evidence for convergent and discriminant validity, with EPSI scale scores correlating more strongly with scores on measures of theoretically similar constructs than with scores on theoretically dissimilar constructs (e.g., EPSI Cognitive Restraint and EDE-Q Restraint vs. EPSI Cognitive Restraint and positive affect). Finally, the eight-factor structure of the EPSI has been replicated across patient and nonpatient samples (Forbush et al. 2013), as well as in male and female samples (Forbush et al. 2014). In sum, the existing data provide promising preliminary support for the validity of the EPSI as a measure of a wide range of eating disorder pathology.

Special Populations and Issues

Given the preponderance of data suggesting that individuals with eating disorders are heterogeneous with regard to gender, race/ethnicity, age, body mass index, and so forth, it seems obvious that the psychometric properties of eating disorder assessments need to be examined in similarly heterogeneous samples. However, the vast majority of eating disorder assessments have been developed and validated in samples of young white females. This most likely reflects the outdated stereotype that eating disorders are problems confined to young, affluent, white women (see also Chapter 7, "Eating Problems in Special Populations"). Unfortunately, without psychometric data on eating disorder measures in more diverse samples, it is impossible to know whether the gathered data are accurate or useful in assessing symptom levels or assigning diagnoses among males and ethnic and racial minorities. Without psychometric data characterizing eating disorder pathology among diverse samples, it is challenging to make appropriate recommendations for treatment planning, insurance reimbursement, and research funding.

There is evidence to suggest that fundamental differences between groups could impact response patterns on eating disorder assessments. For example, evidence suggests that there may be differences between males and females with regard to body ideals, which subsequently may translate into different symptom presentations (Darcy and Lin 2012). As a result, males have been found to score lower than females on measures of "traditional" eating disorder constructs (e.g., EDI Drive for Thinness, EPSI Body Dissatisfaction) but to score higher on measures of "nontraditional" eating disorder constructs (e.g., EPSI Muscle Building [Forbush et al. 2014; Stanford and Lemberg 2012]; see also Chapter 6). Similarly, research suggests that individuals from diverse cultures may not endorse stereotypic eating disorder pathology (e.g., fat phobia) but may engage in alternative forms of eating disorder pathology (e.g., use of herbal purgatives) that are not typically included in current eating disorder assessments (see also Chapter 7). The addition of culturally relevant constructs to the EDE-Q has been found to substantially increase the accuracy with which eating disorder cases are identified (Becker et al. 2010).

Additional considerations may need to be made when assessing children, adolescents, and young adults (see also Chapter 11, "Diagnosis of Feeding and Eating Disorders in Children and Adolescents"). For example, several common eating disorder symptoms are fairly abstract constructs (e.g., overvaluation of shape and weight, loss of control over eating), and assessments of these constructs may require cognitive skills (e.g., abstract reasoning, metacognition) that may not be fully developed in younger respondents (Bravender et al. 2011). Consistent, blanket denial of all symptoms on eating disorder assessments appears to be more common in younger samples (e.g., Berg et al. 2012), and it is possible that this finding may be due, in part, to the advanced cognitive requirements of instruments described in this chapter.

Finally, some constructs may be more difficult to assess in particular samples. For example, given the physiological changes associated with bariatric surgery, the assessment of binge eating in postoperative bariatric surgery patients often needs to be modified (see also Chapter 5, "Assessment of Eating Disorders and Problematic Eating Behavior in Bariatric Surgery Patients"). In sum, given these considerations, current eating disorder assessments may overestimate, underestimate, or misrepresent eating disorder pathology in heterogeneous samples.

Conclusion

Given certain limitations of reliability and validity, additional psychometric data on the EDE-Q, EDI-3, and EPSI are needed. Very few reliability or stability studies have been conducted on any of the multidimensional eating disorder measures, and the majority of research has been conducted using nonclinical samples of women. With regard to the EDE-Q, the inability to replicate the original (or any) factor model must be addressed, with particular attention given to the possibility that a general, underlying dimension exists. Additionally, given the mixed findings, further research is needed on the validity of the EDE-Q as a diagnostic instrument. With regard to the EDI, additional research is needed to both replicate and expand on the psychometric data that currently exist. Despite substantive changes to the EDI-3, little research has examined the psychometric properties of the revised measure. As a result, few conclusions can be made about the replicability or validity of the EDI-3 as a measure of eating disorder pathology. With regard to the EPSI, given that the majority of the control samples have been college students, it may be useful for future research to examine the psychometric properties of this instrument in the general population. Sensitivity, specificity, and receiver operator characteristic analyses could also be conducted to determine whether the EPSI could be used to identify cases of eating disorders. The psychometric properties of all three of these instruments need to be examined in more heterogeneous populations and also should be compared across gender, race/ethnicity, age, and other populations, such as in bariatric surgery patients.

So which "all-in-one" measures should the busy eating disorder professional use? On the basis of our review of the literature, we believe that each of the three measures has numerous advantages as well as certain limitations. We have three main recommendations to help guide clinicians in selecting self-report tools in their practice. First, in the context of tracking client symptom change over time, it is beneficial to select a self-report measure that has strong test-retest reliability, stability, and a replicable factor structure (otherwise, change in the clients' scale scores could reflect the instability of the measure rather than true change). The EDI-3 and EPSI demonstrated good evidence for test-retest reliability and are excellent tools for measuring changes in response to behavioral and pharmacological interventions (although readers should be cautioned that few data on long-term stability are currently available for the EPSI). Notably, an advantage of the EPSI for tracking symptom change is that it possesses well-defined scales and a replicable factor structure relative to the EDI-3. For example, the EPSI assesses purging and binge eating separately, rather than combined together on the same scale, and thereby provides a more nuanced measure of change in specific eating disorder symptomatology.

Second, if one is primarily interested in assessing core constructs delineated in the transdiagnostic model of eating disorders (Fairburn 2008), we recommend the EDE-Q because its scales are well aligned with the six core maintaining features of eating disorders that are targeted in Fairburn's cognitive-behavior therapy for eating disorders. (We refer the interested reader to Chapter 15, "Treatment of Other Eating Problems, Including Pica and Rumination," for more information on Fairburn's transdiagnostic cognitive-behavior therapy approach.) Finally, given that the EPSI has a male-specific Muscle Building scale and was developed and validated in male populations, we recommend using the EPSI to assess eating disorder psychopathology with male clients.

Regardless of their individual choices, clinicians have a number of excellent self-report tools from which to select, and our main recommendation is that eating disorder professionals use one or more of the measures that we have described to assess client outcomes rather than omit assessment altogether. As we mentioned in the introduction of this chapter, assessment can significantly improve client outcomes, which we believe is well worth the time and effort.

Key Clinical Points

- Regular assessment of clients' mental health symptoms has been shown to improve therapeutic outcomes across a range of therapeutic modalities and client types.
- There is support for the validity of all three self-report questionnaires—the Eating Disorder Inventory (EDI), the Eating Disorder Examination Questionnaire (EDE-Q), and the Eating Pathology Symptoms Inventory (EPSI)—to distinguish between cases and noncases of eating disorders. However, the extent to which there is support for the factor structure of these three questionnaires varies substantially.
- The EPSI is a recently developed self-report measure of eating disorder symptoms that has shown good reliability and validity in preliminary studies.
- The EDE-Q is the only one of the three questionnaires that can be used diagnostically; however, empirical support for the validity of the EDE-Q as a diagnostic measure is mixed.

- The majority of research on the psychometric properties of self-report questionnaires has been conducted in heterogeneous samples; therefore, little data are available to support the validity of these three questionnaires in specific populations, such as males, adolescents, or ethnic and racial minorities.

References

Aardoom JJ, Dingemans AE, Slof Op't Landt MCT, et al: Norms and discriminative validity of the Eating Disorder Examination Questionnaire (EDE-Q). Eat Behav 13(4):305–309, 2012 23121779

American Psychiatric Association: Diagnostic and Statistical Manual of Mental Disorders, 4th Edition, Text Revision. Washington, DC, American Psychiatric Association, 2000

Bardone-Cone AM, Boyd CA: Psychometric properties of eating disorder instruments in black and white young women: internal consistency, temporal stability, and validity. Psychol Assess 19(3):356–362, 2007 17845127

Becker AE, Thomas JJ, Bainivualiku A, et al; HEALTHY Fiji Study Group: Validity and reliability of a Fijian translation and adaptation of the Eating Disorder Examination Questionnaire. Int J Eat Disord 43(2):171–178, 2010 19308995

Berg KC, Stiles-Shields EC, Swanson SA, et al: Diagnostic concordance of the interview and questionnaire versions of the Eating Disorder Examination. Int J Eat Disord 45(7):850–855, 2012 21826696

Berg KC, Swanson SA, Stiles-Shields EC, et al: Response patterns on interview and questionnaire versions of the Eating Disorder Examination and their impact on latent structure analyses. Compr Psychiatry 54(5):506–516, 2013 23375185

Bravender TD, Bryant-Waugh R, Herzog DB, et al: Classification of eating disturbance in children and adolescents, in Developing an Evidence-Based Classification of Eating Disorders: Scientific Findings for DSM-5. Edited by Striegel-Moore RH, Wonderlich SA, Walsh BT, et al. Arlington, VA, American Psychiatric Publishing, 2011, pp 167–184

Burlingame GM, Lambert MJ, Reisinger CW, et al: Pragmatics of tracking mental health outcomes in a managed care setting. J Ment Health Adm 22(3):226–236, 1995 10144458

Clark LA, Watson D: Constructing validity: basic issues in objective scale development. Psychol Assess 7(3):309–319, 1995

Clausen L, Rosenvinge JH, Friborg O, et al: Validating the Eating Disorder Inventory-3 (EDI-3): a comparison between 561 female eating disorders patients and 878 females from the general population. J Psychopathol Behav Assess 33(1):101–110, 2011 21472023

Comrey AL: Factor-analytic methods of scale development in personality and clinical psychology. J Consult Clin Psychol 56(5):754–761, 1988 3057010

Cooper Z, Fairburn C: The Eating Disorder Examination: a semi-structured interview for the assessment of the specific psychopathology of eating disorders. Int J Eat Disord 6:1–8, 1987

Crowther J, Lilly R, Crawford P, et al: The stability of the Eating Disorder Inventory. Int J Eat Disord 12:97–101, 1992

Darcy AM, Lin IH-J: Are we asking the right questions? A review of assessment of males with eating disorders. Eat Disord 20(5):416–426, 2012 22985238

Elder KA, Grilo CM, Masheb RM, et al: Comparison of two self-report instruments for assessing binge eating in bariatric surgery candidates. Behav Res Ther 44(4):545–560, 2006 15993381

Engelsen BK, Laberg JC: A comparison of three questionnaires (EAT-12, EDI, and EDE-Q) for assessment of eating problems in healthy female adolescents. Nord J Psychiatry 55(2):129–135, 2001 11802911

Fairburn CG: Cognitive Behavior Therapy and Eating Disorders. New York, Guilford, 2008

Fairburn CG, Beglin SJ: Assessment of eating disorders: interview or self-report questionnaire? Int J Eat Disord 16(4):363–370, 1994 7866415

Forbush KT, Wildes JE, Pollack LO, et al: Development and validation of the Eating Pathology Symptoms Inventory (EPSI). Psychol Assess 25(3):859–878, 2013 23815116

Forbush KT, Wildes JE, Hunt TK: Gender norms, psychometric properties, and validity for the Eating Pathology Symptoms Inventory. Int J Eat Disord 47(1):85–91, 2014 23996154

Friborg O, Reas DL, Rosenvinge JH, et al: Core pathology of eating disorders as measured by the Eating Disorder Examination Questionnaire (EDE-Q): the predictive role of a nested general (g) and primary factors. Int J Methods Psychiatr Res 22:1–10, 2013 24038315

Garner DM: Eating Disorder Inventory-2: Professional Manual. Odessa, FL, Psychological Assessment Resources, 1991

Garner DM: Eating Disorder Inventory-3 Professional Manual. Odessa, FL, Psychological Assessment Resources, 2004

Garner DM, Olmstead MP, Polivy J: Development and validation of a multidimensional eating disorder inventory for anorexia nervosa and bulimia. Int J Eat Disord 2:15–34, 1983

Grilo CM, Masheb RM, Wilson GT: A comparison of different methods for assessing the features of eating disorders in patients with binge eating disorder. J Consult Clin Psychol 69(2):317–322, 2001a 11393608

Grilo CM, Masheb RM, Wilson GT: Different methods for assessing the features of eating disorders in patients with binge eating disorder: a replication. Obes Res 9(7):418–422, 2001b 11445665

Grilo CM, Henderson KE, Bell RL, et al: Eating Disorder Examination-Questionnaire factor structure and construct validity in bariatric surgery candidates. Obes Surg 23(5):657–662, 2013 23229951

Hatfield D, McCullough L, Frantz SH, et al: Do we know when our clients get worse? An investigation of therapists' ability to detect negative client change. Clin Psychol Psychother 17(1):25–32, 2010 19916162

Hrabosky JI, White MA, Masheb RM, et al: Psychometric evaluation of the Eating Disorder Examination-Questionnaire for bariatric surgery candidates. Obesity (Silver Spring) 16(4):763–769, 2008 18379561

Joiner TE Jr, Walker RL, Pettit JW, et al: Evidence-based assessment of depression in adults. Psychol Assess 17(3):267–277, 2005 16262453

Keel PK, Haedt A, Edler C: Purging disorder: an ominous variant of bulimia nervosa? Int J Eat Disord 38(3):191–199, 2005 16211629

Lambert MJ, Shimokawa K: Collecting client feedback. Psychotherapy (Chic) 48(1):72–79, 2011 21401277

Lambert MJ, Whipple JL, Vermeersch DA, et al: Enhancing psychotherapy outcomes via providing feedback on client progress: a replication. Clin Psychol Psychother 9:91–103, 2002

Loevinger J: Objective Tests as instruments of psychological theory: Monograph Supplement 9. Psychol Rep 3:635–694, 1957

Luce KH, Crowther JH: The reliability of the Eating Disorder Examination–Self-Report Questionnaire Version (EDE-Q). Int J Eat Disord 25(3):349–351, 1999 10192002

Mond JM, Hay PJ, Rodgers B, et al: Temporal stability of the Eating Disorder Examination Questionnaire. Int J Eat Disord 36(2):195–203, 2004a 15282689

Mond JM, Hay PJ, Rodgers B, et al: Validity of the Eating Disorder Examination Questionnaire (EDE-Q) in screening for eating disorders in community samples. Behav Res Ther 42(5):551–567, 2004b 15033501

Peterson CB, Crosby RD, Wonderlich SA, et al: Psychometric properties of the Eating Disorder Examination-Questionnaire: factor structure and internal consistency. Int J Eat Disord 40(4):386–389, 2007 17304585

Reas DL, Grilo CM, Masheb RM: Reliability of the Eating Disorder Examination-Questionnaire in patients with binge eating disorder. Behav Res Ther 44(1):43–51, 2006 16301013

Reese RJ, Toland MD, Slone NC, et al: Effect of client feedback on couple psychotherapy outcomes. Psychotherapy (Chic) 47(4):616–630, 2010 21198247

Smith GT, McCarthy DM, Anderson KG: On the sins of short-form development. Psychol Assess 12(1):102–111, 2000 10752369

Stanford SC, Lemberg R: A clinical comparison of men and women on the Eating Disorder Inventory-3 (EDI-3) and the Eating Disorder Assessment for Men (EDAM). Eat Disord 20:379–394, 2012

Stice E, Fisher M, Lowe MR: Are dietary restraint scales valid measures of acute dietary restriction? Unobtrusive observational data suggest not. Psychol Assess 16(1):51–59, 2004 15023092

Stice E, Cooper JA, Schoeller DA, et al: Are dietary restraint scales valid measures of moderate- to long-term dietary restriction? Objective biological and behavioral data suggest not. Psychol Assess 19(4):449–458, 2007 18085937

Tasca GA, Illing V, Lybanon-Daigle V, et al: Psychometric properties of the Eating Disorders Inventory-2 among women seeking treatment for binge eating disorder. Assessment 10(3):228–236, 2003 14503646

Thiel A, Paul T: Test–retest reliability of the Eating Disorder Inventory 2. J Psychosom Res 61(4):567–569, 2006 17011367

Urbina S: Essentials of reliability, in Essentials of Psychological Testing (Essentials of Behavioral Sciences Series; Kaufman AS, Kaufman NL, series eds). Hoboken, NJ, Wiley, 2011, pp 117–150

Watson D: Stability versus change, dependability versus error: issues in the assessment of personality over time. J Res Pers 38:319–350, 2004

Wear R, Pratz O: Test-retest reliability for the eating disorder inventory. Int J Eat Disord 6(6):767–769, 1987

Wilson GT, Nonas CA, Rosenblum GD: Assessment of binge eating in obese patients. Int J Eat Disord 13(1):25–33, 1993 8477274

10 Use of the Eating Disorder Assessment for DSM-5

Deborah R. Glasofer, Ph.D.
Robyn Sysko, Ph.D.
B. Timothy Walsh, M.D.

This chapter provides an overview of the Eating Disorder Assessment for DSM-5 (EDA-5; Sysko et al. 2015), a novel semistructured interview for the diagnosis of feeding and eating disorders described in DSM-5 (American Psychiatric Association 2013). The chapter includes information relevant to researchers–namely, a review of the development and the psychometrics of the EDA-5 and essential principles of the instrument's administration–and, beginning with the section "Instrument Structure and Content," a step-by-step guide for clinicians intending to use the measure as part of routine practice. The EDA-5 is an electronic assessment (available freely at www.eda5.org), and we recommend that readers access the application while reviewing this chapter as an aid for learning about the instrument's structure and content.

 We gratefully acknowledge Jonathan Cohen (Rivington Digital) and Alim Razak for their assistance in the development of the EDA-5 Web site and electronic application.

Eating Disorder Assessment for DSM-5 Overview

With the publication of DSM-5, the category of feeding and eating disorders was revised from the DSM-IV (American Psychiatric Association 1994) disorders. As described in Chapter 1, "Classification of Eating Disorders," some of the changes from DSM-IV were modest (e.g., reducing the frequency of binge eating and/or purging behaviors for the diagnosis of bulimia nervosa [BN]) and others were major (e.g., merging feeding and eating disorders into one category, recognizing binge-eating disorder [BED]). Given the differences between DSM-IV and DSM-5 criteria for feeding and eating disorders, the utility of existing diagnostic assessment tools is quite limited. Thus, as described in detail by Sysko et al. (2015), we chose to develop and validate the EDA-5 as an interview guide to assess for *current* DSM-5 feeding and eating disorders in adults.

The EDA-5 was designed to focus specifically on assessment of the DSM-5 criteria and was not aimed at a broader assessment of other psychopathological features associated with eating disorders, such as the intensity of concerns over shape or weight. As described in Chapter 9, "Self-Report Assessments of Eating Pathology," such facets of eating problems can be conveniently evaluated through the use of self-report measures. Therefore, the EDA-5 differs significantly from some other interview-based measures, such as the Eating Disorder Examination (EDE; Fairburn et al. 2008), which assesses both the DSM criteria for eating disorders and a range of psychopathological features characteristic of individuals with these problems (see also Chapter 8, "Assessment Measures, Then and Now"). The EDE requires extensive training and an extended amount of time to administer; thus, its use has largely been relegated to specialized care settings (e.g., eating disorders clinics). The Structured Clinical Interview for DSM-5 (SCID-5), another interview-based measure, is intended to determine whether an individual meets criteria for any DSM-5 disorder (First et al. 2015). Although it assesses the presence of an eating disorder, it does not ask about pica or rumination disorder and does not attempt to determine with precision the individual's body mass index (BMI) or the particular frequencies of a range of behavioral disturbances such as objective and subjective binge-eating episodes. Although the SCID-5 includes a module on avoidant/restrictive food intake disorder (ARFID), this section is optional and therefore may not be routinely administered. The EDA-5, in contrast, 1) provides a comprehensive assessment of DSM-5 feeding and eating disorder criteria, 2) requires minimal interviewer training, and 3) reduces participant burden. We hope that this instrument will be helpful to practitioners ranging broadly in professional degree, specialty, and experience and will be useful across a range of general clinical settings (e.g., primary care, community mental health centers) to determine when an individual's symptoms are sufficient to suggest the need for a referral to specialist services.

Development and Psychometrics

To date, two studies have evaluated the utility of the EDA-5 in treatment-seeking adults across multiple sites (for details, see Sysko et al. 2015). The first study compared the diagnostic validity of a paper-and-pencil version of the EDA-5 to the EDE and evaluated the test-retest reliability of diagnoses from the EDA-5. High rates of agreement were found between diagnoses using the EDA-5 and the EDE ($\kappa=0.74$ across diagnoses, $n=64$), with κ ranging from 0.65 for other specified feeding or eating disorder/unspecified feeding or eating disorder (OSFED/USFED) to 0.90 for BED. For a randomly selected subgroup of study participants, the EDA-5 was readministered by a new interviewer 7–14 days following the initial assessment. The test-retest κ coefficient was 0.87 across diagnoses, which would be considered excellent to almost perfect; diagnostic agreement was achieved in 19 of 21 cases (90.5%).

In light of feedback from interviewers about the complexity of the interview's skip rules, an electronic application ("app") of the EDA-5, with automated skip rules, was created. The second study compared the diagnostic validity of the EDA-5 app to an interview by an experienced clinician. A high rate of agreement was observed between diagnosis by EDA-5 and experienced clinician ($\kappa=0.83$ across diagnoses, $n=71$). Across individual diagnostic categories, κ ranged from 0.56 for OSFED/USFED to 0.94 for BED.

In both studies, information was collected on interview duration (i.e., participant and interviewer burden) and acceptability of the new measure. The EDA-5 required significantly less time to complete than the EDE. The electronic application of the EDA-5 significantly shortened the length of time needed to administer the interview from the first to the second study, from an average of 19.3 ± 5.6 minutes (range of 5–34 minutes) in the former study to 14.0 ± 6.2 minutes (range of 5–30 minutes) in the latter investigation. Among those who reported a preference for the EDA-5 or the EDE, a larger proportion of individuals preferred the EDA-5 (54.1%) over the EDE (31.1%) [$\alpha^2(2)=14.3$, $P=0.001$].

The results of these preliminary investigations are encouraging. However, these studies, despite their strengths (e.g., the successful administration of the EDA-5 by interviewers with varying degrees of clinical experience), also had several limitations (see Sysko et al. 2015), including a lack of data on the assessment of the feeding disorders (i.e., ARFID, rumination disorder, pica). Thus, additional validation (and replication) studies are warranted.

Principles of Administration

The EDA-5 assesses feeding and eating disorders *in adults* according to the DSM-5 criteria. It is intended for use by clinicians and researchers in a variety of disciplines (e.g., nursing, psychology, social work), and it assumes familiarity with the feeding and eating disorder diagnoses. The questions are posed to assess a *current* problem–that is, a problem within the last 3 months rather than a problem that may have existed in the past.

EDA-5 questions closely mirror the DSM-5 feeding and eating disorder criteria but are worded to aid the assessment process. The interviewer must exercise clinical judgment in answering all questions. It is appropriate to use whatever clinical information is available, including the individual's answers to questions, the interviewer's observations of the individual, and ancillary sources of information such as other treatment providers, close family members, and, as appropriate, people within the individual's community. Interviewers are strongly advised to obtain objective information (i.e., clinician-measured height and weight) whenever possible.

Instrument Structure and Content

The EDA-5 was designed as a semistructured assessment tool. During the administration of the EDA-5 app, each screen adheres to a similar format: section name, symptom being assessed (i.e., individual DSM-5 criterion), example probe to query patient, and answers (Figure 10–1).

Instructions to the interviewer, and clarifications when necessary, are indicated on screen in *italics*. The individual DSM-5 criterion or portions of the criterion to be assessed are provided in the symptom portion of the screen. The probe section provides suggested questions the interviewer may use in determining the presence or absence of the symptom. Interviewers begin by using the probes provided, but clinical judgment should be employed to determine whether follow-up questions are needed to clarify responses. Suggested follow-up questions are sometimes included to enhance standardization and assist those interviewers who are less familiar with the assessment of feeding and eating disorders. In some cases, items

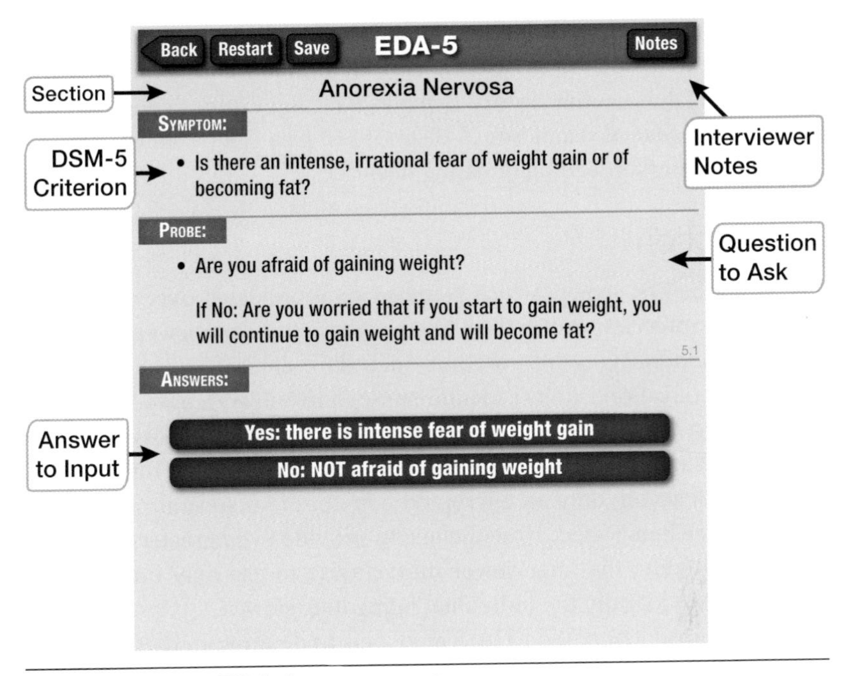

FIGURE 10–1. EDA-5 screen structure.

contain text boxes for data entry (e.g., frequency/type of purging behaviors). The answers section at the bottom of each screen contains a button or buttons with the available options for answers. Following a logical flow diagram based on the DSM-5 criteria, the EDA-5 chooses the next screen to present based on the answer provided. At the top right-hand corner of each screen, there is a "Notes" button. By pressing this button, the interviewer may add comments. Additional comments can be added to those previously entered, and all comments will be available to print in the final report at the conclusion of the interview.

The interview is divided into the following sections, which are more completely described in subsequent subsections: Introduction, Anorexia Nervosa (AN), Binge Eating and Compensatory Behaviors, Bulimia Nervosa (BN), Binge-Eating Disorder (BED), Avoidant/Restrictive Food Intake Disorder (ARFID), Rumination Disorder, Pica, and Other Specified Feeding or Eating Disorder (OSFED). Consistent with DSM-5, the EDA-5 adheres to diagnostic "trumping" rules. Thus, although the electronic version includes content to diagnose all feeding and eating disorders, once criteria for a condition are met, the criteria for other disorders will, in general, not be assessed. For example, if an individual meets criteria for AN, the BN section will be skipped because a diagnosis of AN supersedes that of BN. Questions in the Binge Eating and Compensatory Behaviors and the Pica sections are included for all interviewees. Symptom information from the Binge Eating and Compensatory Behaviors section is required in order to rule in or out several diagnoses. A diagnosis of pica can be assigned in the presence of another feeding or eating disorder.

Introduction

Following the first screen, which contains an abbreviated overview of the EDA-5, the interview proceeds to a page where the interviewer is cued to input basic identifying information, including date of interview, interviewer identification, subject identification, and subject's age. This is the only place in the EDA-5 where identifying information is contained. The EDA-5 does not transmit the information obtained over the Internet and is capable of saving only an encrypted copy of the final summary report on the device being used. Nonetheless, to provide even greater assurance of confidentiality, the interviewer may choose to use only initials (or a code name) to identify the individual being interviewed.

In the introduction, the EDA-5 next aims to determine whether a clinically significant disturbance in eating is, in fact, present. Interviewers are guided first to ask about any problems with eating and then to obtain an overview of the individual's pattern of eating. In the presence of a feeding or eating disturbance (indicated by a positive response to either of the first two symptoms), the interviewer next determines whether the feeding or eating problem is clinically significant (i.e., functionally impairing or distressing). If the disturbance in feeding or eating has resulted in functional impairment or in significant distress (a nearly universal feature outlined in DSM-5 for *all* mental conditions), the interview continues; otherwise, the EDA-5 ends because it has been determined that a clinically significant eating problem is not present. Of particular importance within the realm of feeding and eating disorders, some individuals may minimize their symptoms, and therefore the EDA-5 reminds interviewers that in assessing such individuals, it may be particularly useful to obtain information from others knowledgeable about the individual's symptoms.

The interviewer is asked to input the individual's height and weight, from which the EDA-5 calculates current BMI (kg/m^2). Wherever possible, interviewers should obtain objective measurements, ideally by weighing the individual and measuring his or her height. If the interviewer indicates that the individual is currently underweight, the interviewer will be directed to complete additional questions as part of the AN section. For responses that indicate the individual is currently normal weight, overweight, or obese, interviewers are asked to provide the individual's lowest weight in the past 3 months. If the individual has been underweight within this time frame, the EDA-5 will proceed to the other questions in the AN section. Although DSM-5 does not specify the amount of time an individual should be at a normal weight to be considered recovered from AN or to be assigned another feeding or eating disorder, the EDA-5 uses a 3-month time frame, because this time frame is also used to assess the average frequencies of binge eating and purging. If the interviewer indicates that the individual is not currently and has not been underweight in the last 3 months, the EDA-5 proceeds to the Binge Eating and Compensatory Behaviors section.

Anorexia Nervosa

If the individual endorses current or recent (prior 3 months) low weight, interviewers will be directed to the AN section of the EDA-5. Because restriction of energy intake leading to significantly low body weight (Criterion A for AN in DSM-5) is assessed prior to entering this section, the first question assesses fear of weight gain or becoming fat (Criterion B) (Figure 10–1). Next, all individuals are asked about the presence of behaviors that might interfere with efforts to gain weight (Criterion B). Such behaviors include cutting back on calories or amounts or types of food, exercising, and vomiting after eating. If the individual endorses any of these behaviors, the interviewer may select "Yes: there is persistent behavior to avoid weight gain" (Figure 10–2) and proceed to the next item. This question is aimed solely at determining whether Criterion B is satisfied. More detailed questions about such behaviors are reviewed in the Binge Eating and Compensatory Behaviors section of the EDA-5.

If the individual does not endorse a specific behavior, the interviewer probes in a more open-ended manner: "Do you do anything else that might make it hard for you to gain or maintain weight?" Examples of clinically significant behaviors that might reasonably interfere with weight gain include spitting out food and inappropriate use of stimulants (e.g., as appetite suppressants). If the individual denies both a fear of weight gain and persistent actions that might interfere with weight gain, Criterion B is not satisfied, and the interviewer is guided to the Binge Eating and Compensatory Behaviors section. If the individual endorses either of these items, the interview continues with the remainder of the AN section.

The AN section concludes with items assessing 1) body image distortion, 2) an overemphasis on weight or shape in self-evaluation, and 3) denial of the seriousness of current or recent low weight status. If the individual views his or her body realistically (e.g., does not consider being

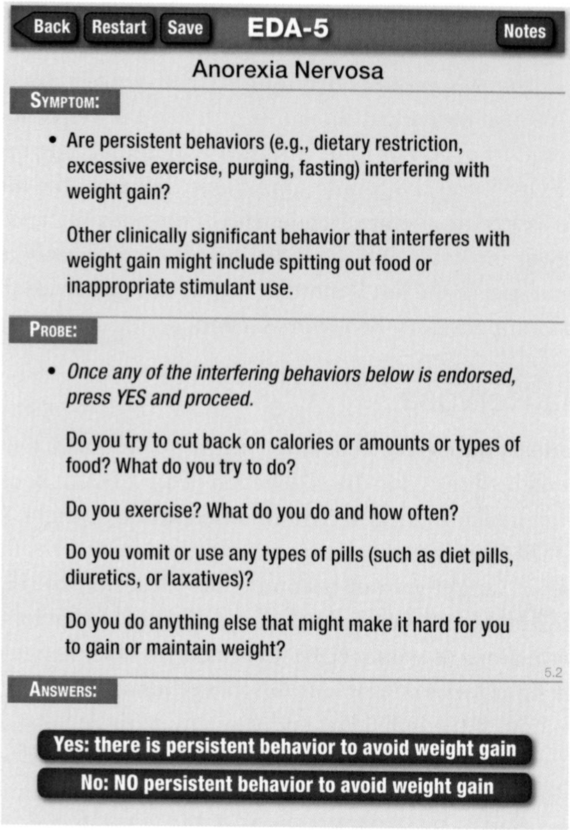

Back | Restart | Save | **EDA-5** | Notes

Anorexia Nervosa

SYMPTOM:

- Are persistent behaviors (e.g., dietary restriction, excessive exercise, purging, fasting) interfering with weight gain?

  Other clinically significant behavior that interferes with weight gain might include spitting out food or inappropriate stimulant use.

PROBE:

- *Once any of the interfering behaviors below is endorsed, press YES and proceed.*

  Do you try to cut back on calories or amounts or types of food? What do you try to do?

  Do you exercise? What do you do and how often?

  Do you vomit or use any types of pills (such as diet pills, diuretics, or laxatives)?

  Do you do anything else that might make it hard for you to gain or maintain weight?

5.2

ANSWERS:

Yes: there is persistent behavior to avoid weight gain

No: NO persistent behavior to avoid weight gain

FIGURE 10–2. EDA-5 anorexia nervosa sample item.

significantly underweight as the way he or she should look), does not feel that his or her self-worth is unduly influenced by weight or body shape, and is aware of the seriousness of being underweight, an AN diagnosis is not assigned. Alternatively, if one or more of these symptoms are endorsed, the individual meets criteria for AN diagnosis. Once the individual meets criteria for this disorder, or for any of the other disorders subsequently assessed, a pop-up window visible to the interviewer indicates that a diagnosis has been assigned (Figure 10–3). After the AN section, the interviewer will be guided into the Binge Eating and Compensatory Behaviors section.

Binge Eating and Compensatory Behaviors

The Binge Eating and Compensatory Behaviors section poses questions about the presence, type, and frequency of aberrant eating episodes and of

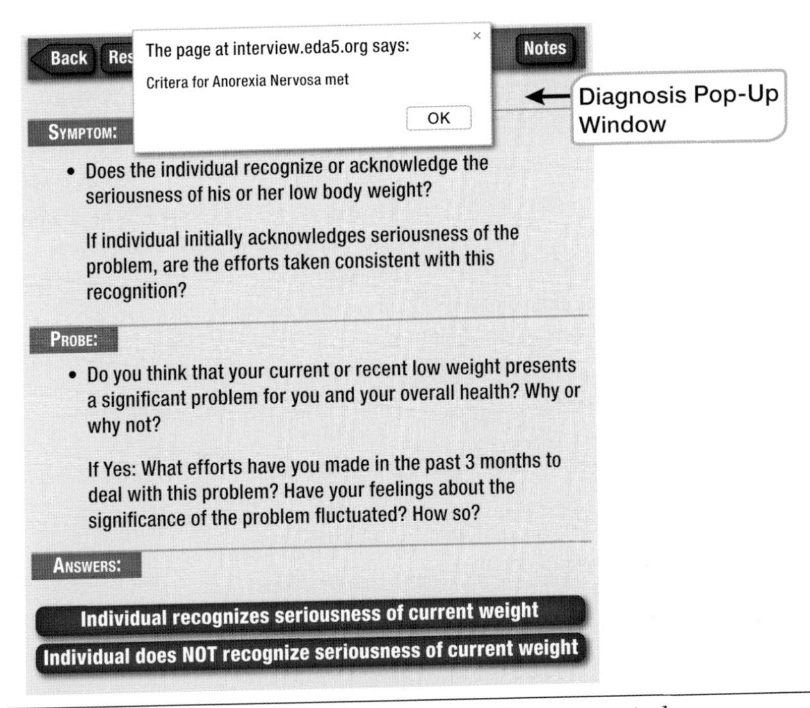

FIGURE 10–3. Example of EDA-5 diagnosis pop-up window.

abnormal behaviors to compensate for eating. Consistent with Criterion A for both BN and BED, the questions in this EDA-5 section focus first on the assessment of *objective binge episodes* (OBEs); these are referred to as *binge-eating episodes* in DSM-5, which are defined as discrete eating episodes characterized by a loss of control in which an amount of food is consumed that is definitely larger than most individuals would eat in a similar period of time under similar circumstances. DSM-5 is silent on whether OBEs are required for individuals with AN to be designated as having the binge-eating/purging subtype of AN. In constructing the EDA-5, we decided that the presence of recurrent OBEs and/or purging within the last 3 months, operationalized as occurring at least once per month on average, would satisfy the requirements of this subtype. In the service of collecting information of clinical utility in assessing other individuals with eating disorders, the EDA-5 also assesses the frequency of *subjective binge episodes* (SBEs), defined as aberrant eating episodes in which the individual describes eating a normal, for the context, or small amount of food (for examples, see Table 10–1) but experiences a sense of loss of control over eating. SBEs are not specifically referred to in DSM-5 but may be of clinical significance.

TABLE 10–1. Examples of objectively and subjectively large amounts of food

Objectively large	Subjectively large
2 pints of ice cream	½ pint of ice cream, 2 (1 inch × 1 inch) brownies
10 apples	5 carrot sticks, 2 tablespoons of peanut butter, ½ cup of nuts, 1 individual yogurt
2 boxes of waffles, 1 pound of pasta, 8 ounces of cheese, 1 box of chocolate donuts	2 bowls of cereal
1 family-size bag of chips	2 individual yogurts, ½ grapefruit, 3 waffles
4 peanut butter sandwiches, 2 bananas	6-inch sub sandwich, 2 snack-size bags of chips
10 muffins, 10 bagels, 20 pats of butter, 20 pats of jelly, 20 pats of cream cheese, 1 piece of fruit	2 muffins
>2 bags of frozen vegetables	1 bag of frozen vegetables
4 slices of pizza, 1 calzone	3 slices of pizza
2 Big Macs, 2 orders of large fries, milk shake	2 Big Macs
½ of an 8-inch two-layer cake with frosting	1 piece of pie, 10 Oreo cookies

Note. This table provides *examples* of objectively large versus subjectively large amounts of food. It is therefore possible that a smaller amount of food than delineated might be considered an objective binge episode or that a larger amount of food than delineated might be considered a subjective binge episode. If a determination of size is ambiguous, consultation with other interviewers is recommended.

The Binge Eating and Compensatory Behaviors section concludes by evaluating purging behaviors and excessive exercise. Frequent purging behavior or excessive exercise satisfies Criterion B of BN and excludes a diagnosis of BED (BED Criterion E). Purging behavior (but not excessive exercise) also satisfies the criterion for the binge-eating/purging subtype of AN. The intended function of purging and excessive exercise behaviors (e.g., weight control, compensation for binge eating) is evaluated in this section. Binge-eating and/or purging subtype and frequency are stored by the EDA-5 and, at the conclusion of the interview, summarized in a report that can be printed or saved on the device in encrypted form. (For more details, see "Notes and Results" section later in this chapter.)

Loss of Control: Is It a Binge?

OBEs and SBEs both require that individuals endorse a sense of loss of control during the episode of eating. Although loss of control must be present for an eating episode to be characterized as a binge, assessing loss of control can be challenging for a variety of reasons (Blomquist et al. 2014; Fairburn et al. 2008; Latner et al. 2014). For example, some individuals describe a dissociative or "numbing" quality during or following the binge episodes that may make it difficult to recall or evaluate their psychological experience when they were eating. After binge eating has persisted for some time, individuals may report that their binge-eating episodes are no longer characterized by an acute feeling of loss of control (and that sometimes these episodes are even planned in advance) but rather by behavioral indicators of impaired control, such as difficulty resisting binge eating or difficulty stopping a binge once it has begun. The impairment in control associated with binge eating is not absolute; for example, an individual may continue binge eating while the telephone is ringing but cease eating if a roommate or spouse unexpectedly enters the room. An episode may or may not be planned in advance and is usually (but not always) characterized by rapid consumption. The binge eating often continues until the individual is uncomfortably, or even painfully, full.

The EDA-5 Binge Eating and Compensatory Behaviors section begins with a series of probes to help the interviewer ascertain the presence of the psychological experience of feeling out of control while eating (Figure 10–4).

Because loss of control while eating can be difficult to assess, the interviewer may need to present illustrative metaphors or examples to confirm that the individual understands the construct being assessed. Potentially useful probes include the following:

1. Another way of thinking about this is to imagine a ball sitting atop a hill. Once it starts rolling, it keeps going and going. In the past 3 months, have you had an experience of eating and feeling like you could not stop, like you just kept going and going? (This is adapted from the child version of the EDE [Bryant-Waugh et al. 1996, per Tanofsky-Kraff et al. 2004].)
2. Think of a car parked on a steep incline with no emergency brake; it starts going slowly down the hill and then picks up speed and does not stop. In the past 3 months, have you ever felt like this while eating?
3. In the past 3 months, have you ever been interrupted during an episode of eating and felt like you could not stop thinking about going back to eating? What happened when the interruption ended (e.g., did you return to eating)?

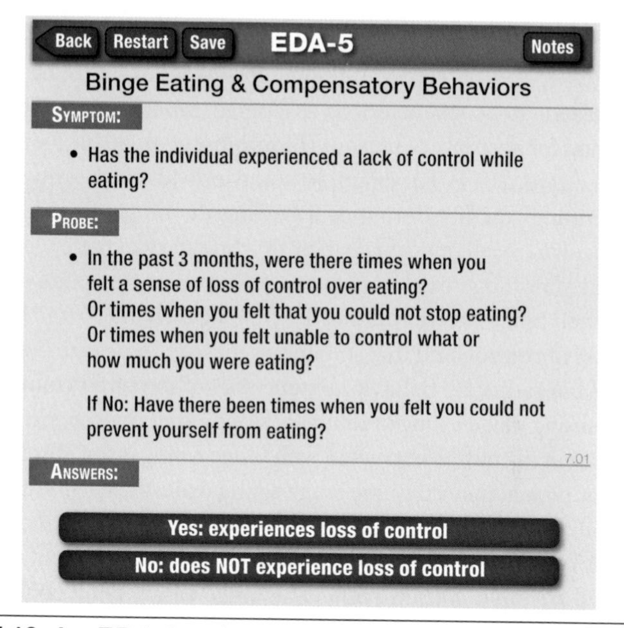

FIGURE 10–4. EDA-5 probes assessing loss of control while eating.

If the individual denies loss of control in the past 3 months, the interviewer will proceed next to a series of questions regarding purging behavior. If loss of control is endorsed, the interviewer will then be guided to assess the size of the binge episodes during which the loss of control is experienced.

It's a Binge! Is It Large or Small?

The EDA-5 next queries about OBEs, episodes in which the individual describes feeling out of control and eating what would clearly be a large amount of food (Figure 10–5). If OBEs are endorsed, the interviewer is asked to note, in the text box provided, the type and amount of food typically consumed during a binge episode.

The context in which the eating occurred must be evaluated; for example, what would be regarded as excessive consumption at a typical meal might be considered normal during a meal eaten for a celebration or holiday (e.g., Thanksgiving, Fourth of July). Examples of amounts of food that would meet the threshold of objectively large, developed on the basis of ratings from our clinical staff, are provided in Table 10–1 as a guideline for EDA-5 interviewers.

If the first example provided by the individual is *not* a clearly large amount of food, the interviewer might ask for a second example of "the

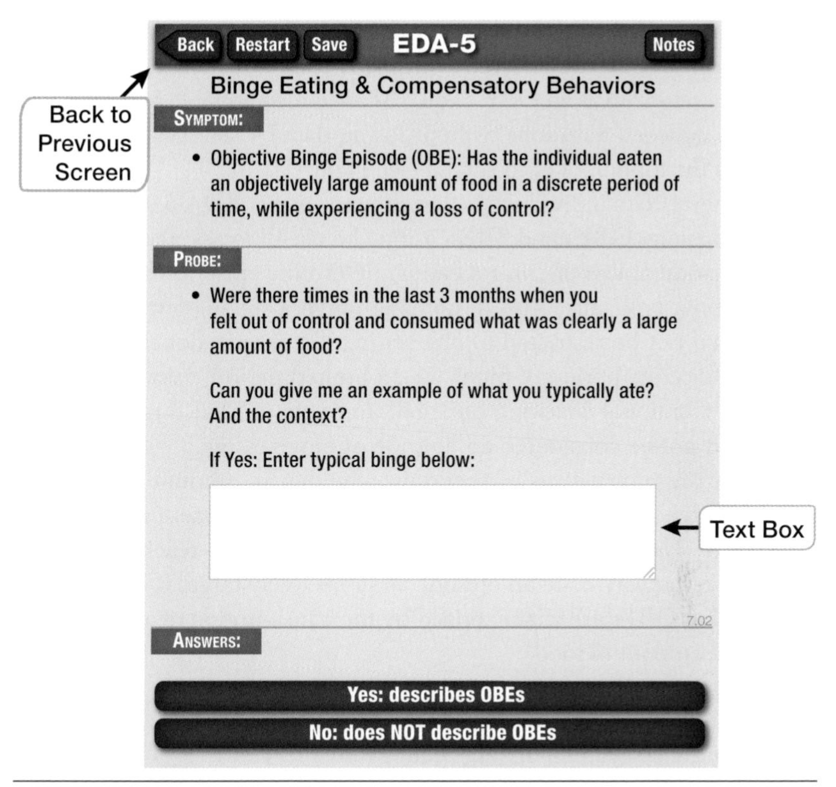

FIGURE 10–5. EDA-5 objective binge episode assessment.

largest amount of food that you recall eating in the last 3 months, while experiencing a loss of control." If the individual denies OBEs, the interviewer is guided next to a series of questions about smaller binge episodes. However, if OBEs are endorsed, the frequency of such episodes must be obtained before proceeding.

The EDA-5 Binge Eating and Compensatory Behaviors section next asks about SBEs. As with OBEs, if SBEs are described, the interviewer is asked to note the type and amount of food in a typical episode. If this type of eating episode is not described as having occurred in the past 3 months, the interviewer is guided to a series of questions about purging behaviors. However, if SBEs are endorsed, the frequency of such episodes must be obtained before proceeding.

Other Common Challenges in Assessing Binge Eating

Because some individuals have difficulty recalling or distinguishing among different binge episodes, information gathered about typical episodes does not always occur in the sequence with which the EDA-5 proceeds. In such cases, the interviewer may want to take notes and input the information into the EDA-5 only once it is clear whether the episode is better characterized as an OBE or an SBE. It is also possible to move back and forth between questions without losing data by selecting the "Back" button on the top left of each screen (see Figure 10–5).

In general, if an individual is struggling to answer EDA-5 items related to distinguishing OBEs and SBEs, it may be useful to ask about the most recent episode of loss-of-control eating, determine episode size, and then inquire about typicality. Also of note, although a single episode of binge eating need not be restricted to one setting, these episodes should occur within a "discrete period of time" (i.e., a limited period, usually less than 2 hours). Continual snacking on small amounts of food throughout the day would not be considered an episode of binge eating.

When the interviewer is uncertain whether an amount of food described is objectively large, he or she should 1) use the examples provided in Table 10–1 as guidelines, 2) confer with colleagues to reach consensus, or 3) conservatively code an episode as subjectively large. It is important to recall that OBEs are characterized by the consumption of an *unambiguously* large amount of food.

Probing About Compensatory Behaviors

Following the assessment of binge eating, the interviewer is directed to ask about the use of inappropriate purging behaviors, including self-inducted vomiting or misuse of laxatives, diuretics, or other medications (e.g., diet pills, stimulants) (Figure 10–6). Indicators of misuse include 1) using the purging behavior explicitly to compensate for binge eating, 2) using a prescription medicine without medical supervision, 3) using greater quantities of the medicine than recommended, and 4) using the medicine more frequently than recommended. If purging is endorsed, information will next be collected on the frequency and types of behaviors present in the 3 months prior to assessment. If the individual denies use of purging behaviors, the interviewer proceeds to ask about excessive exercise.

The EDA-5 guides the interviewer to determine whether exercise is excessive or inappropriate by asking about several possible concerns (Figure 10–7). Exercise may be viewed as excessive if it interferes with daily functioning (e.g., the individual avoids family responsibilities), persists despite significant injury or other medical complications, becomes overly compulsive (e.g., the individual feels excessive guilt if unable to exercise), or is clearly an inappropriate level of physical activity given

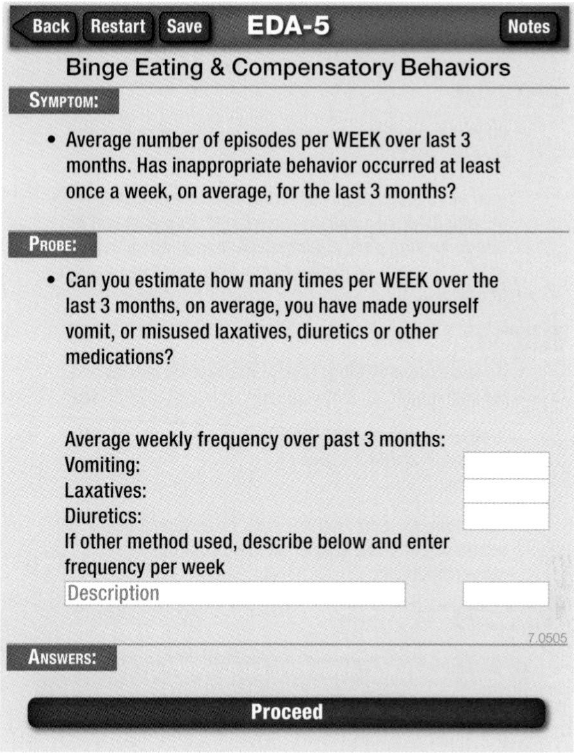

Back Restart Save **EDA-5** Notes

Binge Eating & Compensatory Behaviors

SYMPTOM:

- Average number of episodes per WEEK over last 3 months. Has inappropriate behavior occurred at least once a week, on average, for the last 3 months?

PROBE:

- Can you estimate how many times per WEEK over the last 3 months, on average, you have made yourself vomit, or misused laxatives, diuretics or other medications?

Average weekly frequency over past 3 months:
Vomiting:
Laxatives:
Diuretics:
If other method used, describe below and enter frequency per week
Description

7.0505

ANSWERS:

Proceed

FIGURE 10–6. EDA-5 assessment of purging behaviors.

weight status (i.e., the individual is underweight). In instances in which indicators of misuse are not clear, additional potentially useful probes include the following:

1. Do you (or would you) continue to exercise if you are (were) ill or injured?
2. Have you canceled or missed important social plans because you could not tolerate skipping the exercise?
3. Is your exercise routine the primary determinant of how you arrange your work or school schedule?
4. How easy or difficult is it for you to take days off from your exercise regimen?
5. How much do you vary the routine in type or duration of exercise? How easy or difficult would varying the routine have been in the past 3 months?

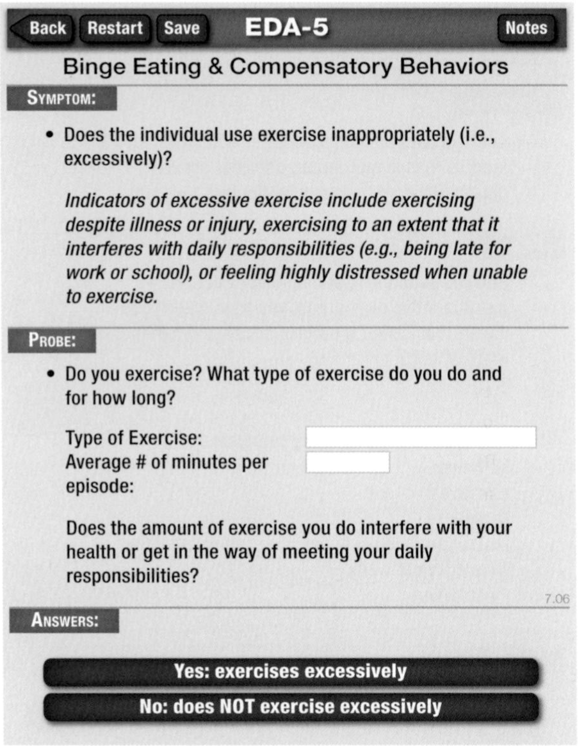

Back Restart Save **EDA-5** Notes

Binge Eating & Compensatory Behaviors

SYMPTOM:

- Does the individual use exercise inappropriately (i.e., excessively)?

Indicators of excessive exercise include exercising despite illness or injury, exercising to an extent that it interferes with daily responsibilities (e.g., being late for work or school), or feeling highly distressed when unable to exercise.

PROBE:

- Do you exercise? What type of exercise do you do and for how long?

Type of Exercise:
Average # of minutes per episode:

Does the amount of exercise you do interfere with your health or get in the way of meeting your daily responsibilities?

7.06

ANSWERS:

Yes: exercises excessively

No: does NOT exercise excessively

FIGURE 10–7. EDA-5 questions on inappropriate exercise.

Data fields are provided for the interviewer to note the individual's preferred type(s) of exercise and the average duration of a typical exercise session (Figure 10–7). If the behavior described is determined to be excessive by the interviewer, he or she asks questions about the frequency of the behavior.

If the individual endorses purging behavior, excessive exercise, or both, the interviewer is guided to assess the purpose of these behaviors–that is, whether they are intended to control weight or to compensate specifically for binge-eating episodes. If neither purging behavior nor excessive exercise is noted, then the end of the Binge Eating and Compensatory Behaviors section has been reached.

Assessing Frequency of Behaviors

Each series of questions about the frequency of OBEs, SBEs, purging behaviors, and excessive exercise follows the same structure (see example in Figure 10–8). The interviewer is first guided to obtain a weekly frequency estimate for the 3 months prior to assessment (Figure 10–8A). Because DSM-5 employs a threshold of at least once a week to meet the criteria for binge eating in BN and BED, and for purging behavior in BN, the EDA-5 focuses on determining whether the frequencies of the behaviors endorsed early in the interview are at or below this threshold. However, the EDA-5 obtains information on frequency even if it is less than once weekly, because this information may be of clinical importance and may suggest the presence of a subthreshold disorder (e.g., OSFED). If a threshold of at least once per week is met, the interviewer will be asked to note the average weekly frequency in a text box on the following screen (Figure 10–8B). If the threshold of at least once per week is *not* met, the interviewer will be guided to ask about monthly frequency. If a threshold of at least once per month is met, then the interviewer will be asked to note the average monthly frequency in a text box on the following screen. If the threshold of at least once per month is *not* met, the EDA-5 will retain the information regarding the presence of particular behaviors but will not probe for additional frequency information.

As previously noted, information collected in the Binge Eating and Compensatory Behaviors section determines subtyping of AN cases as well as the next appropriate section to which the interviewer should be guided (e.g., BN, ARFID). If a diagnosis of AN has been met and the subtype determined, the next section to be accessed is the Pica section. If symptoms consistent with BN (i.e., OBEs and purging behaviors of at least once per week) or BED (i.e., OBEs of at least once per week) are endorsed in this section, the interviewer will be guided accordingly. In all other instances, the next section to be accessed is the ARFID section.

Bulimia Nervosa

Assuming that the individual is *not* underweight (either currently or in the past 3 months) and has endorsed at least one OBE per week on average and at least one episode of inappropriate compensatory behavior (e.g., vomiting, laxatives, excessive exercise) per week on average in the last 3 months, the interviewer is directed to the BN section of the EDA-5. This section contains one item assessing overreliance on weight or shape for self-evaluation (Figure 10–9).

If this symptom is endorsed, the individual meets criteria for a BN diagnosis, and a pop-up window indicates to the interviewer that a diagnosis has been reached. The EDA-5 then proceeds to the Pica section. If the individual does not meet criteria for BN, the interviewer is guided to the ARFID section.

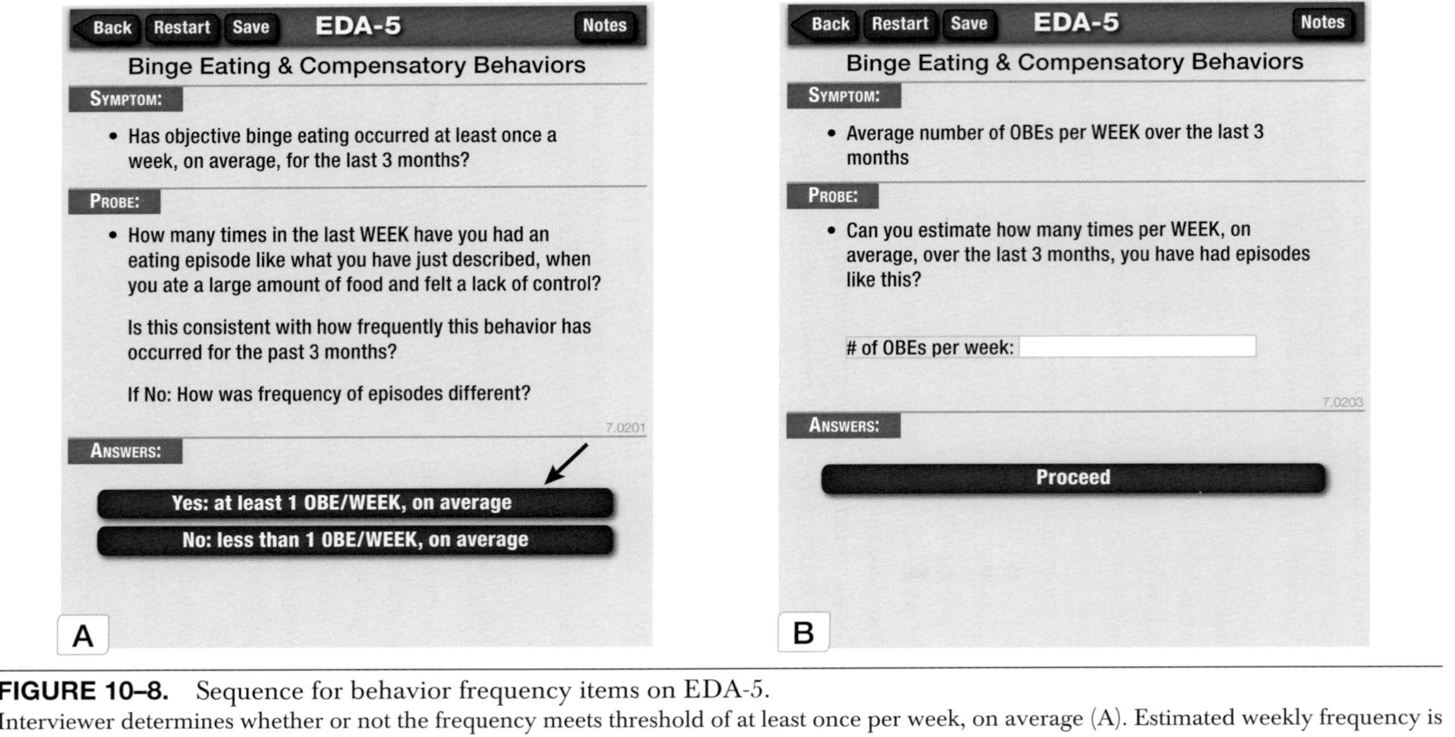

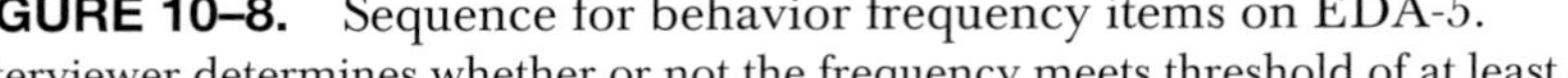

FIGURE 10–8. Sequence for behavior frequency items on EDA-5.
Interviewer determines whether or not the frequency meets threshold of at least once per week, on average (A). Estimated weekly frequency is entered (B).

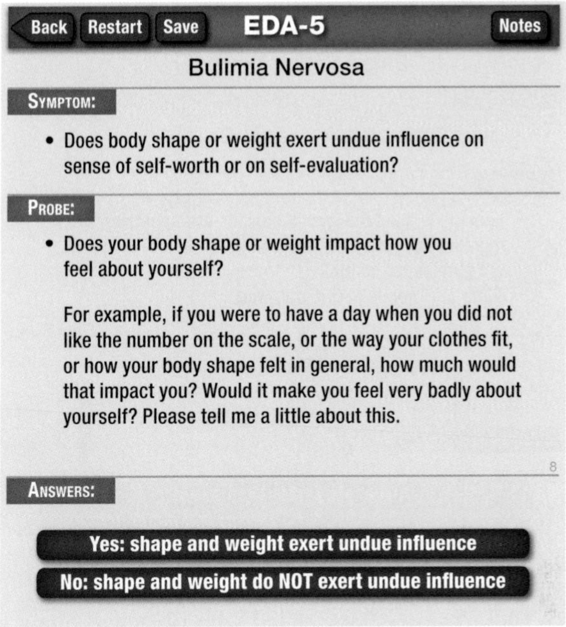

Back Restart Save **EDA-5** Notes

Bulimia Nervosa

SYMPTOM:

- Does body shape or weight exert undue influence on sense of self-worth or on self-evaluation?

PROBE:

- Does your body shape or weight impact how you feel about yourself?

For example, if you were to have a day when you did not like the number on the scale, or the way your clothes fit, or how your body shape felt in general, how much would that impact you? Would it make you feel very badly about yourself? Please tell me a little about this.

8

ANSWERS:

Yes: shape and weight exert undue influence

No: shape and weight do NOT exert undue influence

FIGURE 10–9. EDA-5 questions on overvaluation of shape and weight.

Binge-Eating Disorder

Assuming that the individual is *not* underweight (either currently or in the past 3 months), has endorsed at least one OBE per week on average, and denies frequent inappropriate compensatory behavior in the 3 months prior to assessment, the interviewer is directed to the BED section of the EDA-5. The next several items assess features typically associated with OBEs (e.g., eating more rapidly than normal, eating in the absence of hunger). For each probe, the interviewer is encouraged to anchor the individual to the OBE example described in the Binge Eating and Compensatory Behaviors section (see Figures 10–5 and 10–10). Per the DSM-5 criteria, if the individual endorses at least three of the five features and endorses significant distress about the binge episodes, the individual meets criteria for a BED diagnosis; a pop-up window indicates that a diagnosis has been reached. Regardless of whether or not a diagnosis of BED is assigned, the interviewer is guided next into the ARFID section of the EDA-5.

It may be surprising that the EDA-5 assesses for the presence of ARFID even after an individual's symptoms have satisfied the criteria for BED. A brief description of the trumping rules embedded in the feeding and eating disorders section of DSM-5 is required in order to explain the

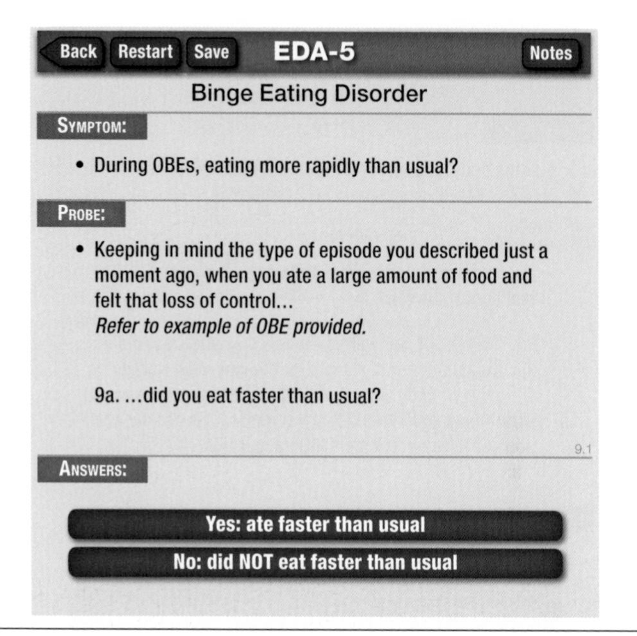

FIGURE 10–10. Feature(s) associated with objective binge episodes in EDA-5.

rationale. In DSM-5, a current diagnosis of AN excludes a diagnosis of any other feeding or eating disorder except pica (in the DSM-5 scheme, individuals with any other disorder can also receive a diagnosis of pica). Similarly, if criteria for AN are not met but criteria for BN are satisfied, the diagnosis of BN excludes all other disorders except pica. A diagnosis of AN, BN, BED, or ARFID excludes a diagnosis of rumination disorder. However, DSM-5 does *not* provide explicit guidance on whether a diagnosis of ARFID should exclude a diagnosis of BED or vice versa. In reality, it is difficult to imagine that an individual's symptoms would simultaneously involve both frequent binge eating and the level of clinically significant restriction of food intake required for ARFID. Nonetheless, because the DSM-5 criteria do not exclude this possibility, the criteria for ARFID are assessed in the EDA-5 even after a diagnosis of BED has been made; if the criteria for ARFID are satisfied, the EDA-5 will also assign that diagnosis.

Avoidant/Restrictive Food Intake Disorder

The EDA-5 gateway item for the ARFID section is the presence of severe food restriction or avoidance that has resulted in nutritional problems

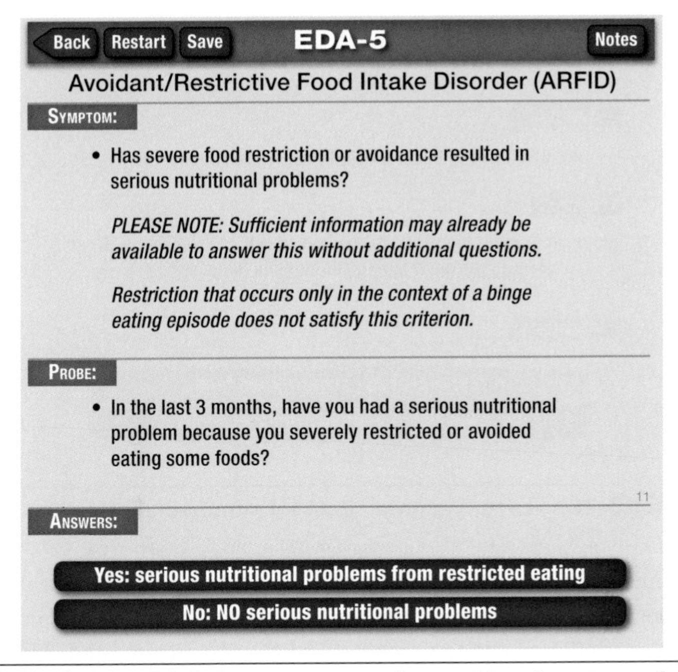

FIGURE 10–11. EDA-5 gateway item for avoidant/restrictive food intake disorder (ARFID).

(Figure 10–11). At this juncture, a note reminds the interviewer that "sufficient information may already be available to answer this without additional questions." This reminder is included because, as described in the previous paragraph, depending on the symptoms that have thus far been endorsed by the individual (i.e., subthreshold BN or BED symptoms), the transition into the ARFID section can be awkward.

If the first ARFID symptom is denied (or not met on the basis of information already obtained) and neither a BN nor BED diagnosis was previously assigned, then the interviewer is guided into the Rumination Disorder section. If serious nutritional problems as a result of highly restrictive eating are present, the interviewer is guided to ask four additional probes to assess 1) significant weight loss, 2) related significant medical problems, 3) need for nutritional supplements (e.g., Ensure, Sustacal, Boost) or enteral feeding (e.g., the use of a tube inserted into the stomach), and 4) resultant psychosocial impairment. If one or more of these symptoms are endorsed, the interviewer continues with the remainder of the ARFID items. If all of these symptoms are denied, the interviewer is guided to the Rumination Disorder section.

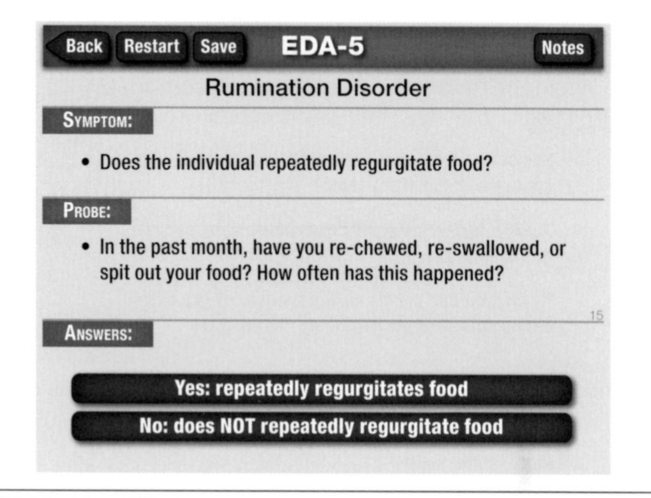

FIGURE 10–12. EDA-5 gateway item for rumination disorder.

To meet criteria for a diagnosis of ARFID, the individual's eating disturbance must not be better explained by a lack of available resources, by culturally sanctioned eating practices, or by a concurrent medical or mental condition. It should be noted that many individuals with ARFID have (or have had) a problem that contributes to the restrictive eating, such as medical illnesses affecting the gastrointestinal tract (e.g., regional enteritis, gluten intolerance, food allergies) or other mental disorders (e.g., autism spectrum disorder). An important question is whether the restrictive eating problem is so severe that it requires clinical attention in addition to that routinely needed to address the other disorder.

If ARFID is diagnosed, a pop-up window indicates to the interviewer that a diagnosis has been reached, and the EDA-5 directs the interviewer to the Pica section. If ARFID criteria are not met, the interviewer is directed to the Rumination Disorder section.

Rumination Disorder

The Rumination Disorder section of the EDA-5 requires an initial assessment of the presence of repeated regurgitation of food via re-chewing, re-swallowing, or spitting out of food (Figure 10–12). If this behavior is absent, the interviewer proceeds to the Pica section. If such behavior is present, the interviewer is guided to determine if it is best accounted for by another medical or mental condition, such as esophageal reflux or intellectual disability. Rumination disorder frequently occurs in association with medical problems such as esophageal reflux; the critical question, in this instance,

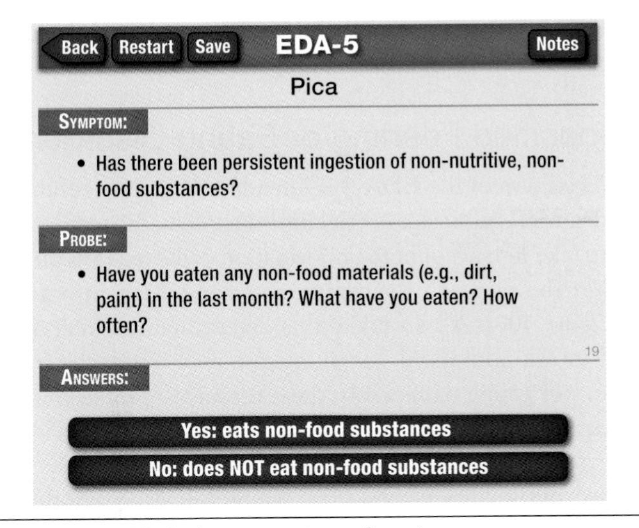

FIGURE 10–13. EDA-5 gateway item for pica.

is whether or not the reflux is sufficient to explain the symptoms of rumination.

If there is no alternate problem associated with this behavior (or if the alternate is not a sufficient explanation of the symptoms described) and if the severity of the behavior warrants specialized clinical attention (e.g., nutritional counseling, targeted psychotherapy), a diagnosis of rumination disorder is indicated by a pop-up window. Whether or not a diagnosis of rumination disorder is assigned, the next section presented is the Pica section.

Pica

Pica, characterized by the repeated ingestion of nonnutritive substances, can occur with any of the other feeding and eating disorders. Thus, all individuals are asked about at least the gateway item for this section of the EDA-5 (Figure 10–13). Because the EDA-5, in its current form, is an adult assessment, the eating of nonnutritive substances is assumed to be inappropriate to the individual's developmental level. When individuals endorse this behavior, interviewers must confirm 1) that this is not part of a culturally sanctioned or normative practice and 2) that if the behavior occurs in the setting of an associated medical or mental condition (e.g., pregnancy, intellectual disability), it is severe enough to merit specialized clinical attention. In these cases, a diagnosis of pica is assigned and is indicated in a pop-up window.

At this juncture in the interview, if a feeding and eating disorder diagnosis has been made, the interviewer will be provided with a summary form of EDA-5 results (see "Notes and Results" section below). If no feeding or eating disorder diagnosis has thus far been assigned, the interviewer will be guided into the OSFED section.

Other Specified Feeding or Eating Disorder

The OSFED section of the EDA-5 is intended to capture residual feeding and eating disorder diagnoses. A brief introduction to the section advises interviewers to take into account the information collected thus far and to decide whether the cluster of symptoms endorsed fits into an OSFED category (Figure 10–14A). To make this determination, interviewers will likely need to ask additional questions, possibly about the individual's weight history or eating patterns. In these instances, probes might include the following:

1. What has your highest weight been within the last 3 months?
2. How much weight, if any, have you lost in the last 3 months? 6 months? Year?
3. Do you eat at night, long after dinner or after you have slept for a while? How often has this occurred in the last 3 months? What do you remember about these types of eating episodes?

On the following screen, the interviewer will be asked to choose the most appropriate diagnosis based on the data and the interviewer's clinical impression (Figure 10–14B). Because DSM-5 does not provide diagnostic criteria for any of these disorders and because an individual may have symptoms consistent with more than one OSFED, the clinician must use his or her judgment to decide which category is most appropriate.

One option in the OSFED section of the EDA-5 is "other (unspecified) feeding or eating disorder." The interviewer assigns this diagnosis when an individual has an unspecified but clinically significant constellation of feeding and eating disorder symptoms that do not meet either the criteria for any of the formally recognized feeding and eating disorders or the descriptions provided in the OSFED section of the EDA-5.

Notes and Results

Interviewer Notes

The EDA-5 allows for the interviewer to take notes as needed by using the "Notes" button at the top right-hand corner of each screen (see Figure 10–1). New comments are added to those previously entered, and all comments are

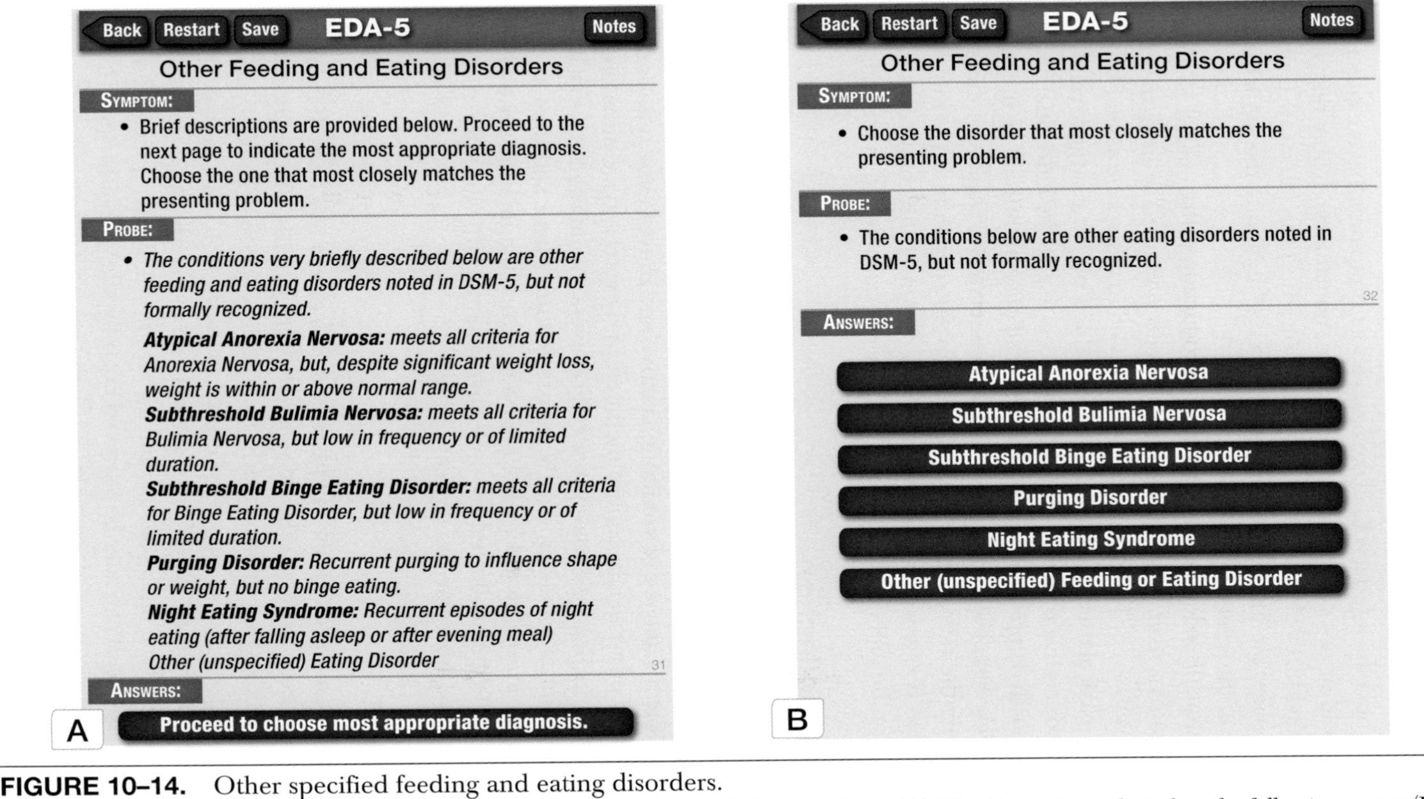

FIGURE 10–14. Other specified feeding and eating disorders.
Brief descriptions of other feeding and eating disorders are provided to guide the interviewer (A). The diagnosis is selected on the following screen (B).

printed in the final report at the conclusion of the interview (see "Output" section below). The notes area is meant to be used by the interviewer throughout the interview to make notes about symptoms that are either subthreshold or not clearly diagnostic but are, nonetheless, highly relevant to the individual's clinical presentation. To return to the interview from the Notes page, the interviewer presses the "Save" button at the top left-hand corner of the screen.

Upon completion of the EDA-5, the interviewer is guided to a final comments screen, in which the interviewer is reminded to enter additional notes as desired. The notes space can be used to remark on salient features of the particular case (e.g., if the individual is a bariatric surgery candidate or postoperative patient) or interview process (e.g., if the individual had difficulty with comprehension of items or recall of symptoms). If an individual has been diagnosed with an OSFED, the interviewer might use this space to clarify the rationale for his or her diagnostic decision. If the individual has been diagnosed with USFED, a description of the condition's symptoms can be noted in this space. All notes will be included in the output.

Data Collection

The following data are collected and stored by the EDA-5 for output on the Results screen (Figure 10–15): Interview (demographics), BMI, Binge Eating (typical OBE items and OBEs per week), specific compensatory behaviors (frequency of vomiting; laxative and diuretic use; type and frequency of other weight-control methods; and exercise type, duration, and frequency), Diagnosis, and Notes. Interviewers should remember that this information is *not* electronically transferred anywhere and item-by-item responses are *not* stored by the interview. Once the interviewer exits the EDA-5, the data collected are no longer retained. However, the report itself may be stored on the device.

Output

Output from the interview can be recorded in one of two ways. If the interviewer selects "print" on the Results screen (Figure 10–15), the interviewer will be guided to a reformatted EDA-5 Results screen (Figure 10–16) that can be printed if a printer is accessible to the device. Alternatively, if the interviewer selects "Save," he or she is asked to log in to an account previously established on the device, and the report will be encrypted and stored on the device. It can later be retrieved but only after the interviewer logs in with the username and password he or she previously entered.

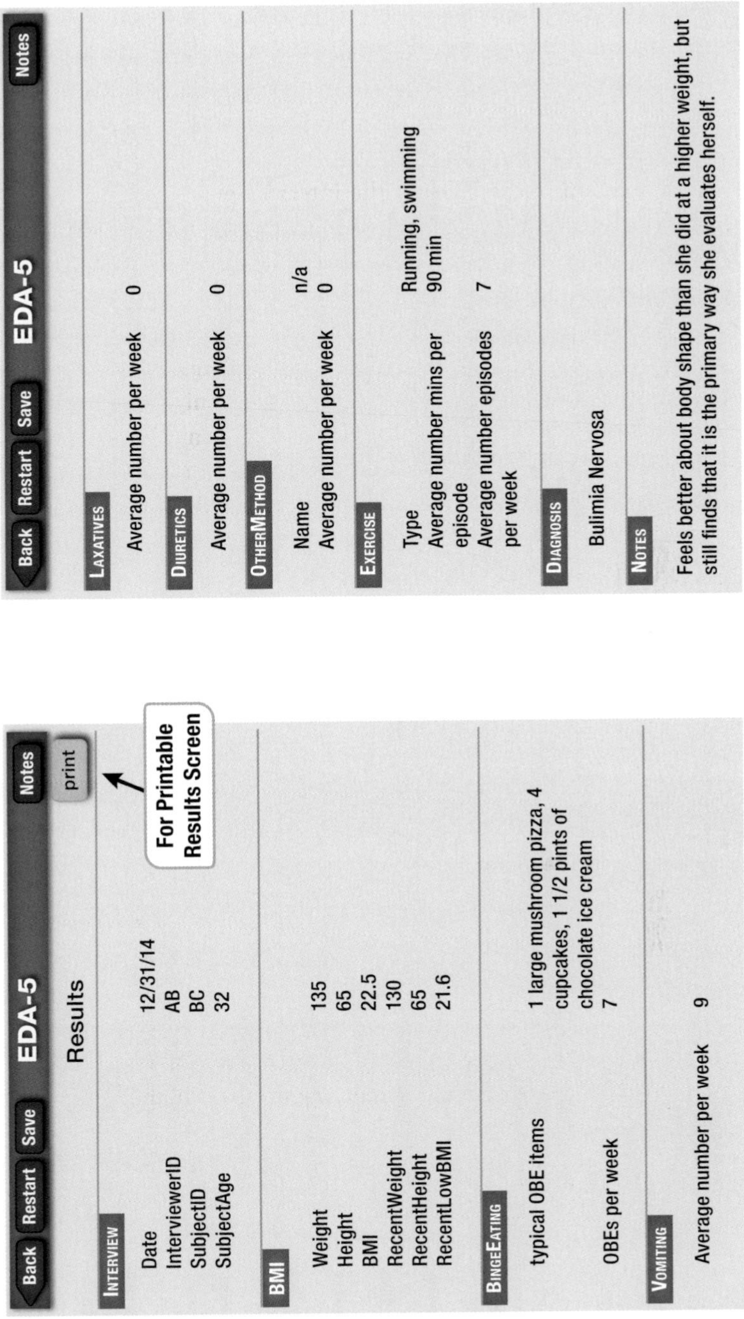

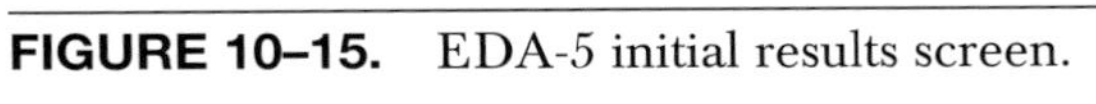

FIGURE 10–15. EDA-5 initial results screen.

EDA-5 Results

Interview		
	Date	12/31/14
	InterviewerID	AB
	SubjectID	BC
	SubjectAge	32
BMI		
	Weight	135
	Height	65
	BMI	22.5
	RecentWeight	130
	RecentHeight	65
	RecentLowBMI	21.6
BingeEating		
	typical OBE items	1 large mushroom pizza, 4 cupcakes, 1 1/2 pints of chocolate ice cream
	OBEs per week	7
Vomiting		
	Average number per week	9
Laxatives		
	Average number per week	0
Diuretics		
	Average number per week	0
OtherMethod		
	Name	n/a
	Average number per week	0
Exercise		
	Type	Running, swimming
	Average number mins per episode	90 min
	Average number episodes per week	7
Diagnosis		
	Bulimia Nervosa	
Notes		

Feels better about body shape than she did at a higher weight, but still finds that it is the primary way she evaluates herself.

FIGURE 10–16. EDA-5 printable results form.

Future Directions

We hope that the first version of the EDA-5 provides an acceptable, accurate tool for the diagnosis of DSM-5 feeding and eating disorders. We are well aware that in this original form, the EDA-5 does not fit all professionals' needs. Depending on the setting, for example, interviewers may prefer a long-form version of the measure (i.e., without trumping rules) or a measure that assesses past feeding and eating disorder diagnoses (such as tools described in Chapter 8, "Assessment Measures, Then and Now").

It is also apparent that several more substantial adaptations of the original EDA-5 warrant development and rigorous study. For example, a broad categories system of diagnosis (i.e., focusing on shared features or symptom clusters of feeding and eating conditions) was proposed as a potentially useful diagnostic scheme to reduce the number of cases classified as eating disorder not otherwise specified using DSM-IV (Sysko and Walsh 2011a, 2011b; Walsh and Sysko 2009). This type of classification system appears to virtually eliminate the need for a residual diagnostic category (Machado et al. 2013; Nakai et al. 2013; Sysko and Walsh 2011a, 2011b). The utility of this system in reducing the number of cases designated as DSM-5 OSFED and USFED could be evaluated if the EDA-5 is adapted for broad categories assessment.

To be used across a variety of different populations, the EDA-5 must also undergo adaptation. Perhaps the most straightforward of these changes would be translation of the measure into other languages so that it can be used across cultures and countries to enhance accuracy and standardization of feeding and eating disorder diagnoses. In addition, the EDA-5 would benefit from modest changes to make it more palatable to and appropriate for younger populations, akin to adjustments made to the EDE for use with children (Bryant-Waugh et al. 1996) (see Chapter 11, "Diagnosis of Feeding and Eating Disorders in Children and Adolescents").

Conclusion

The EDA-5 is a novel measure providing comprehensive assessment of DSM-5 feeding and eating disorder criteria while reducing participant burden and requiring minimal interviewer training. It is our hope that this semistructured interview will address some of the limitations of prior assessments and will prove helpful to practitioners ranging broadly in professional background, specialty, and experience across a variety of clinical and research settings.

Key Clinical Points

- The Eating Disorder Assessment for DSM-5 (EDA-5) assesses *current* feeding and eating disorders *in adults* according to the DSM-5 criteria. It is intended for use by clinicians and researchers in a variety of disciplines (e.g., nursing, psychology, social work), and it assumes familiarity with the DSM-5 feeding and eating disorder diagnoses.
- In contrast to other available semistructured diagnostic interviews, the EDA-5 requires minimal interviewer training and reduces participant burden.
- In its current electronic application form, the EDA-5 uses automated skip rules to mirror DSM-5's diagnostic "trumping" rules.
- The EDA-5 collects and retains information about frequency of behavioral symptoms of feeding and eating conditions; however, it is not aimed at a broader assessment of associated psychopathological features, such as the intensity of concerns over shape or weight.
- In initial psychometric studies, the EDA-5 demonstrated high rates of diagnostic agreement with the Eating Disorder Examination (EDE) and with clinician interview. In addition, test-retest reliability of the EDA-5 was excellent. The EDA-5 required significantly less time to complete than the EDE.
- Although further study of the measure's ability to diagnose feeding disorders is warranted and further development of the measure so that it might be used across a variety of populations is needed, the EDA-5 is a promising new diagnostic instrument for the assessment of DSM-5 feeding and eating disorders.

References

American Psychiatric Association: Diagnostic and Statistical Manual of Mental Disorders, 4th Edition. Washington, DC, American Psychiatric Association, 1994

American Psychiatric Association: Diagnostic and Statistical Manual of Mental Disorders, 5th Edition. Arlington, VA, American Psychiatric Association, 2013

Blomquist KK, Roberto CA, Barnes RD, et al: Development and validation of the Eating Loss of Control Scale. Psychol Assess 26(1):77–89, 2014 24219700

Bryant-Waugh RJ, Cooper PJ, Taylor CL, et al: The use of the Eating Disorder Examination with children: a pilot study. Int J Eat Disord 19(4):391–397, 1996 8859397

Fairburn CG, Cooper Z, O'Connor M: Eating Disorder Examination, Edition 16.0D, in Cognitive Behavior Therapy and Eating Disorders. Edited by Fairburn CG. New York, Guilford, 2008, pp 265–308

First MB, Williams JBW, Karg RS, et al: Structured Clinical Interview for DSM-5 Disorders, Research Version (SCID-5-RV). Arlington, VA, American Psychiatric Association, 2015

Latner JD, Mond JM, Kelly MC, et al: The Loss of Control over Eating Scale: development and psychometric evaluation. Int J Eat Disord 47(6):647–659, 2014 24862351

Machado PP, Gonçalves S, Hoek HW: DSM-5 reduces the proportion of EDNOS cases: evidence from community samples. Int J Eat Disord 46(1):60–65, 2013 22815201

Nakai Y, Nin K, Teramukai S, et al: Comparison of DSM-IV diagnostic criteria versus the Broad Categories for the Diagnosis of Eating Disorders scheme in a Japanese sample. Eat Behav 14(3):330–335, 2013 23910776

Sysko R, Walsh BT: Does the Broad Categories for the Diagnosis of Eating Disorders (BCD-ED) scheme reduce the frequency of eating disorder not otherwise specified? Int J Eat Disord 44(7):625–629, 2011a 21997426

Sysko R, Walsh BT: Rethinking the nosology of eating disorders, in Developing an Evidence-Based Classification of Eating Disorders: Scientific Findings for DSM-5. Edited by Striegel-Moore RH, Wonderlich SA, Walsh T, et al. Arlington, VA, American Psychiatric Association, 2011b, pp 3–17

Sysko R, Glasofer DR, Hildebrandt T, et al: The Eating Disorder Assessment for DSM-5 (EDA-5): development and validation of a structured interview for feeding and eating disorders. Int J Eat Disord 48(5):452–463, 2015 25639562

Tanofsky-Kraff M, Yanovski SZ, Wilfley DE, et al: Eating-disordered behaviors, body fat, and psychopathology in overweight and normal-weight children. J Consult Clin Psychol 72(1):53–61, 2004 14756614

Walsh BT, Sysko R: Broad Categories for the Diagnosis of Eating Disorders (BCD-ED): an alternative system for classification. Int J Eat Disord 42(8):754–764, 2009 19650083

11 Diagnosis of Feeding and Eating Disorders in Children and Adolescents

Natasha A. Schvey, Ph.D.
Kamryn T. Eddy, Ph.D.
Marian Tanofsky-Kraff, Ph.D.

Eating disorders affect nearly 3% of adolescents in the United States (Swanson et al. 2011), whereas associated psychopathology, such as undue influence of shape and weight (Neumark-Sztainer et al. 2002), loss of control over eating (Tanofsky-Kraff et al. 2008a), unhealthy weight-control practices (Neumark-Sztainer et al. 2012), and compensatory behaviors (Solmi et al. 2014), is increasingly common among both male and female youths (Ackard et al. 2007; Field et al. 2014). Disordered eating attitudes and behaviors are associated with numerous physical and psychological consequences, including depression, substance use, and

---

The opinions or assertions contained herein are the private ones of the authors and are not to be construed as official or reflecting the views of the Department of Defense, the Henry M. Jackson Foundation, or the Uniformed Services University of the Health Sciences.

poorer overall health (Field et al. 2012). Furthermore, unhealthy weight-control behaviors in youths are significant risk factors for the development of full-threshold eating disorders, and binge eating and loss-of-control eating in youth predict weight gain and excess adiposity (Goldschmidt et al. 2013), placing children at risk for a host of psychological and physical comorbidities (Dixon 2010). Importantly, research has consistently shown that eating disturbances tend to begin in childhood and adolescence (Tanofsky-Kraff et al. 2004); therefore, early detection of aberrant eating behaviors and cognitions is crucial for both prevention and treatment. Because childhood and adolescent eating symptoms commonly persist into adulthood (Goldschmidt et al. 2014; Kotler et al. 2001) and overweight youths are up to 20 times more likely to be overweight adults (Field et al. 2005), the assessment and diagnosis of feeding and eating disorders in youths and adolescents are critical (see also Chapter 3, "Eating Problems in Children and Adolescents").

The assessment of eating disorder symptoms in youths presents unique challenges, such as the child's or adolescent's unfamiliarity with key constructs (Bravender et al. 2007; Neumark-Sztainer and Story 1998); the lack of concordance between self-report, parent-report, and interview assessments (Field et al. 2004; Shomaker et al. 2013; Tanofsky-Kraff et al. 2003); the need for clarification of certain terms, such as *dieting,* which may be subject to interpretation (Neumark-Sztainer and Story 1998); and the selection of developmentally appropriate definitions and criteria (e.g., determination of what constitutes an "objectively large amount of food" for a growing child). Although measures of eating disorder symptoms and associated features developed for adults have been used unaltered with pediatric and adolescent samples, we focus in this chapter exclusively on measures that have been specifically developed or adapted for use in youths. We assembled our list, which is not exhaustive, by searching scholarly databases for terms related to child and adolescent feeding and eating disorders, diagnostic assessment, and eating pathology. We have included measures that assess eating disorders and eating-related psychopathology specifically in children and adolescents under age 18 years.

DSM-5 (American Psychiatric Association 2013), the most recent edition of the *Diagnostic and Statistical Manual,* was published in 2013. Consequently, at the time this chapter was written, few measures had been developed to assess the diagnostic criteria for feeding and eating disorders, which have undergone changes since DSM-IV (American Psychiatric Association 1994). Moreover, there is a paucity of measures that assess *pica* (the persistent ingestion of nonnutritive items such as dirt and chalk), *rumination disorder* (repeated regurgitation of food), or avoidant/restrictive food intake disorder (ARFID), a reformulation of the DSM-IV diagnosis, "feeding disorder of infancy or early childhood" (see also Chapter 8, "Assessment Measures, Then and Now"). The development of assessment tools to detect these aberrant behaviors in youths is critical for both research and clinical practice. If youths and/or their parents are not queried and assessed for specific symptoms, it is unlikely that the behavior(s) will be detected within clinical or research settings, and thus intervention and treatment may be thwarted and research efforts hindered. At the conclusion of this chapter in the section "Proposed Eating Disorder Assessment for DSM-5 Adaptation for Youths," we propose and discuss a novel assessment tool to address these gaps.

Tools to Assess Eating Disorder Symptoms

Interview Versus Self-Report Methodology

Interview methodology is often considered the optimal means of assessing eating-related psychopathology (Fairburn and Beglin 1994). This is largely because interviews allow for explanation and clarification of complex core features germane to feeding and eating disorders. Additionally, interviews are often considered preferable because of the methodological limitations inherent in self-report measures, such as selection of socially acceptable responses, nonresponse, and lack of clarification for ambiguous terms (e.g., dieting, loss of control). Although concordance between interview and self-report measures is high for unambiguous behaviors, such as laxative misuse, much lower concordance is observed for those behaviors whose definitions are more abstract, such as binge eating and overvaluation of shape (Fairburn and Beglin 1994). Other factors such as literacy level, speaking English as a second language, and cultural differences might impede an individual's comprehension and valid completion of questionnaire measures. In the assessment of children, semistructured interview methods are not reliant on literacy and thus may be appropriate for a wider range of ages and socioeconomic backgrounds. (For more interview methodology, see Chapter 8.)

Despite the advantages of interview methodology, there are also considerable disadvantages, especially among pediatric samples. Interview methods may be costly, because of the extensive training required for assessors as well as the significant amount of time the administration may require (30–60 minutes on average, and potentially longer for children who have difficulty comprehending abstract concepts) (Fairburn and Beglin 1994). In contrast, self-report measures are often brief and require little training or qualification for assessors. Also, interview methods are not feasible in the collection of nationally representative data and therefore may be less practical for large-scale research samples. Furthermore, certain behaviors, such as purging and binge eating, may be considered shameful by the respondent, who may be less likely to endorse such behaviors in a face-to-face interview (Lavender and Anderson 2009); this potential issue is especially salient for adolescents, who may be particularly self-conscious and sensitive to the perceived judgment of others. As a result, the assessor must take into account the purpose of the assessment, characteristics of the respondent, and practical considerations when selecting the most appropriate measure. The use of more than one type of assessment is typically recommended to best capture complex eating pathology and associated features (Tanofsky-Kraff 2008).

Interview Measures

Eating Disorder Examination Adapted for Children

To date, the most commonly used interview measure for the assessment of eating pathology in youths is the Eating Disorder Examination adapted for children (ChEDE; Bryant-Waugh et al. 1996). Adapted from the 61-item Eating Disorder Examination (EDE; Fairburn and Cooper 1993), the ChEDE was first piloted in a sample of children ages 7–14 seeking treatment in an eating disorders clinic. The ChEDE, like the EDE, is a semistructured interview, a format that facilitates an interactive assessment wherein a child's questions can be answered, age-related differences may be addressed, and key concepts (e.g., loss of control) can be explained in full until the child demonstrates comprehension. Additionally, follow-up queries can be posed to the child for improved specificity and accuracy. The ChEDE yields four subscale scores–Dietary Restraint, Eating Concern, Shape Concern, and Weight Concern–and a global score, all of which range from 1 to 6 (with higher scores indicative of greater pathology). The ChEDE may be used diagnostically to determine the presence of anorexia nervosa (AN), bulimia nervosa (BN), binge-eating disorder (BED), or other specified feeding or eating disorder (OSFED), as well as to further elucidate subthreshold eating pathology, such as undue influence of shape or weight or compensatory behaviors.

Training for administration of the ChEDE is ideally conducted by trained postgraduates in the field of pediatric eating disorders and entails reviewing the criteria for eating disorders and discussing each item on the interview. Audiotaped interviews are listened to and co-rated by trainees. Trainees then practice administering the ChEDE with simulated patients, observe an actual ChEDE administration, and ultimately administer the ChEDE under observation and supervision. Training continues until interrater reliability between trainee and trainer reaches 95%. To ensure fidelity, ongoing supervision is provided and all ChEDE administrations are audiotaped so that ambiguous responses may be reviewed in regular meetings. Additional information on training for the ChEDE is described elsewhere (Tanofsky-Kraff et al. 2004, 2007a).

One primary adaptation that differentiates the ChEDE from the EDE is the use of a card sort task to assess overvaluation of shape and weight, which may be an abstract and difficult concept for children to grasp. In the card sort task, children are asked to write down "those things that are important to you in how you see yourself or think about yourself" and sort the items in order of importance. The child is then asked to indicate where on this list shape and weight would fit. Additionally, for the ChEDE, certain items have been rephrased to better assess intent as opposed to behavior. For instance, although a child may wish to abstain from food for a period of 8 hours or more, he or she may be unable to do so because of parental supervision. To assess this possibility, the original ChEDE asks, "Would you have done ____ if you *could* have?" (Bryant-Waugh et al. 1996). Recent iterations of the ChEDE, however, have opted out of this modification (Tanofsky-Kraff et al. 2007a). The interviewer should use his or her discretion in determining whether to assess both behavior and intent.

The ChEDE queries respondents primarily regarding the 4 weeks preceding administration to assess present functioning. Because DSM-5 diagnostic criteria for both BN and BED require a duration of 3 months, the respondent is also asked to recall certain feelings and behaviors (e.g., meal skipping, binge episodes) during this time span. Owing to difficulty in recall for children, parents may be enlisted to help with this task. Specifically, a parent or guardian may fill in a 3-month calendar with significant events and scheduled activities (e.g., holidays, birthdays, after-school clubs) to cue the child's memory.

The ChEDE enables the categorization of eating episodes into four different types: objective bulimic episodes, subjective bulimic episodes, objective overeating without the experience of loss of control, and no episode. To ascertain the presence of an eating episode, the interviewer asks respondents about the "largest" amount of food they have consumed within the past 28 days. To assist respondents with recollecting types and amounts of food consumed in a given episode, a book of photographed food portions may be employed as a visual aid (Hess 1997). It is recommended that determination of whether an ambiguously large amount of food is "objectively large" be made by consensus of the research team.

Whereas DSM-5 diagnostic criteria for BED in adults specify that binge-eating episodes must be objectively large, extant research indicates that the presence of loss of control, rather than amount of food consumed, may be the more salient feature of a binge episode in youths (Shomaker et al. 2010). Furthermore, because it may be difficult to determine what constitutes an objectively large amount of food in children and adolescents who reach puberty and physical maturation at different rates, the presence of loss of control is often a more accurate proxy for a binge-eating episode in youths. Therefore, it is critical to assess both objective binge-eating episodes and subjective binge-eating episodes; in the latter, the child experiences loss of control while consuming a subjectively large amount of food.

The ChEDE has been used to assess children as young as age 6 years (Tanofsky-Kraff et al. 2003) and may be used through late adolescence. The ChEDE has demonstrated excellent psychometric properties, including interrater reliability, internal consistency, and discriminant validity in both clinical and research samples (Bryant-Waugh et al. 1996; Tanofsky-Kraff et al. 2004). Administration typically takes 1 hour, although 1½ hours may be more realistic for younger children, youths with attention deficits, or youths who struggle to comprehend abstract concepts. At the onset of the interview, youths are informed that they may take breaks as needed (e.g., to use a restroom or stretch). Breaks may also be suggested at the interviewer's discretion if a child begins to lose focus.

Supplemental Sections to the Eating Disorder Examination Adapted for Children

To bolster the ChEDE's specificity and utility, two supplemental sections have been added: the Standard Pediatric Eating Episode Interview (SPEEI) (Tanofsky-Kraff et al. 2007a) and the Age of Onset of any Eating-Disordered Behavior, Overweight, and Dieting (Tanofsky-Kraff et al. 2005). Both have demonstrated feasibility in pediatric and adolescent samples.

Administered following the overeating section of the ChEDE, the SPEEI queries respondents about the behavioral, physical, emotional, and contextual aspects of a specified eating episode. The SPEEI is used to assess critical features of a binge episode, such as negative affect, prior caloric restriction, and shame following eating. If a child endorses more than one aberrant eating episode, only one is selected as the target for the SPEEI (Tanofsky-Kraff et al. 2007a). The SPEEI is a useful clinical and research tool to further assess antecedents to, subjective experience during, and emotional and physical consequences of a binge episode.

The Age of Onset of any Eating-Disordered Behavior, Overweight, and Dieting supplement to the ChEDE (Tanofsky-Kraff et al. 2005) provides additional temporal information pertaining to loss of control over eating, dieting, and overweight onset. Children are queried regarding the onset, duration, and nature of dieting attempts and weight-control behaviors; the age at which they became overweight; and the age at which they first experienced loss of control, regardless of the amount of food consumed.

Children's Binge Eating Disorder Scale

The Children's Binge Eating Disorder Scale (C-BEDS; Shapiro et al. 2007) is a brief seven-item interview assessment of BED and subthreshold binge behaviors, such as eating in response to negative affect. This measure may be a useful instrument for assessing both threshold and subsyndromal binge eating in youths. Additionally, the child-friendly terminology and brevity make it a viable screening tool for the presence of binge behaviors in youths. Because the C-BEDS employs provisional diagnostic criteria and has not yet been validated in large, diverse samples, it would benefit from additional psychometric testing and validation. This measure is useful in assessing specific behaviors and cognitions associated with binge eating in a brief interview format wherein difficult concepts may be explained and elaborated upon.

Self-Report Measures

Although semistructured interviews are often considered the gold standard method of assessment in youths (Tanofsky-Kraff et al. 2003), existing research indicates that methods of assessment, such as self-report questionnaires, that do not involve direct questioning by an interviewer may yield higher and potentially more valid rates of eating pathology, the open expression of which may be blunted during face-to-face interviews (Lavender and Anderson 2009). Although self-report measures have utility in clinical and research settings, they may require supplemental objective and/or parent-report data. Selection of measures may vary depending on the purpose of assessment; for instance, some assessments are diagnostic, whereas others may be more useful in elucidating accompanying symptoms and subsyndromal behaviors (see also Chapter 9, "Self-Report Assessments of Eating Pathology").

Diagnostic Measures

To diagnostically assess eating disorders in youths, well-validated adult measures, such as the Eating Disorder Examination Questionnaire (EDE-Q; Fairburn and Beglin 1994) and the Questionnaire on Eating and Weight Patterns (QEWP; Spitzer et al. 1993), have been adapted and validated for use in pediatric populations to determine the presence of AN, BN, BED, and OSFED. The EDE-Q has not yet been adapted for DSM-5; the QEWP adaptation for DSM-5 was recently published (Yanovski et al. 2015).

The Youth Eating Disorder Examination Questionnaire (YEDE-Q; Goldschmidt et al. 2007), adapted from the EDE-Q (Fairburn and Beglin 1994), was designed for diagnostic use with child and adolescent samples. The specific modifications were modeled after those used in the ChEDE (Bryant-Waugh et al. 1996), wording was adapted for a third-grade reading level, and examples and pictures are provided. The YEDE-Q, which was piloted in a sample of overweight youths ages 12–17 years, demonstrated agreement with the ChEDE on subscale scores and assessment of binge episodes (Goldschmidt et al. 2007). The YEDE-Q may be used diagnostically to determine presence of AN, BN, BED, and OSFED, as well as to assess subthreshold disordered thoughts and behaviors. The YEDE-Q may be effectively used in place of more cumbersome and time-intensive assessment methods.

The Questionnaire on Eating and Weight Patterns–Adolescent Version (QEWP-A; Johnson et al. 1999) is an adaptation of the QEWP that may be used diagnostically to assesses the presence of BED and BN in youths. It assesses both behavioral and cognitive features and may also be accurate in detecting subthreshold or prodromal BED and BN. The measure, piloted in a sample of individuals ages 10–18 years, demonstrated concurrent validity and stability. See Yanovski et al. (2015) for the QEWP-A DSM-5 adaptation. Table 11–1 summarizes details about diagnostic measures of feeding and eating disorders in youths.

Nondiagnostic Measures

Several adult measures have also been adapted for use with children to assess nondiagnostic markers of eating pathology, such as dieting, food preoccupation, compensatory behaviors, and concerns about becoming overweight. The Children's Eating Attitudes Test (ChEAT; Maloney et al. 1988), adapted from the Eating Attitudes Test (EAT; Garner and Garfinkel 1979), reliably assesses food preoccupation, dieting, eating-related attitudes, and fear of becoming overweight in youths age 8 or older. The measure has demonstrated strong test-retest and internal reliability, and administration takes approximately 35 minutes. Scores are comparable to those observed in adult samples (Maloney et al. 1988).

The Eating Disorder Inventory–Child (EDI-C; Garner 1991) is an adaptation of the Eating Disorder Inventory (EDI; Garner et al. 1983), a nondiagnostic, multiscale assessment of symptoms commonly associated with AN and BN. The measure consists of 91 forced-choice items, which form 11 subscales: three assess thoughts and behaviors related to eating, shape, and weight; five capture psychological traits associated with eating pathology (e.g., perfectionism, interoceptive awareness); and the rest assess traits commonly observed in eating disorder patients (e.g., impulse regulation).

TABLE 11–1. Tools to assess eating disorder symptoms: child assessments

Measure	Type of assessment	Symptoms assessed	Age (years)	Number of items/duration	Citation
Diagnostic measures					
Children's Binge Eating Disorder Scale (C-BEDS)	Interview	Binge-eating disorder and subthreshold binge behaviors	5–13	7	Shapiro et al. 2007
Eating Disorder Examination Adapted for Children (ChEDE)	Interview	Anorexia nervosa, bulimia nervosa, binge-eating disorder, other specified feeding or eating disorders	7–14	36/1 hour	Bryant-Waugh et al. 1996
Questionnaire on Eating and Weight Patterns–Adolescent Version (QEWP-A)	Questionnaire	Binge-eating disorder, bulimia nervosa	10–18	12	Johnson et al. 1999
Youth Eating Disorder Examination Questionnaire (YEDE-Q)	Questionnaire	Anorexia nervosa, bulimia nervosa, binge-eating disorder, other specified feeding or eating disorders	12–17	39	Goldschmidt et al. 2007
Nondiagnostic measures					
Children's Eating Attitudes Test (ChEAT)	Questionnaire	Food preoccupation, dieting, eating-related attitudes	8–13	35 minutes	Maloney et al. 1988
Dutch Eating Behavior Scale (DEBQ)	Questionnaire	Eating in response to negative affect, eating in response to external cues, restraint	7–12	37	van Strien et al. 1986
Eating Disorder Inventory–Child (EDI-C)	Questionnaire	Associated symptoms of anorexia nervosa and bulimia nervosa	9–16	91	Garner 1991
Kids' Eating Disorders Survey (KEDS)	Questionnaire	Body dissatisfaction, restriction, binge eating, compensatory behaviors	9–16	14	Childress et al. 1992

TABLE 11–1. Tools to assess eating disorder symptoms: child assessments *(continued)*

Measure	Type of assessment	Symptoms assessed	Age (years)	Number of items/duration	Citation
Tools to assess associated features					
Eating in the Absence of Hunger for children and adolescents (EAH-C)	Questionnaire	Eating in response to emotional and environmental cues	6–19	14	Tanofsky-Kraff et al. 2008b
Emotional Eating Scale for children and adolescents (EES-C)	Questionnaire	Eating in response to emotional cues	8–18	25	Tanofsky-Kraff et al. 2007c
Perception of Teasing Scale (POTS)	Questionnaire	Weight- and appearance-based teasing	10–18	49	Thompson et al. 1995
Yale Food Addiction Scale for Children (YFAS)	Questionnaire	Food addiction	4–16	25	Gearhardt et al. 2013

The primary factors derived from the EDI-C are drive for thinness, affective instability, self-esteem, overeating, and maturity fears. The EDI-C has been administered to child and adolescent samples (Eklund et al. 2005), although the scale's length may pose a challenge for younger respondents.

The Kids' Eating Disorders Survey (KEDS; Childress et al. 1992) is a self-report nondiagnostic measure that assesses body dissatisfaction, restriction, binge eating, and compensatory behaviors. The KEDS was piloted among respondents ages 9–16 and has demonstrated adequate test-retest reliability (Childress et al. 1993). For an assessment of body dissatisfaction, youths are provided with eight figure drawings and asked to indicate which most resembles their current shape or weight and which resembles what they "would most want to look like." Children are also provided with descriptions of sample binge episodes and asked to indicate whether they have consumed a similar or greater amount in a period of 2 hours. This item, designed to measure binge eating, does not assess loss of control, the hallmark feature of binge eating (Shomaker et al. 2010). Therefore, determination of a binge cannot be made from this measure alone. Furthermore, the sample binge episodes provided may prove difficult for children to extrapolate from in the event that dissimilar foods were consumed during an eating episode. This measure may be most appropriate for assessment of body dissatisfaction, dieting, and compensatory behaviors among school-age children. (See Table 11–1 for a summary of nondiagnostic measures of eating-related psychopathology.)

Tools to Assess Associated Features of Eating Disorder Symptoms

Children and adolescents presenting with disordered eating are a heterogeneous population; therefore, additional indices of eating-related cognitions and behaviors are warranted. Furthermore, certain pathological behaviors and features (e.g., eating in response to negative affect) may precede full-threshold eating disorders and weight problems; therefore, it is critical to assess for aberrant eating attitudes and behaviors in youths. To further elucidate the associated features commonly observed among youths presenting with eating pathology, several measures have been adapted and developed. Four measures that assess associated features specifically pertaining to eating and weight pathology are listed in Table 11–1. Indices (e.g., Children's Depression Inventory) that assess more general psychopathology are beyond the scope of this chapter.

Eating in Response to External and Affective Cues

Environmental cues and affective states can precipitate eating, even in the absence of physiological hunger. Eating in the absence of hunger has been well documented among children and adolescents (Tanofsky-Kraff et al. 2008b) and is associated with loss-of-control eating, dysregulation of hunger and satiety cues, and excess body weight. Questionnaires have been developed for use with children and adolescents to specifically assess eating in the absence of hunger (Tanofsky-Kraff et al. 2008b), eating in response to affective states (Tanofsky-Kraff et al. 2008b)and environmental cues (Tanofsky-Kraff et al. 2007c), and food addiction (Gearhardt et al. 2013) (see details in Table 11–1).

Weight-Based Teasing

The experience of weight-related teasing in youth predicts poor body image, unhealthy eating behaviors, binge eating, and disordered eating cognitions (Puhl and Latner 2007). Therefore, it is critical to assess the experience of weight-based victimization among overweight youths, who are particularly vulnerable to both weight-based teasing and the onset of aberrant eating behaviors. Overweight and obese youths face pervasive stigmatization by peers, teachers, health care providers, and parents. As a result, overweight youths may suffer psychological, interpersonal, and physical health consequences. To measure weight-based and physical appearance–based teasing in youths, the Perception of Teasing Scale (POTS; Thompson et al. 1995) was developed to retrospectively assess teasing that occurred between ages 5 and 16 years.

An additional measure of weight-based victimization, Experiences of Weight-Based Victimization, has been developed for research purposes in adolescent populations (Puhl and Luedicke 2012). This measure identifies the perpetrator, nature, and duration of weight-based teasing, as well as the target's response. Weight-based teasing is useful to assess in both clinical and research settings because it is common among youths of all weight strata (Puhl and Luedicke 2012) and is significantly predictive of unhealthy weight-control practices, binge eating, and disordered eating thoughts and behaviors (Puhl and Latner 2007).

Parent-Report Measures

Because some youths, particularly younger children, may struggle to conceptualize and describe complex emotions and behaviors (e.g., eating in response to negative affect) and may need assistance with the recall and chronology of eating behaviors, parent-report measures may be particularly valuable when assessing disordered eating. Consequently, a number of parent-report measures have been developed to assess feeding and eating disturbances in youths (Table 11–2).

Despite the utility of parent report in providing information that may be beyond the scope of a child's understanding, memory, or insight, informant discrepancies are common among various clinical assessments of psychopathology in youths (De Los Reyes and Kazdin 2005). For instance, parent and child reports of disordered eating demonstrate greatest concordance when no eating pathology is present; the two reports have been shown to lack concordance in the presence of eating pathology (Johnson et al. 1999).

In a large cross-sectional study of nearly 8,000 adolescent-parent dyads, parents and children were generally discordant in symptom reports (Swanson et al. 2014). As in prior studies, parents were less likely than their children to report the children's bulimic behaviors. Additionally, despite pronounced sex differences in self-report measures (adolescent girls are two to four times more likely than male age-mates to report binge eating), parent-report measures did not differ according to the sex of the child (Swanson et al. 2014). Parent-report measures were, however, predictive of body mass index and were also more likely than child measures to accurately report thinness (Swanson et al. 2014). Additionally, parent report may be more reliable for abstract concepts, such as eating in the absence of hunger (Shomaker et al. 2013). Thus, parent-report measures may be useful in identifying youths at risk for low weight, as well as inappropriate weight gain over time. Objective measurement of a child's weight is optimal, although if it is not feasible, parent report is probably preferable to child self-report, because children's estimates of their own weight are frequently inaccurate (Sarafrazi et al. 2014). It is likely, however, that parent-report measures grossly underestimate the presence of secretive binge and compensatory behaviors; therefore, caution should be used when relying solely on parent-report measures.

Parent-Report Interview Measures

Several parent-report interview measures exist to assess general psychopathology in youths. Table 11–2 lists these measures, including the Diagnostic Interview Schedule for Children–Parent Version (DISC-P; Shaffer et al. 1993), the Schedule for Affective Disorders and Schizophrenia for School-Age Children (KSADS; Kaufman et al. 1997), the Development and Well-Being Assessment (DAWBA) parent interview (Goodman et al. 2000), and the Composite International Diagnostic Interview parent interview

TABLE 11–2. Tools to assess eating disorder symptoms: parent reports

Measure	Type of assessment	Symptoms assessed	Age (years)	Citation(s)
Parent-report measures for children and adolescents				
Diagnostic Interview Schedule for Children–Parent Version (DISC-P)	Interview	Comprehensive psychiatric evaluation (with Eating Disorder subsection)	8–19	Fisher et al. 1993; Shaffer et al. 1993
Schedule for Affective Disorders and Schizophrenia for School-Age Children (KSADS)	Interview	Comprehensive psychiatric evaluation (with Eating Disorder subsection)	7–17	Kaufman et al. 1997
Development and Well-Being Assessment (DAWBA) parent interview	Interview	Comprehensive psychiatric evaluation (with Eating Disorder subsection)	5–16	Goodman et al. 2000
Composite International Diagnostic Interview (CIDI) parent interview	Interview	Comprehensive psychiatric evaluation (with Eating Disorder subsection)		Robins et al. 1988
Questionnaire on Eating and Weight Patterns–Parent Version (QEWP-P)	Questionnaire	Binge eating and purging	10–18	Johnson et al. 1999
Eating in the Absence of Hunger (EAH-P)	Questionnaire	Eating in response to emotional and environmental cues	6–19	Shomaker et al. 2013; Tanofsky-Kraff et al. 2008b
Parent-report measures for younger pediatric samples				
Children's Eating Behaviour Questionnaire (CEBQ)	Questionnaire	Eating style	2+	Wardle et al. 2001
Child Feeding Questionnaire (CFQ)	Questionnaire	Feeding practices, food acceptance, proneness to obesity	2–11	Birch et al. 2001

(CIDI; Robins et al. 1988). To date, these measures have not generally been adapted to reflect DSM-5 diagnostic criteria. These measures may be used in full for a comprehensive psychiatric evaluation, or only the "Eating Disorder" subsection may be administered. Of note, however, certain parent-report measures of eating pathology have demonstrated lack of sensitivity (Fisher et al. 1993), which may reflect parents' inability to infer children's emotions (e.g., *fear* of gaining weight) or may be the result of secrecy surrounding certain behaviors. This discordance is consistent with other parent-report measures (Swanson et al. 2014) and underscores the need for both child and parent report (or child report alone) for the diagnosis and classification of eating pathology.

Parent-Report Questionnaire Measures

Additional parent-report measures include parent versions of the Questionnaire on Eating and Weight Patterns (QEWP-P; Spitzer et al. 1993) and of the Eating in the Absence of Hunger questionnaire (EAH-P; Tanofsky-Kraff et al. 2008b). Notably, the QEWP demonstrates high concordance between child self-report and parent report in the presence of no diagnosis (82% agreement); however, concordance is significantly reduced when the child reports subthreshold binge eating (15.5%) or BED (25%) (Johnson et al. 1999). This difference may be due to the secrecy and shame associated with binge eating and suggests that parents' reporting of sensitive behaviors may be insufficient in the assessment of adolescent eating and weight pathology. In contrast, the parent version of the EAH demonstrated significantly greater construct validity than the child report, perhaps because of the abstract nature of the construct of interest (Shomaker et al. 2013).

Parent-Report Measures for Younger Pediatric Samples

Although the utility of parent-report measures in the assessment of adolescents is unclear (Johnson et al. 1999; Swanson et al. 2014), parent reports are necessary in the evaluation of younger pediatric samples. Parent-report measures that assess eating and feeding behaviors in children as young as age 2 years have been developed. These include the Children's Eating Behaviour Questionnaire (CEBQ; Wardle et al. 2001), which assesses dimensions of eating style (e.g., satiety responsiveness, fussiness, emotional overeating), and the Child Feeding Questionnaire (CFQ; Birch et al. 2001), which measures feeding practices, food acceptance, and proneness to obesity in youths ages 2–11 years (see Table 11–2). These scales may have important predictive utility because problematic eating in early childhood is a risk factor for the onset of eating disorders (Jacobi et al. 2004).

Alternative Methods of Assessing Eating Pathology and Associated Features in Youths

Given the myriad challenges facing clinicians and researchers assessing aberrant eating in youths–for instance, limited recollection of foods consumed, lack of insight regarding affective states, and the discordance of parent-report measures–several novel methods have been developed for more thorough and ecologically valid assessments. Although these methods may be more cumbersome and costly, they provide objective data that may contribute substantially to the understanding of eating behaviors in youths.

Feeding Paradigms

Retrospective dietary recall may pose a challenge even for adult respondents and recall may be unreliable or invalid among youths (McPherson et al. 2000); laboratory feeding paradigms enable researchers to examine eating behavior in a controlled setting. Using well-established paradigms and test meals, energy intake and macronutrient content of both binge and regular meals can be ascertained in the laboratory (Tanofsky-Kraff et al. 2007b). Additionally, researchers can precisely assess both premeal and postmeal affect, rather than relying on retrospective report. Laboratory feeding studies have been adapted for youths and have been critical in the investigation of binge and eating behaviors in youths who are lean and those who are overweight (Mirch et al. 2006; Tanofsky-Kraff et al. 2009).

Ecological Momentary Assessment

Ecological momentary assessment (EMA) has been used in adult populations to gather random and event sampling of food intake, food-related cognitions, and affect in natural settings and shows promise for use in pediatric and adolescent samples (Hilbert et al. 2009; Ranzenhofer et al. 2014; Shingleton et al. 2013) (see Chapter 12, "Application of Modern Technology in Eating Disorder Assessment and Intervention"). Feasibility of EMA has been demonstrated in children as young as age 7 years (Silk et al. 2011). When EMA is conducted with children, child-specific cellular phones or personal digital assistants are provided and participants are trained in their use. Notably, EMA may detect individuals who denied presence of loss of control in clinical interviews and thereby may serve as an important method of detecting false-negative loss-of-control eaters (Hilbert et al. 2009). The data garnered from this method may elucidate the antecedents to binge-eating and aberrant eating episodes and help to establish the temporal relationship among mood (Hilbert et al. 2009), interpersonal difficulties (Ranzenhofer et al. 2014), and eating behaviors.

Neuropsychological Assessments

Neuropsychological and neurobiological tools may have utility in identifying neural markers and correlates of eating disorders in youths (Eddy and Rauch 2011). Additionally, neuropsychological methods may be used to identify children who are at risk for binge eating and obesity. Because neural response to food-related stimuli develops in youth, functional magnetic resonance imaging and neuropsychological assessments may be helpful in determining neural mechanisms involved in the development and maintenance of eating and weight disorders (e.g., Lock et al. 2011; Marsh et al. 2011). Review of the literature pertaining to the neurobiology of adolescent eating disorders is beyond the scope of this chapter.

Proposed Eating Disorder Assessment for DSM-5 Adaptation for Youth

To date, the only comprehensive diagnostic tools developed for the detection of DSM-5 feeding and eating disorders are the EDE Version 17.0D (Fairburn et al. 2014) and the Eating Disorder Assessment for DSM-5 (EDA-5; Sysko et al. 2015). The EDA-5 (described in Chapter 10, "Use of the Eating Disorder Assessment for DSM-5") lends itself well to a child-specific adaptation. An adaptation of the EDA-5 for use with child and adolescent populations could be disseminated in both clinical and research settings and would provide diagnostic information pertaining to binge eating, compensatory behaviors, dietary restraint, ARFID, pica, and rumination disorder, in addition to the range of OSFED subtypes, such as night eating syndrome and purging disorder. This computerized assessment, administered by an interviewer via computer or mobile device, has been shown to minimize participant burden (Sysko et al. 2015). This format may be particularly useful with children and adolescents, in whom sustained attention can vary widely. For use of the EDA-5 with youths, the language should be modified in accordance with prior measures (e.g., the ChEDE [see subsection "Interview Measures" within this chapter]), to aid in comprehension. Additional information and elaboration should be provided pertaining to abstract constructs; for instance, "loss of control" should be described in more detail with the use of metaphor (e.g., "the example of a ball rolling down a hill, going faster and faster" [Tanofsky-Kraff et al. 2004]). As described in Chapter 10, the adult version of the EDA-5 employs the DSM-5 trumping rules (e.g., a current diagnosis of AN excludes any other feeding or eating disorder, with the exception of pica); however, in pediatric and adolescent samples, it will be important to administer the full battery so that every category of feeding and eating disorder is assessed. In the assessment of younger children, it is also important to obtain supplemental information from parents. For instance, parental report may be necessary to document any medical problems or nutritional deficiencies resulting from low energy intake. Although the digitized format of the assessment will likely reduce time and burden for respondents, it does require that a member of the clinical or research team administer the interview.

Conclusion

The assessment and diagnosis of feeding and eating disorders in youths are complex and merit a holistic approach. Although the prevalence of full-threshold eating disorders among youths is estimated at approximately 3% (Swanson et al. 2011), subthreshold eating behaviors and cognitions, such as binge and loss-of-control eating, dietary restriction, and preoccupation with shape and weight, are quite common among child and adolescent samples (Ackard et al. 2007; Eddy et al. 2010; Tanofsky-Kraff et al. 2004). Therefore, the early detection and diagnosis of disordered eating and related psychopathology are vital in preventing the onset of full-threshold eating disorders and obesity during child and adolescent development. To better assess feeding and eating pathology in youths, several measures, both interviews and self-reports, have been developed or adapted from adult measures.

Relatively few children meet full DSM-5 criteria for eating and feeding disorders; however, many endorse problematic eating behaviors and cognitions that may be prodromal or increase risk for full-syndrome eating disorders. Therefore, it is strongly recommended that children be assessed both for the diagnostic criteria and for subthreshold features of feeding and eating disorders, such as loss-of-control eating and hyperresponsivity to food cues; where feasible, interview assessments and self-report measures should be administered in tandem. Alternative methods, such as feeding paradigms or EMA, may prove useful in assessing in vivo eating behaviors and affect.

Although the utility of parent-report measures remains indeterminate, and some argue that diagnosis can be made based on child report alone (Johnson et al. 1999; Swanson et al. 2014), parents can play a crucial role in assisting their child with recall and providing relevant information such as weight status and medical sequelae. Parent report may be less reliable, however, for the assessment of potentially shameful behaviors, such as binge eating and purging. Because self-reported weight may not be an accurate proxy for measured weight in youths (Sarafrazi et al. 2014) and dietary recall may pose a challenge for younger respondents (McPherson et al. 2000), objective measures of eating behavior and weight should be collected whenever feasible.

Owing to the relatively recent release of DSM-5, few measures exist that assess the revised diagnostic criteria and newly added categories. In fact, the EDA-5 is the only available tool to assess pica, rumination disorder, and ARFID, in addition to AN, BN, and BED. Therefore, this is an area in need of future research and clinical effort. More specifically, research should focus on measurement development to assess DSM-5 diagnostic criteria and categories of feeding and eating disorders in both youths and adults.

Key Clinical Points

- Well-validated interview and questionnaire assessments of eating disorder symptoms have been adapted for pediatric populations.
- Clinicians and researchers are advised to assess diagnostic criteria as well as associated behaviors, cognitions, and risk factors.
- Interview methods are considered the optimal means of assessing eating-related psychopathology, although training and administration may be cumbersome.
- Self-report measures may augment respondent candor and incur less participant burden.
- Data on the utility of parent-report measures are mixed, although parent report may be necessary for younger children and for estimates of weight and medical sequelae.
- The administration of multiple assessments (e.g., interview and self-report) is recommended.
- Adaptations of measures to assess DSM-5 diagnostic criteria are warranted.
- Objective measures of eating behavior and weight should be collected whenever feasible.

References

Ackard DM, Fulkerson JA, Neumark-Sztainer D: Prevalence and utility of DSM-IV eating disorder diagnostic criteria among youth. Int J Eat Disord 40(5):409–417, 2007 17506079

American Psychiatric Association: Diagnostic and Statistical Manual of Mental Disorders, 4th Edition. Washington, DC, American Psychiatric Association, 1994

American Psychiatric Association: Diagnostic and Statistical Manual of Mental Disorders, 5th Edition. Arlington, VA, American Psychiatric Association, 2013

Birch LL, Fisher JO, Grimm-Thomas K, et al: Confirmatory factor analysis of the Child Feeding Questionnaire: a measure of parental attitudes, beliefs and practices about child feeding and obesity proneness. Appetite 36(3):201–210, 2001 11358344

Bravender T, Bryant-Waugh R, Herzog D, et al; Workgroup for Classification of Eating Disorders in Children and Adolescents: Classification of child and adolescent eating disturbances. Int J Eat Disord 40(suppl):S117–S122, 2007 17868122

Bryant-Waugh RJ, Cooper PJ, Taylor CL, et al: The use of the Eating Disorder Examination with children: a pilot study. Int J Eat Disord 19(4):391–397, 1996 8859397

Childress A, Jarrell MP, Brewerton TD: The Kids' Eating Disorders Survey (KEDS): internal consistency, component analysis, and test-retest reliability. Paper presented at the International Conference on Eating Disorders, New York, April 1992

Childress AC, Brewerton TD, Hodges EL, et al: The Kids' Eating Disorders Survey (KEDS): a study of middle school students. J Am Acad Child Adolesc Psychiatry 32(4):843–850, 1993 8340308

De Los Reyes A, Kazdin AE: Informant discrepancies in the assessment of childhood psychopathology: a critical review, theoretical framework, and recommendations for further study. Psychol Bull 131(4):483–509, 2005 16060799

Dixon JB: The effect of obesity on health outcomes. Mol Cell Endocrinol 316(2):104–108, 2010 19628019

Eddy KT, Rauch SL: Neuroimaging in eating disorders: coming of age. Am J Psychiatry 168(11):1139–1141, 2011 22193598

Eddy KT, Le Grange D, Crosby RD, et al: Diagnostic classification of eating disorders in children and adolescents: how does DSM-IV-TR compare to empirically derived categories? J Am Acad Child Adolesc Psychiatry 49(3):277–287, quiz 293, 2010 20410717

Eklund K, Paavonen EJ, Almqvist F: Factor structure of the Eating Disorder Inventory-C. Int J Eat Disord 37(4):330–341, 2005 15856502

Fairburn CG, Beglin SJ: Assessment of eating disorders: interview or self-report questionnaire? Int J Eat Disord 16(4):363–370, 1994 7866415

Fairburn C, Cooper Z: The Eating Disorder Examination, 12th Edition, in Binge Eating: Nature, Assessment, and Treatment. Edited by Fairburn CG, Wilson GT. New York, Guilford, 1993, pp 317–360

Fairburn CG, Cooper Z, O'Connor M: Eating Disorder Examination, Edition 17.0D. The Center for Research on Dissemination at Oxford. April 2014. Available at: http://www.credo-oxford.com/6.2.html. Accessed March 17, 2015.

Field AE, Taylor C, Celio A, et al: Comparison of self-report to interview assessment of bulimic behaviors among preadolescent and adolescent girls and boys. Int J Eat Disord 35(1):86–92, 2004

Field AE, Cook NR, Gillman MW: Weight status in childhood as a predictor of becoming overweight or hypertensive in early adulthood. Obes Res 13(1):163–169, 2005 15761176

Field AE, Sonneville KR, Micali N, et al: Prospective association of common eating disorders and adverse outcomes. Pediatrics 130(2):e289–e295, 2012 22802602

Field AE, Sonneville KR, Crosby RD, et al: Prospective associations of concerns about physique and the development of obesity, binge drinking, and drug use among adolescent boys and young adult men. JAMA Pediatr 168(1):34–39, 2014 24190655

Fisher PW, Shaffer D, Piacentini JC, et al: Sensitivity of the Diagnostic Interview Schedule for Children, 2nd Edition (DISC-2.1) for specific diagnoses of children and adolescents. J Am Acad Child Adolesc Psychiatry 32(3):666–673, 1993

Garner DM: The Eating Disorder Inventory–C. Lutz, FL, Psychological Assessment Resources, 1991

Garner DM, Garfinkel PE: The Eating Attitudes Test: an index of the symptoms of anorexia nervosa. Psychol Med 9(2):273–279, 1979 472072

Garner DM, Olmstead MP, Polivy J: Development and validation of a multidimensional eating disorder inventory for anorexia nervosa and bulimia. Int J Eat Disord 2:15–34, 1983

Gearhardt AN, Roberto CA, Seamans MJ, et al: Preliminary validation of the Yale Food Addiction Scale for children. Eat Behav 14(4):508–512, 2013 24183146

Goldschmidt AB, Doyle AC, Wilfley DE: Assessment of binge eating in overweight youth using a questionnaire version of the Child Eating Disorder Examination with instructions. Int J Eat Disord 40(5):460–467, 2007 17497710

Goldschmidt AB, Boutelle K, Tanofsky-Kraff M: Binge eating in children and adolescents, part I: classification, correlates, and development, in A Clinician's Guide to Binge Eating Disorder. Edited by Alexander J, Goldschmidt AB, Grange DL. New York, Routledge, 2013, pp 42–53

Goldschmidt AB, Wall MM, Loth KA, et al: The course of binge eating from adolescence to young adulthood. Health Psychol 33(5):457–460, 2014 23977873

Goodman R, Ford T, Richards H, et al: The Development and Well-Being Assessment: description and initial validation of an integrated assessment of child and adolescent psychopathology. J Child Psychol Psychiatry 41(5):645–655, 2000 10946756

Hess MA: Portion Photos of Popular Foods. Chicago, IL, American Dietetic Association and University of Wisconsin-Stout, 1997

Hilbert A, Rief W, Tuschen-Caffier B, et al: Loss of control eating and psychological maintenance in children: an ecological momentary assessment study. Behav Res Ther 47(1):26–33, 2009 19010458

Jacobi C, Hayward C, de Zwaan M, et al: Coming to terms with risk factors for eating disorders: application of risk terminology and suggestions for a general taxonomy. Psychol Bull 130(1):19–65, 2004 14717649

Johnson WG, Grieve FG, Adams CD, et al: Measuring binge eating in adolescents: adolescent and parent versions of the Questionnaire of Eating and Weight Patterns. Int J Eat Disord 26(3):301–314, 1999 10441246

Kaufman J, Birmaher B, Brent D, et al: Schedule for Affective Disorders and Schizophrenia for School-Age Children-Present and Lifetime Version (K-SADS-PL): initial reliability and validity data. J Am Acad Child Adolesc Psychiatry 36(7):980–988, 1997 9204677

Kotler LA, Cohen P, Davies M, et al: Longitudinal relationships between childhood, adolescent, and adult eating disorders. J Am Acad Child Adolesc Psychiatry 40(12):1434–1440, 2001 11765289

Lavender JM, Anderson DA: Effect of perceived anonymity in assessments of eating disordered behaviors and attitudes. Int J Eat Disord 42(6):546–551, 2009 19172594

Lock J, Garrett A, Beenhakker J, et al: Aberrant brain activation during a response inhibition task in adolescent eating disorder subtypes. Am J Psychiatry 168(1):55–64, 2011 21123315

Maloney MJ, McGuire JB, Daniels SR: Reliability testing of a children's version of the Eating Attitude Test. J Am Acad Child Adolesc Psychiatry 27(5):541–543, 1988 3182615

Marsh R, Horga G, Wang Z, et al: An FMRI study of self-regulatory control and conflict resolution in adolescents with bulimia nervosa. Am J Psychiatry 168(11):1210–1220, 2011 21676991

McPherson RS, Hoelscher DM, Alexander M, et al: Dietary assessment methods among school-aged children: validity and reliability. Prev Med 31(2):S11–S33, 2000

Mirch MC, McDuffie JR, Yanovski SZ, et al: Effects of binge eating on satiation, satiety, and energy intake of overweight children. Am J Clin Nutr 84(4):732–738, 2006 17023698

Neumark-Sztainer D, Story M: Dieting and binge eating among adolescents: what do they really mean? J Am Diet Assoc 98(4):446–450, 1998 9550169

Neumark-Sztainer D, Story M, Hannan PJ, et al: Weight-related concerns and behaviors among overweight and nonoverweight adolescents: implications for preventing weight-related disorders. Arch Pediatr Adolesc Med 156(2):171–178, 2002 11814380

Neumark-Sztainer D, Wall M, Story M, et al: Dieting and unhealthy weight control behaviors during adolescence: associations with 10-year changes in body mass index. J Adolesc Health 50(1):80–86, 2012 22188838

Puhl RM, Latner JD: Stigma, obesity, and the health of the nation's children. Psychol Bull 133(4):557–580, 2007 17592956

Puhl RM, Luedicke J: Weight-based victimization among adolescents in the school setting: emotional reactions and coping behaviors. J Youth Adolesc 41(1):27–40, 2012 21918904

Ranzenhofer LM, Engel SG, Crosby RD, et al: Using ecological momentary assessment to examine interpersonal and affective predictors of loss of control eating in adolescent girls. Int J Eat Disord 47(7):748–757, 2014 25046850

Robins LN, Wing J, Wittchen HU, et al: The Composite International Diagnostic Interview: an epidemiologic instrument suitable for use in conjunction with different diagnostic systems and in different cultures. Arch Gen Psychiatry 45(12):1069–1077, 1988 2848472

Sarafrazi N, Hughes J, Borrud L, et al: Perception of weight status in U.S. children and adolescents aged 8–15 years, 2005–2012. NCHS Data Brief (158):1–7, 2014

Shaffer D, Schwab-Stone M, Fisher P, et al: The Diagnostic Interview Schedule for Children-Revised Version (DISC-R), I: preparation, field testing, interrater reliability, and acceptability. J Am Acad Child Adolesc Psychiatry 32(3):643–650, 1993 8496128

Shapiro JR, Woolson SL, Hamer RM, et al: Evaluating binge eating disorder in children: development of the Children's Binge Eating Disorder Scale (C-BEDS). Int J Eat Disord 40(1):82–89, 2007 16958120

Shingleton RM, Eddy KT, Keshaviah A, et al: Binge/purge thoughts in nonsuicidal self-injurious adolescents: an ecological momentary analysis. Int J Eat Disord 46(7):684–689, 2013 23729243

Shomaker LB, Tanofsky-Kraff M, Elliott C, et al: Salience of loss of control for pediatric binge episodes: does size really matter? Int J Eat Disord 43(8):707–716, 2010 19827022

Shomaker LB, Tanofsky-Kraff M, Mooreville M, et al: Links of adolescent- and parent-reported eating in the absence of hunger with observed eating in the absence of hunger. Obesity (Silver Spring) 21(6):1243–1250, 2013 23913735

Silk JS, Forbes EE, Whalen DJ, et al: Daily emotional dynamics in depressed youth: a cell phone ecological momentary assessment study. J Exp Child Psychol 110(2):241–257, 2011 21112595

Solmi F, Sonneville KR, Easter A, et al: Prevalence of purging at age 16 and associations with negative outcomes among girls in three community-based cohorts. J Child Psychol Psychiatry 56(1):87–96, 2014

Spitzer RL, Yanovski JA, Marcus MD: The Questionnaire on Eating and Weight Patterns–Revised (QEWP-R), in Obesity Research, Vol 1. Edited by Yanovski, SZ. New York, New York State Psychiatric Institute, 1993, pp 306–324

Swanson SA, Crow SJ, Le Grange D, et al: Prevalence and correlates of eating disorders in adolescents: results from the National Comorbidity Survey Replication Adolescent Supplement. Arch Gen Psychiatry 68(7):714–723, 2011 21383252

Swanson SA, Aloisio KM, Horton NJ, et al: Assessing eating disorder symptoms in adolescence: is there a role for multiple informants? Int J Eat Disord 47(5):475–482, 2014 24436213

Sysko R, Glasofer DR, Hildebrandt T, et al: The Eating Disorder Assessment for DSM-5 (EDA-5): development and validation of a structured interview for feeding and eating disorders. Int J Eat Disord 48(5):452–463 2015 25639562

Tanofsky-Kraff M: Binge eating among children and adolescents, in Handbook of Childhood and Adolescent Obesity. Edited by Jelalian E, Steele RG. New York, Springer, 2008, pp 42–57

Tanofsky-Kraff M, Morgan CM, Yanovski SZ, et al: Comparison of assessments of children's eating-disordered behaviors by interview and questionnaire. Int J Eat Disord 33(2):213–224, 2003 12616588

Tanofsky-Kraff M, Yanovski SZ, Wilfley DE, et al: Eating-disordered behaviors, body fat, and psychopathology in overweight and normal-weight children. J Consult Clin Psychol 72(1):53–61, 2004 14756614

Tanofsky-Kraff M, Faden D, Yanovski SZ, et al: The perceived onset of dieting and loss of control eating behaviors in overweight children. Int J Eat Disord 38(2):112–122, 2005 16134103

Tanofsky-Kraff M, Goossens L, Eddy KT, et al: A multisite investigation of binge eating behaviors in children and adolescents. J Consult Clin Psychol 75(6):901–913, 2007a 18085907

Tanofsky-Kraff M, Haynos AF, Kotler LA, et al: Laboratory-based studies of eating among children and adolescents. Curr Nutr Food Sci 3(1):55–74, 2007b 19030122

Tanofsky-Kraff M, Theim KR, Yanovski SZ, et al: Validation of the Emotional Eating Scale adapted for use in children and adolescents (EES-C). Int J Eat Disord 40(3):232–240, 2007c 17262813

Tanofsky-Kraff M, Marcus MD, Yanovski SZ, et al: Loss of control eating disorder in children age 12 years and younger: proposed research criteria. Eat Behav 9(3):360–365, 2008a 18549996

Tanofsky-Kraff M, Ranzenhofer LM, Yanovski SZ, et al: Psychometric properties of a new questionnaire to assess eating in the absence of hunger in children and adolescents. Appetite 51(1):148–155, 2008b 18342988

Tanofsky-Kraff M, McDuffie JR, Yanovski SZ, et al: Laboratory assessment of the food intake of children and adolescents with loss of control eating. Am J Clin Nutr 89(3):738–745, 2009 19144730

Thompson JK, Cattarin J, Fowler B, et al: The Perception of Teasing Scale (POTS): a revision and extension of the Physical Appearance Related Teasing Scale (PARTS). J Pers Assess 65(1):146–157, 1995 16367650

van Strien T, Frijters JE, Bergers GP, et al: The Dutch Eating Behavior Questionnaire (DEBQ) for assessment of restrained, emotional, and external eating behavior. Int J Eat Disord 5(2):295–315, 1986

Wardle J, Guthrie CA, Sanderson S, et al: Development of the Children's Eating Behaviour Questionnaire. J Child Psychol Psychiatry 42(7):963–970, 2001 11693591

Yanovski SZ, Marcus MD, Wadden TA, et al: The Questionnaire on Eating and Weight Patterns-5: an updated screening instrument for binge eating disorder. Int J Eat Disord 48(3):259–261 2015 25545458

12 Application of Modern Technology in Eating Disorder Assessment and Intervention

Jo M. Ellison, Ph.D.
Stephen A. Wonderlich, Ph.D.
Scott G. Engel, Ph.D.

Technology is becoming ubiquitous in daily life. Statistics regarding the infiltration of mobile devices and Internet access into society are staggering. In the United States, 90% of adults report owning a mobile phone, and 58% of this group own a smartphone (Pew Research Internet Project 2014). These rates are similar to those of other nations, such as South Korea, Japan, Australia, Norway, Sweden, Denmark, the United Kingdom, and the Netherlands, where smartphone ownership rates passed the 50% threshold by 2014. The worldwide smartphone ownership rate is, in fact, still growing, and eMarketer (2014) predicted that the rate would reach 25% in 2015. Home Internet access statistics vary based on the type of Internet subscription surveyed. The U.S. government census suggests that 74.4% of Americans had Internet service in their homes in 2013 (File and Ryan 2014). Approximately 79% of European Union households report having high-speed Internet service (Eurostat 2013). American ownership of smartphones and home Internet connections crosses demographic groups, including those defined by gender, race, ethnicity, and urban versus rural settings. However, certain groups, including young adults and those with more education or higher household income, report greater utilization of such technology (File and Ryan 2014; Pew Research Internet Project 2014).

The evident popularity of technology makes it important for clinicians to consider how they might incorporate it into professional practice. In fact, the health care industry is already capitalizing on the ease of access to technology. In 2013, of the 60% of U.S. adults who reported tracking their weight, diet, or exercise regimen, 21% reported that they used technology to track these data (Fox 2013). The purpose of this chapter is to provide clinicians with information about the practical application of technology in both the assessment and treatment of eating disorders. Several areas of recent technological development and empirical study fall under this large umbrella; however, our focus in this chapter is on those areas most relevant to clinical practice with individuals with eating disorders. We discuss ecological momentary assessment (EMA) in terms of its use in the scientific study of these conditions and as a possible clinical tool for data collection. We review ecological momentary intervention (EMI), another portable strategy that has emerged in conjunction with EMA and that can be useful in delivering interventions to individuals as they go about daily routines. We then discuss the utility and effectiveness of Web-based and telemedicine treatments. Finally, we offer a practical examination of how clinicians can integrate portable technology into practice.

Ecological Momentary Assessment

Largely due to the limitations of retrospective self-report, including memory limitations and cognitive biases, researchers are increasingly relying on innovative real-time approaches to data collection to improve the validity of their data (Smyth et al. 2001). EMA involves the use of portable devices, including personal digital assistants (PDAs) and mobile phones, that enable intensive assessment of an individual's states and behaviors in naturalistic settings and in close approximations of real time.

EMA has been used successfully in the study of depression (aan het Rot et al. 2012), substance use disorders (Shiffman 2009), psychotic disorders (Oorschot et al. 2009), borderline personality disorder (Ebner-Priemer et al. 2006), and eating disorders (Smyth et al. 2001). In addition to reducing retrospective recall bias, EMA is advantageous in that it collects data in the natural environment and thus avoids the artificiality of laboratory settings (Smyth et al. 2001). Furthermore, intensive and repeated assessment of

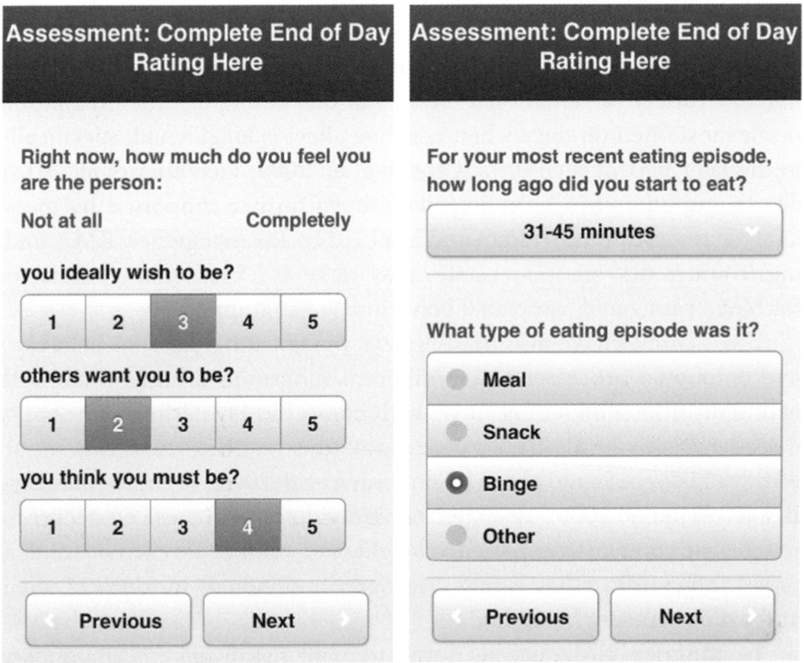

FIGURE 12–1. Example ecological momentary assessment mood rating and eating episode rating.
Source. Reprinted with permission from Real Time Assessment in the Natural Environment (ReTAINE), http://retaine.org.

clinical variables, over hours, days, and weeks, allows for the examination of relationships among various environmental or psychological factors and objective behaviors. For example, EMA can examine theoretically meaningful causal variables (e.g., stressful events, emotional states) and various behavioral outcome variables (e.g., alcohol consumption, binge eating, exercising) in a manner that carefully accounts for the temporal order of events, thus potentially clarifying cause and effect. Figure 12–1 provides two screen shots of an EMA questionnaire that could be viewed and completed on a mobile device.

There has been a dramatic increase in the use of EMA for the study of eating disorders in the past decade (Wonderlich 2010). This body of research has improved understanding of various causal factors (e.g., ecological factors, stress, emotion) involved in eating disorders. For example, an early EMA study of bulimia nervosa (BN) revealed that bulimic symptoms are most likely to occur on weekends and between the hours of 7 and 9 P.M. (Smyth et al. 2009). EMA studies have also shown that negative emotional states increase while positive emotional states decrease before various eating disorder behaviors in anorexia nervosa (AN; Engel et al. 2013), BN (Smyth et al. 2007), and binge-eating disorder (BED; Goldschmidt et al. 2012). Other data suggest that individuals with AN and BN experience a marked variety of "emotional days," but that eating disorder symptoms occur most often on days when negative affect is heightened, specifically in the later part of such days (Crosby et al. 2009; Lavender et al. 2013). These and other EMA findings have been further supported by meta-analytic research (Haedt-Matt and Keel 2011). Taken together, EMA findings confirm that emotional states may serve as a momentary risk factor for binge eating and associated behaviors (e.g., purging).

EMA studies have also fruitfully examined eating disorder behaviors and emotional processes across different subgroups of individuals with eating disorders, including those with comorbid borderline personality disorder (Selby et al. 2012), posttraumatic stress disorder (Karr et al. 2013), a history of child abuse (Wonderlich et al. 2007), or multi-impulsive BN (Myers et al. 2006). As expected, individuals with these co-occurring psychiatric conditions experience heightened emotional reactivity and, at times, differ from other eating-disordered individuals in terms of affect and eating disorder behavior.

In summary, EMA has been used to make significant contributions to the empirical study of eating disorders in the last decade. Existing studies highlight the momentary relationship of emotional states and eating disorder behavior and have implications for maintenance models of eating disorders. Furthermore, these data suggest that clinicians may benefit from examining momentary processes surrounding eating disorder behaviors, in terms of both conceptualizing individual cases and devising clinical interventions to interrupt decision making in affect-laden moments preceding and following a given behavior. In line with this recommendation, a new treatment for BN (i.e., integrative cognitive-affective therapy) is based on momentary models of bulimic behavior derived from EMA studies and has been shown to effectively reduce bulimic symptoms in a randomized controlled trial (RCT) (Wonderlich et al. 2014). Future EMA studies are needed to further elucidate the temporal nature of eating disorder behaviors in ways that can inform effective clinical applications of the results.

Ecological Momentary Intervention

Heron and Smyth (2010) refer to ecological momentary interventions as the delivery of interventions to people as they go about their daily lives. This definition suggests that EMI may be relatively unstructured (e.g., an individual is reminded to complete food logs) or highly structured (e.g., a smoker receives explicit instructions at times of day that have been empirically demonstrated to be high risk). EMI may include response-contingent interventions (e.g., delivering a text message with explicit instructions after a patient reports increasing levels of negative affect via EMA) or non-response-contingent interventions (e.g., delivering a text message at previously determined times of day, such as at mealtimes in weight loss protocols). EMI has been implemented in several areas of psychology and behavioral medicine, including smoking cessation (Rodgers et al. 2005), physical activity promotion (King et al. 2008), and substance use treatment (Weitzel et al. 2007). It has been successfully used by a wide range of individuals (from teenagers to the elderly) who have significantly different levels of technological sophistication (Heron and Smyth 2010).

The study of EMI in eating disorder samples has been relatively limited. Early noncontrolled pilot studies (Bauer et al. 2003; Shapiro et al. 2010) suggested that text message interventions may have small effects on reducing eating disorder symptoms in posthospitalization aftercare studies, particularly for individuals with less severe forms of eating disorders. In an RCT comparing a text message–based EMI with treatment as usual in adults with BN, patients in the text messaging condition provided weekly symptom reports over 16 weeks following hospital discharge and received tailored feedback based on their symptom status (Bauer et al. 2012). Individuals in the treatment-as-usual condition were discharged from inpatient treatment and received no follow-up contact beyond additional outpatient care sought on their own. Those in the text messaging condition were significantly more likely to achieve remission of eating disorder symptoms than individuals in the treatment-as-usual condition.

Although the empirical database for EMI and eating disorders remains undeveloped, obesity researchers have more extensively evaluated the utility of this modality of intervention. Findings suggest that EMI is a promising strategy to produce clinically significant weight loss in overweight and obese adults (e.g., Coons et al. 2012; Rao et al. 2011). The inclusion of handheld technology, in particular, has been associated with significantly more weight loss among obese individuals than more traditional programs that rely on behavioral weight loss strategies without EMI (e.g., Burke et al. 2011; Haapala et al. 2009; Patrick et al. 2009). For example, in an RCT involving overweight individuals seeking weight loss, Burke et al. (2011) compared three self-monitoring and recording systems: 1) paper record, 2) a PDA with dietary and exercise software, and 3) a PDA with the same software plus a daily message delivered on the PDA. In this 2-year investigation, participants who received information on their PDA plus a daily message were the most likely to have achieved a 5% weight loss when assessed at 6-month follow-up.

Overall, it seems that EMI confers more benefit if it includes a more comprehensive intervention or is offered as an adjunct to an in-person treatment. This pattern was recently replicated in a study comparing an in-person group-based weight loss intervention with a treatment that offered the same intervention plus a PDA to record food consumption, record activity level, and provide decision-support strategies (i.e., 15-minute coaching calls from a paraprofessional every 2 weeks to review data and assist the individual in establishing calorie and activity goals; Spring et al. 2013). The group receiving the intervention plus the PDA lost more weight than the group receiving the in-person intervention as a stand-alone treatment; this pattern was maintained at each of several follow-up assessments. The authors highlight that the delivery of EMI was shown to be effective while using relatively minimal amounts of paraprofessional time, supporting the utility of EMI as an adjunctive strategy. Furthermore, this study was conducted in a primary care facility through the Veterans Affairs system, suggesting that such interventions can be delivered effectively in non-specialty-based settings.

It may yet be premature to draw conclusions about the effectiveness of mobile phones and similar devices as weight loss tools (Rao et al. 2011), and more research is certainly warranted in feeding and eating disorder populations. However, existing applications of EMI (e.g., Spring et al. 2013) suggest that the intervention holds promise in comprehensive primary care–based weight management programs and possibly in improving dissemination and implementation of evidence-based interventions.

Web-Based Prevention and Treatment of Eating Disorders

In eating disorders, the effectiveness and feasibility of technology-based interventions that do not rely on momentary transactions between a patient (providing data) and a computer (processing the patient's data) have also been of interest. These Web-based platforms, focusing on prevention and/or treatment, allow individuals to log on to a standardized and often comprehensive program that includes assessment, education, and provision of various interventions.

Web-Based Prevention and Intervention Programs

A clear benefit of online platforms for eating disorder prevention is the relative ease with which larger numbers of young people can be targeted (Bauer 2014). This area of study is changing rapidly, and scientifically based conclusions may lag behind technological advances. Consequently, the following study review serves as a general discussion of online prevention and intervention programs available at the time of publication. At this time, most studies focus exclusively on prevention in female populations.

The Web-based format of prevention and treatment programs changes slightly depending on the specific intervention. Some provide stand-alone materials and activities without clinician interaction, some offer asynchronous message boards for group or individual clinical contact, and others provide synchronous discussions and messaging for group and individual clinical contact.

Several programs focus on prevention by enrolling females who may be at risk for developing an eating disorder because they have elevated shape and weight concerns. How a given program works with respect to prevention varies. Student Bodies, for example, is a Web-based prevention program developed and studied by Taylor et al. (2006) that presents psychoeducational materials and involves brief e-mail–based interactions between clinicians and participants. This intervention, compared with no intervention, has been shown to significantly reduce weight and shape concerns, and subsequent analyses suggest that improvements are maintained (Beintner et al. 2012). Other prevention programs, including the Body Project and its online version, eBody Project (Stice et al. 2012), use an approach based on cognitive-dissonance theory. Namely, these programs aim to help individuals reduce their drive to pursue a thin body type by engaging in a variety of activities in which the thin ideal is critiqued. The online version of the program did not significantly differ from the in-person version on major outcome variables, including body dissatisfaction, thin-ideal internalization, eating disorder symptoms, and negative affect (Stice et al. 2012). The effects of the eBody Project on eating disorder pathology faded more quickly than those of the Body Project, but the online version still produced greater and more enduring reduction in risk for large weight gain at 1- and 2-year follow-ups (Stice et al. 2014). Taken together, these studies indicate that online prevention programs can have an impact, even when their scope is limited to psychoeducation or reduction of thin-ideal internalization.

More comprehensive online treatment programs are also available. Set Your Body Free (Paxton et al. 2007) is one such program; it employs multiple modalities and has been used with individuals reporting significant body dissatisfaction as well as those reporting current disordered eating behaviors. It has been shown to reduce problematic eating attitudes and behaviors, body dissatisfaction, avoidant tendencies, body comparison, and internalization of the thin ideal (Paxton et al. 2007). Another program, adapted for adolescent girls and titled My Body, My Life: Body Image Program for Adolescent Girls, appears similarly effective for this population (Heinicke et al. 2007). Finally, ProYouth is a Web-based prevention/intervention program that helps to find the appropriate level of treatment for the individual depending on the severity of his or her symptoms. This program operates in seven European Union countries and delivers treatment content through a variety of modalities, at varying levels of intensity, essentially personalizing the intervention based on each individual's unique symptom pattern. For example, online, synchronous chat sessions are offered to participants either in group or individual format (ProYouth 2013). Initial investigations indicated that, as the developers intended, participants at high risk for an eating disorder generally used more intensive modules than did those participants at "moderate risk" (Lindenberg et al. 2011). ProYouth is currently operational and open to public enrollment in the participating countries (Bauer 2014).

Overall, such online prevention and intervention programs appear to be comparable in effectiveness to traditional face-to-face options and certainly more effective than no intervention. Retention for these platforms appears high, suggesting that this modality is appealing to program participants who may not have sought other treatments (Bauer 2014). Additionally, Web-based treatments may show promise as cost-effective methods of reducing the rate of onset of eating disorders. One limitation related to online prevention programs is their current state of limited availability to the general public. Although manuals for many traditional face-to-face prevention programs have been published, the online versions are not readily available to those outside specific academic research settings. As the technology and empirical support for these interventions increase, it seems reasonable to assume that greater access will follow.

Web-Based Individual Therapy

The use of technology in the active treatment of individuals with eating disorder diagnoses has been attempted in different ways. Web-based treatment delivered to individual patients differs from traditional face-to-face treatment and from telemedicine in that Web-based treatment does not include an audiovisual interaction between clinician and patient. Web-based individual treatment involves communicating via electronic messages and viewing online materials (e.g., information modules, videos).

Web-based individual therapy for eating disorders has been studied in multiple countries with generally positive results. To date, cognitive-behavioral therapy (CBT) is the most widely studied Web-based individual treatment approach (Aardoom et al. 2013; Dölemeyer et al. 2013). The amount of actual therapist contact time in such treatments is similar to that in face-to-face treatments, averaging once a week, although the amount of time interacting with the patient each week may differ based on mode of delivery (e.g., e-mail vs. synchronous chat; Dölemeyer et al. 2013). In three studies evaluating Web-based CBT–guided self-help interventions (Carrard et al. 2011; Ljotsson et al. 2007; Sánchez-Ortiz et al. 2011), treatment targeted individuals with binge eating for a duration varying from 12 weeks to 6 months. Treatment content was presented in sequential online modules, with additional weekly electronic communication with a clinician. All three studies reported significant symptom reduction in treatment subjects compared with wait-list control subjects at rates comparable to those of previous face-to-face guided self-help trials (Carrard et al. 2011; Ljotsson et al. 2007; Sánchez-Ortiz et al. 2011).

Overall, patients in Web-based CBT trials appear to improve over time, report notable reductions in global eating disorder symptoms (e.g., concerns over eating, restraint, weight, and shape) and binge-eating behaviors, and tend to maintain these improvements after treatment ends (Dölemeyer et al. 2013; Shingleton et al. 2013). Symptom improvement extends to comorbid depression and anxiety, as well as to overall quality of life (Dölemeyer et al. 2013).

Individuals who are likely to respond best to Web-based treatment include those who struggle with binge eating (rather than simple food restriction; Aardoom et al. 2013) and those who are willing to engage maximally with the technology (i.e., adhere to the modules and engage in more "sessions"). Higher levels of online contact with a therapist yield higher rates of symptom reduction (Shingleton et al. 2013).

Although Web-based CBT appears promising, with initial studies indicating benefits roughly comparable to the effects of face-to-face treatments (e.g., Wagner et al. 2013), more studies comparing Web-based treatments with other active treatments (i.e., not simply using a wait-list control comparison) are required to better appreciate how robust the effects of this modality of intervention might be (Aardoom et al. 2013).

Web-Based Relapse Prevention Following Intensive Treatment

Given the high relapse rates among patients with eating disorders (Steinhausen 2002; Steinhausen and Weber 2009), the possibility of using Web-based interventions in aftercare to reduce the risk of recurrence of these conditions is appealing. As described in the section "Ecological Momentary Intervention," Bauer et al. (2012) found that treatment as usual with added text message–based EMI, provided to individuals with BN following completion of an inpatient treatment, was associated with sustained and significantly improved remission of eating disorder symptoms compared with treatment as usual without EMI. To date, however, little other research has been done in this area. In Germany, one research group has developed a Web-based relapse prevention program, VIA, and studied its use in individuals following completion of inpatient AN treatment (Fichter et al. 2012). VIA includes nine monthly sessions of CBT-informed content provided through self-monitoring, monthly real-time chat sessions hosted by a clinician, and the possibility of e-mail with a readily available therapist. Compared with participants receiving treatment as usual, those receiving the online intervention demonstrated a greater increase in body mass index and improvements in eating disorder behaviors, suggesting a more favorable course of the disorder over time (Fichter et al. 2012). Compared with control subjects and partial completers, participants who completed all sessions of VIA reported significantly better continued health improvement throughout the intervention and during follow-up periods; completers were also significantly less likely to be readmitted for inpatient treatment during the follow-up period (Fichter et al. 2013). VIA is now available to hospital systems that have a German-speaking population and a specialized eating disorder treatment unit for any patients with AN or BN as their level of care steps down following discharge from the inpatient program (M. Fichter, personal communication, August 2014). In light of these promising results, future studies of Web-based relapse prevention programs are warranted.

Patient Acceptability of Web-Based Eating Disorder Treatment

Many clinicians are concerned about how Web-based treatments might impact the therapeutic relationship. Evidence suggests that the association between the therapist-client relationship and outcomes is not as strong in online-only treatments as it is in traditional face-to-face treatments (Cavanagh and Millings 2013). In other words, the mechanism of change in Web-based treatments, while likely still involving aspects of relational factors, may differ from that in traditional therapy. Research suggests that to improve outcomes in Web-based psychological treatments, the clinician must encourage active engagement in the treatment and provide a supportive yet accountable environment for the patient. Additionally, the technology itself is often built with therapeutic relationships in mind, with technology-based messages and reminders that are designed to be supportive and motivational (Cavanagh and Millings 2013).

As one might expect, some patients report liking the flexibility and convenience of Web-based treatments, whereas other patients describe negative impressions of the impersonal nature of online eating disorder treatment interactions. It seems important to balance concerns about the therapeutic relationship in Web-based treatments with the potential for such treatments to assist patients who 1) experience barriers to treatment access (e.g., lack of transportation), 2) learn material well when it is presented in a variety of formats (e.g., visual and verbal information combined), and/or 3) are reluctant to seek help due to shame about their eating disorder symptoms (Paxton and Franko 2010). In a study of opinions about prevention programs, potential participation in a face-to-face, group-based eating disorder prevention program was offered to a sample of undergraduate women. Individuals scoring higher on weight concerns were likely to report that the group format was a deterrent to participation, suggesting that an online intervention might be more appealing to those with greater weight and shape concerns (Atkinson and Wade 2013). Dropout rates in Web-based CBT interventions for eating disorder behavior appear similar to those in Web-based treatments studied in other fields, suggesting average levels of acceptability for individuals with eating disorders (Aardoom et al. 2013; Dölemeyer et al. 2013). Carrard et al. (2011) reported that the dropout rate from their Internet-guided self-help treatment for BED was similar to rates from other face-to-face guided self-help treatments for BED but also reported a higher dropout rate among those participants who had higher levels of shape concern and a higher drive for thinness. Overall, studies that have examined patient views of Web-based treatments report mixed findings; however, there is evidence that these treatments can be effective with no suggestion of harm when implemented properly (Robinson and Serfaty 2003). Thus, it appears that continued study of these interventions is warranted, not only using symptom-based outcome measures but also using metrics of patient perception of the treatment and its outcomes.

Telemedicine

Telemedicine refers to face-to-face treatment between an individual patient and a clinician that is delivered via camera and/or audiovisual technology. According to the American Telemedicine Association (ATA), over 12,000 citations can be found in PubMed (the freely accessible U.S. National Library of Medicine MEDLINE database) regarding telemedicine. Broadly, the ATA reports that telemedicine is cost-effective, improves the health care provided, and is generally well liked by patients (American Telemedicine Association 2013). In a review of 65 studies looking at live videoconferencing psychotherapy for a variety of mental health concerns and a variety of patients, evidence revealed similar outcomes to traditional face-to-face treatments and good acceptability ratings by patients. The studies included in the review were predominantly using individual therapy sessions (71%) with adults (86%), and the treatments were largely cognitive-behavioral in nature (45%). The highest percentage of studies focused on the treatment of psychological trauma disorders (21%). The conclusions of the review suggest a great need for continued study of telemedicine and a need to improve the measures used to assess patient experience and outcome in order to obtain more information about how telemedicine is viewed by patients (Backhaus et al. 2012). One of the largest bodies of literature on telemedicine exists within the field of psychiatry. Broad findings from literature reviews suggest that consultation, diagnosis, medication management, assessment, and therapeutic treatments for psychological conditions have not been found to be significantly different when done via videoconferencing versus face-to-face contacts. Additionally, the benefits to rural, elderly, prisoner, military, and other hard-to-reach populations have been great, often with reduced cost to clinics. Also, few differences were found in adherence to treatment, attendance, and overall patient responses, suggesting that telemedicine is seen as acceptable and satisfactory to patients (Monnier et al. 2003; O'Reilly et al. 2007).

Findings from the limited amount of eating disorder telemedicine treatment research replicate the findings described above. Mitchell et al. (2008) found that CBT provided via telemedicine is as effective as face-to-face CBT and also provides the added benefit to rural populations of intervention without the need for transportation. Additional analyses of this data set suggest that telemedicine can be delivered at a substantial cost savings when compared with having therapists or patients travel, frequently across long distances, for face-to-face treatment (Crow et al. 2009). Of note, although therapists demonstrated a preference for face-to-face treatment over telemedicine, in that they were more critical of the quality of therapeutic relationships in telemedicine-based treatment, patients had no significant preference for one type of treatment over the other (Ertelt et al. 2011).

It has been several years since telemedicine has been actively compared with a traditional face-to-face intervention in the eating disorder field. The findings likely would be even more robust currently, because the ease of access to teleconferencing software and facilities has greatly improved, as have Internet connection speeds and clarity of webcam images, making the experience more seamless and lifelike (Shingleton et al. 2013). Additionally, the young adult and adolescent populations that are potential recipients of such care are more familiar with such technology and have wider access to it than ever before, making it likely a more feasible care option.

Technological Innovation and the Treatment of Eating Disorders: A Practical Discussion

Given the preponderance of mobile technologies and the ease of Internet access, it makes sense that clinicians treating eating disorders would want to integrate technology into their practices. This sentiment may be especially true of clinicians working with young adult and adolescent patients, who are already heavily invested in and excited about technology. There are a number of different ways to integrate technology into practice, whether it is through interventions that take place completely over the Internet, that use technology as an adjunct to face-to-face treatment, or that rely on some combination of different traditional interventions with technology. Incorporating different types of technology into practice can be difficult in terms of feasibility, knowledge and comfort with technology, licensure and liability coverage, and other legal concerns. While the research discussed previously highlights the potential value of using mobile technologies, the Internet, and telemedicine in clinical practice, it is important to address a number of practical issues and concerns relevant to the practicing eating disorder clinician.

Integrating Mobile Technology and Practice

Mobile technologies (e.g., EMA, EMI) represent important contributions to the field of mental health and have been important in eating disorder research through improving models of disorder onset and maintenance; however, incorporating the technology itself into clinical practice can be challenging because of its complexity. Collecting large amounts of momentary data without the technical and statistical assistance available at research facilities is not likely feasible or useful for the typical clinician. However, using technology to collect the data for treatment seems to be the most obvious way for a clinician to integrate clinical treatments and mobile health technologies. For example, the clinician can simply replace elements of interventions or homework (e.g., meal planning, food records, relaxation exercises) with appropriate smartphone applications. Another example of a simple integration of technology into clinical interventions would be taking photographs of handouts or capturing information discussed in session on a mobile device so that the participant can have access to this information during difficult moments between sessions. Web sites that provide this type of information in formats that are easy to view on mobile devices would also be helpful. Patients could bookmark or create icons for these Web sites and easily access the information when needed.

Applications, or *apps*, are programs available for download or purchase on a number of different types of mobile devices, including mobile phones and tablets. The content and purpose of such apps vary widely, and a number of different apps are currently available that attempt to modify various types of behavior relevant to an eating disorder clinician. The most common apps in this category focus on simple monitoring of eating behavior and meal planning. Many apps encourage restrictive eating and emphasize weight loss; consequently, such apps may be contraindicated for most patients with eating disorders. Some apps allow for goals of weight gain or weight maintenance and may be more applicable to patients with eating disorders. SparkPeople and MyFitnessPal are among the more popular producers of these types of applications. Some more sophisticated apps may collect data about other elements of eating, such as food micronutrient content, timing of meals, and speed of eating meals. Among these types of apps, there are many free options, and some that require a purchase fee.

We discuss two apps that seem particularly relevant for possible integration into eating disorder treatment, largely because they allow individuals to set behavioral goals and then compare actual outcome with the goals. Recovery Record and Rise Up+Recover are specifically produced for use by eating disorder patients and are meant to be used in conjunction with face-to-face treatment. Both apps are free to download onto a mobile device.

Recovery Record describes itself as useful in the treatment of full and subthreshold eating disorders and body image disturbances (Recovery Record 2014). Patients using Recovery Record can use templates to create a meal plan and set goals for eating and other behaviors (e.g., weighing, body checking, coping strategies); individuals can also personalize their goals, timelines, and reminders. Messages are sent to the user if planned meals appear to have been skipped, to remind the individual to record certain data, or to remind him or her of a particular goal. To tailor questions and messages, patients indicate which types of behaviors or emotional states are most relevant to them. The app also allows for connection with a treatment team by syncing a clinician app with the patient app, enabling meal plans and other information to be viewed by the treatment provider. The clinician can also send messages and feedback to the patient through the app. The app's Web site is very user friendly and meant to help orient patients and clinicians (Recovery Record 2014).

Rise Up+Recover allows for logging of meals, emotional states, various behaviors (including substance use), and coping skills. The app enables patients to export PDF summaries of their logged information, which can then be sent to a clinician. This app has been recently translated into German and Spanish, and there is also a podcast, *Recovery Warriors,* that is produced weekly by the makers of the app. The podcast and discussion boards are easily accessible through the app and focus on sharing the experiences of others struggling with eating disorders and the presentation of scientific findings from the eating disorder field. The focus of the app is toward patients, and the Web site is a source for accessing podcasts, music, book recommendations, and more; however, there is less emphasis on how to help clinicians use the app (Recovery Warriors 2014).

Recommending apps for patient use in conjunction with eating disorder treatment implies that from a legal perspective, such apps are part of the clinician's therapeutic intervention. Thus, it behooves the clinician to be very familiar with the apps (both the way they work and the research behind them) before recommending their use (Kramer et al. 2015).

Additionally, wearable ambulatory devices that capture movement, sleep, and other physiological data may be useful in eating disorder treatment. A variety of types of ambulatory devices can be found at health and recreation retailers or larger online retailers, often listed under keywords such as "fitness tracker" or "activity tracker." Popular makers of these types of wearable devices include Fitbit, Misfit, Jawbone, and Nike, among many others. These types of devices monitor biometric data, generally limited to movement (walking/exercise), movement during sleep, and heart rate. The devices also transfer collected data via wireless Internet or Bluetooth to a companion app for the device; some of the apps allow one to set goals and monitor progress toward those goals (Taylor 2014).

Although these technologies might not be as easily applicable for patients with AN and BN diagnoses because of the potential for misuse in driven/compelled exercising or caloric restriction, treatment of BED may be well served by the addition of a behavioral-activation component offered by these products. A meta-analysis evaluating the efficacy of mobile health technology in increasing physical activity found generally positive results, suggesting the potential clinical utility of such technologies in achieving behavioral change (Fanning et al. 2012). Kim and Park (2012) created a model containing several factors that predict perceived usefulness of mobile health technologies; perceived usefulness, in turn, is thought to influence actual use of such devices and, ultimately, behavioral change. The most potent factors that were found to predict perceived usefulness of mobile health devices were the individual's sense of his or her potential for health deterioration, his or her engagement in social competition, and his or her perceived sense of self-efficacy with the technological system. Despite the lack of specific studies examining the efficacy of adjunctive use of mobile health technology in eating disorder treatments, broad results from behavioral change literature suggest that if properly motivated to use such technology, individuals can successfully use such devices or apps to change behaviors.

Ethical and Professional Issues

Kramer et al. (2015) present a thorough discussion of legal and regulatory concerns related to the use of technology in clinical practice. They suggest that an important issue related to apps is data storage among those apps that allow for transmission of information between patient and clinician. The same data storage issues are relevant to clinicians using e-mails or text messages to communicate with clients. When data are transmitted, even if the clinician was not expecting or did not endorse the information transfer, the burden is placed on the "entity" that is covered by the Health Insurance Portability and Accountability Act (HIPAA) to ensure that data are handled appropriately (i.e., the clinician is responsible). Once the clinician receives electronic patient data, the data should be moved into the patient record and then deleted from the mobile device or e-mail so that the data are no longer stored on virtual databases or other servers. Mobile technology tends to use less secure networks that are more susceptible to third-party interception, and although higher levels of security are available for use, one cannot be sure that the patient is using such security measures. Although there are no specific guidelines set for HIPAA compliance in terms of mobile phone data management, it is best for clinicians to thoroughly review these issues and find encryption apps or virtual private network (VPN) systems that are HIPAA compliant and provide secure transfer and storage of information. Additionally, it is important for clinicians to draw boundaries in terms of length or frequency of such electronic communications with patients in order to create consistent expectations and to avoid a dramatic increase in clinician demand and burden. Confidentiality may also be boosted by suggesting that patients use pseudonyms or nondescript e-mail addresses separate from work or home e-mail accounts to reduce the risk of an accidental information breach (Paxton and Franko 2010).

Extensive forethought is required to create risk-management policies for situations in which patients indicate imminent risk to themselves or others via electronic communications. For example, with e-mails, the clinician can set an automatic reply to all e-mails reminding the individual to call 911 in the case of emergency and stating that e-mail is monitored at a particular and limited frequency. However, text messaging or synchronized apps do not necessarily have the same automatic-reply features, and therefore, both written and verbal consent procedures may need to be more comprehensive and documentation more thorough (Kramer et al. (2015). There is some benefit to electronic communication in that the conversations between patient and clinician are already documented verbatim. For example, in chat rooms used for synchronous individual or group therapy sessions, a full transcript is typically available. Full transcripts and digital, time-stamped records can also be helpful to clinicians. In the case of eating disorder treatment, there is added risk of patient medical deterioration of which clinicians using Web-based treatment may not be aware. Clinicians may want to add elements to consent procedures that include releases to communicate with a local health care provider or family member in the case of geographically isolated patients (Paxton and Franko 2010). Telemedicine also has the added complication of duty-to-warn laws when there may not be clinical supervision of the patient wherever he or she is located at the time of the telemedicine intervention. Therefore, it is important to create risk-management plans that reflect the laws of the states in which the telemedicine is being practiced. To address these laws, the clinician needs to be thorough when providing informed consent to patients, highlighting differences between states when using telemedicine as well as discussing potential differences in the risk of confidentiality breaches in telemedicine and in traditional face-to-face treatment (Kramer et al. 2015). Overall, it is important to have thorough risk-management protocols when engaging in electronic communication with patients and to continually remind patients of the policies of the practice.

Telemedicine, despite being well supported in scientific literature, has not been standardized in many health care and legal systems. Therefore, when considering the incorporation of telemedicine into clinical practice, the clinician needs to recognize the lack of standardized procedures, equipment, and ethical guidelines (Valdagno et al. 2014). One issue to think about is whether the clinician and patient will be within the geographical boundaries of the clinician's licensing body. In the United States, state licensure boards exist to protect the interests of their citizens, and thus they prefer that all clinicians who provide services to their citizens be licensed in their state. Obtaining multiple state licensures can become problematic because of increased financial and administrative strain on the providers (Kramer et al. 2015). Some states are moving toward changing licensing laws to increase ease of use of telemedicine; such legal changes would be especially important in states with large rural populations. If U.S. clinicians are interested in getting state or neighboring-state licensure boards and legislatures to discuss these issues, the ATA provides a great deal of information about political precedent and strategies for clinicians to use in communication with their representatives and legislators about these issues (American Telemedicine Association 2013).

Different state laws pertaining to issues of clinical practice and mental health also may be significant to clinicians incorporating technology into practice. Kramer et al. (2015) caution clinicians to be very familiar with HIPAA guidelines as well as state privacy laws that might apply to use of different technologies. They also suggest that clinicians take the time to get basic training in the use of these technologies to help troubleshoot and to cut down on mistakes that might cause breaches in confidentiality (Kramer et al. 2015). Often clinics and a patient's home will differ in versions of software, Internet browsers, webcam and microphone accessories, and Internet speeds, which can increase the potential for technical difficulties and frustrations for both patient and clinician. Thus, the more the clinician can be helpful in mitigating these problems, the more therapy can be successfully conducted.

Liability insurance is a rapidly changing issue and a potential area of concern for clinicians practicing telemedicine or other technology-based treatment. It is important for clinicians to ask their liability insurance providers about the level of coverage provided through a policy and to run through potential scenarios with them to ensure adequate protection. It may be advisable to obtain written clarification on coverage areas in liability insurance when existing policy language is not written to clarify telemedicine applications (Kramer et al. 2015). Medicare recently created standards related to credentialing and privileging providers in the use of telemedicine, and it is hoped that these policies will continue to improve federal standards for technology-based treatment over time (American Telemedicine Association 2013). It can be helpful both legally and professionally for clinicians to create relationships with other clinicians who are providing telemedicine or other technology-based treatments as a resource for ongoing consultation (Kramer et al. (2015).

Conclusion

To date, a variety of different technologies have been employed in eating disorder assessment and practice; these include EMA, EMI, Web-based prevention programs, Web-based individual treatment, Web-based relapse prevention programs, and telemedicine. Some technologies have been used primarily in areas of research (e.g., EMA), and their clinical applicability is not well developed. Many technologies are on the cusp of broader application yet are still in the stage of development and efficacy trials; therefore, although they may be available for research participants, they are not widely available to clinicians in practice (e.g., prevention programs or online versions of individual treatment). Other technologies are ready for implementation, to be used as adjuncts to traditional interventions (e.g., apps) or as new methods of implementing existing treatments (e.g., Web-based or telemedicine-based implementation of individual therapy). A clear area in need of additional research is telemedicine-based intervention in eating disorders; additionally, technology exists that would allow clinicians to begin to use this method of treatment, after addressing potential administrative and licensing concerns.

The findings on efficacy of technology-based interventions for eating disorders lag behind the access to such technology. A major problem in researching technology and clinical practice is the rapid rate of technology development compared with the slower rate of research validation and dissemination. The average amount of time it takes for RCTs to be conducted and the evidence to be published is 5.5 years (Kumar et al. 2013). This lag time is too great to keep up with technology; the programs or devices being tested in such trials will be obsolete by the time the evidence supporting their use is established. Additionally, in the world of apps and Web-based content, frequent updates and minor changes are often necessary for such programs to remain competitive or even usable. Thus, the exact versions of apps and devices that have gone through rigorous research are likely not the same apps and devices that were used at the start of the research process. Although the rate of technological innovation and the rate of the research process appear to be diametrically opposed, solutions are being proposed to improve the compatibility of these systems.

One proposed solution involves the use of new research designs, such as repeated measures designs, that allow for greater statistical power using smaller participant numbers so that studies may be completed more quickly and efficiently. Another avenue would be to reduce the research and development on the front end of RCTs. The National Institutes of Health hopes to increase the effectiveness of mobile health research in this way by sharing resources and data collection. The solution involves a network that gives researchers access to the underlying structure of these technologies and to databases already collected. Thus, new mobile health technologies may be built more quickly, will not need to be created from scratch, and instead will build on existing, previously studied platforms. Also, data could be combined with or supplemented by existing databases, so that these types of studies and developments are not conducted in isolation, taking years to disseminate and apply in the clinic (Kumar et al. 2013). Open mHealth is a nonprofit group that advertises its "open architecture" to help jump-start creative ideas and implementation. By providing information and resources on how to create mobile apps and other ambulatory assessment programs, Open mHealth seeks to reduce production time and get research started quickly, building on the past success of other researchers (Open mHealth 2014). Additionally, the National Institutes of Health funds the Patient Reported Outcomes Measurement Information System (PROMIS), which provides clinicians with Internet access to previously established and tested self-report health measures for adults and children. The purpose is to create stronger networks of data that use the same outcome measures to make results more comparable and application to clinical settings easier. The measures and scoring information are provided at their Web site (PROMIS Network 2011).

It is important to note that as technology rapidly changes and evolves, empirical studies documenting the utility and effectiveness of technology-enhanced eating disorder treatment will be a step behind newer, emerging technologies. For example, many more technologies are available to you, the reader, than were available at the time this chapter was written. Overall, utilizing technology in clinical practice is appealing to clinicians and patients and can help to enhance treatment, overcome barriers to treatment, and increase the scope of interventions. Using technology in clinical practice also comes with unique challenges and requires careful planning and documentation in order to protect clinicians and patients. The future of the integration of technology and psychological treatment is exciting and full of promise, with increasing opportunities to involve clinicians and patients in improving research and to apply research findings.

Key Clinical Points

- Ecological momentary assessment has been used extensively in empirical research on eating disorders, but its clinical application remains largely undeveloped.
- Increasing numbers of clinicians and researchers are developing ecological momentary intervention strategies for the treatment of obesity; these types of interventions for use in the treatment of eating disorders are still in early stages of development.
- Prevention-oriented technologies have been shown to be somewhat effective in reducing the risk of eating disorder onset, but translating these into everyday clinical practice is rare.
- Web-based individual treatments of eating disorders can effectively target eating disorder symptoms; however, availability of such programs to the general public is still somewhat limited outside of several countries in the European Union. Similarly, technology-based aftercare strategies to reduce the risk of relapse have been shown to be effective but are not yet readily available to clinicians.
- Although "apps" that may complement clinical practice are increasingly available, typically these have not been empirically studied.

- Telemedicine is expanding dramatically in psychiatry and psychology in general, and it has been shown to be potentially effective in eating disorder treatment. This technology has significant, immediate implications for eating disorder treatment.

References

aan het Rot M, Hogenelst K, Schoevers RA: Mood disorders in everyday life: a systematic review of experience sampling and ecological momentary assessment studies. Clin Psychol Rev 32(6):510–523, 2012

Aardoom JJ, Dingemans AE, Spinhoven P, et al: Treating eating disorders over the Internet: a systematic review and future research directions. Int J Eat Disord 46(6):539–552, 2013 23674367

American Telemedicine Association: Research outcomes: telemedicine's impact on healthcare cost and quality. April 2015. Available at: http://www.americantelemed.org/docs/default-source/policy/examples-of-research-outcomes---telemedicine's-impact-on-healthcare-cost-and-quality.pdf. Accessed August 3, 2015.

Atkinson MJ, Wade TD: Enhancing dissemination in selective eating disorders prevention: an investigation of voluntary participation among female university students. Behav Res Ther 51:806–816, 2013 24140874

Backhaus A, Agha Z, Maglione ML, et al: Videoconferencing psychotherapy: a systematic review. Psychol Serv 9(2):111–131, 2012 22662727

Bauer S: Challenges in healthcare delivery: the potential of technology-enhanced strategies [PowerPoint slides]. Presentation at the annual meeting of the Academy of Eating Disorders, New York, March 2014

Bauer S, Percevic R, Okon E, et al: Use of text messaging in the aftercare of patients with bulimia nervosa. Eur Eat Disord Rev 11:279–290, 2003

Bauer S, Okon E, Meermann R, et al: Technology-enhanced maintenance of treatment gains in eating disorders: efficacy of an intervention delivered via text messaging. J Consult Clin Psychol 80(4):700–706, 2012 22545736

Beintner I, Jacobi C, Taylor CB: Effects of an Internet-based prevention programme for eating disorders in the USA and Germany–a meta-analytic review. Eur Eat Disord Rev 20(1):1–8, 2012 21796737

Burke LE, Conroy MB, Sereika SM, et al: The effect of electronic self-monitoring on weight loss and dietary intake: a randomized behavioral weight loss trial. Obesity (Silver Spring) 19(2):338–344, 2011 20847736

Carrard I, Crépin C, Rouget P, et al: Randomised controlled trial of a guided self-help treatment on the Internet for binge eating disorder. Behav Res Ther 49(8):482–491, 2011 21641580

Cavanagh K, Millings A: (Inter)personal computing: the role of the therapeutic relationship in e-mental health. J Contemp Psychother 43:197–206, 2013

Coons MJ, Demott A, Buscemi J, et al: Technology interventions to curb obesity: a systematic review of the current literature. Curr Cardiovasc Risk Rep 6(2):120–134, 2012 23082235

Crosby RD, Wonderlich SA, Engel SG, et al: Daily mood patterns and bulimic behaviors in the natural environment. Behav Res Ther 47(3):181–188, 2009 19152874

Crow SJ, Mitchell JE, Crosby RD, et al: The cost effectiveness of cognitive behavioral therapy for bulimia nervosa delivered via telemedicine versus face-to-face. Behav Res Ther 47(6):451–453, 2009 19356743

Dölemeyer R, Tietjen A, Kersting A, et al: Internet-based interventions for eating disorders in adults: a systematic review. BMC Psychiatry 13:207, 2013 23919625

Ebner-Priemer UW, Kuo J, Welch SS, et al: A valence-dependent group-specific recall bias of retrospective self-reports: a study of borderline personality disorder in everyday life. J Nerv Ment Dis 194(10):774–779, 2006 17041290

eMarketer: Worldwide smartphone usage to grow 25% in 2014. June 11, 2014. Available at: http://www.emarketer.com/Article/Worldwide-Smartphone-Usage-Grow-25-2014/1010920. Accessed March 18, 2015.

Engel SG, Wonderlich SA, Crosby RD, et al: The role of affect in the maintenance of anorexia nervosa: evidence from a naturalistic assessment of momentary behaviors and emotion. J Abnorm Psychol 122(3):709–719, 2013 24016011

Ertelt TW, Crosby RD, Marino JM, et al: Therapeutic factors affecting the cognitive behavioral treatment of bulimia nervosa via telemedicine versus face-to-face delivery. Int J Eat Disord 44(8):687–691, 2011 22072405

Eurostat: Internet access and use in 2013. December 18, 2013. Available at: http://ec.europa.eu/eurostat/documents/2995521/5168694/4-18122013-BP-EN.PDF/. Accessed June 10, 2015.

Fanning J, Mullen SP, McAuley E: Increasing physical activity with mobile devices: a meta-analysis. J Med Internet Res 14(6):e161, 2012 23171838

Fichter MM, Quadflieg N, Nisslmüller K, et al: Does Internet-based prevention reduce the risk of relapse for anorexia nervosa? Behav Res Ther 50(3):180–190, 2012 22317754

Fichter MM, Quadflieg N, Lindner S: Internet-based relapse prevention for anorexia nervosa: nine-month follow-up. J Eat Disord 1:23, 2013 24999404

File T, Ryan C: Computer and Internet access in the United States: 2013. November 2014. Available at: http://www.census.gov/hhes/computer/. Accessed March 18, 2015.

Fox S: Tracking for health [Pew Research Center Web site]. January 28, 2013. Available at: http://www.pewinternet.org/2013/01/28/tracking-for-health/. Accessed March 18, 2015.

Goldschmidt AB, Engel SG, Wonderlich SA, et al: Momentary affect surrounding loss of control and overeating in obese adults with and without binge eating disorder. Obesity (Silver Spring) 20(6):1206–1211, 2012 21938073

Haapala I, Barengo NC, Biggs S, et al: Weight loss by mobile phone: a 1-year effectiveness study. Public Health Nutr 12(12):2382–2391, 2009 19323865

Haedt-Matt AA, Keel PK: Revisiting the affect regulation model of binge eating: a meta-analysis of studies using ecological momentary assessment. Psychol Bull 137(4):660–681, 2011 21574678

Heinicke BE, Paxton SJ, McLean SA, et al: Internet-delivered targeted group intervention for body dissatisfaction and disordered eating in adolescent girls: a randomized controlled trial. J Abnorm Child Psychol 35(3):379–391, 2007 17243014

Heron KE, Smyth JM: Ecological momentary interventions: incorporating mobile technology into psychosocial and health behaviour treatments. Br J Health Psychol 15 (Pt 1):1–39, 2010 19646331

Karr TM, Crosby RD, Cao L, et al: Posttraumatic stress disorder as a moderator of the association between negative affect and bulimic symptoms: an ecological momentary assessment study. Compr Psychiatry 54(1):61–69, 2013 22789761

Kim J, Park HA: Development of a health information technology acceptance model using consumers' health behavior intention. J Med Internet Res 14(5):e133, 2012 23026508

King AC, Ahn DK, Oliveira BM, et al: Promoting physical activity through handheld computer technology. Am J Prev Med 34(2):138–142, 2008 18201644

Kramer GM, Kinn JT, Mishkind MC: Legal, regulatory, and risk management issues in the use of technology to deliver mental health care. Cogn Behav Pract 22(3):258–268 2015

Kumar S, Nilsen WJ, Abernethy A, et al: Mobile health technology evaluation: the mHealth evidence workshop. Am J Prev Med 45(2):228–236, 2013 23867031

Lavender JM, De Young KP, Wonderlich SA, et al: Daily patterns of anxiety in anorexia nervosa: associations with eating disorder behaviors in the natural environment. J Abnorm Psychol 122(3):672–683, 2013 23647124

Lindenberg K, Moessner M, Harney J, et al: E-health for individualized prevention of eating disorders. Clin Pract Epidemiol Ment Health 7:74–83, 2011 21687562

Ljotsson B, Lundin C, Mitsell K, et al: Remote treatment of bulimia nervosa and binge eating disorder: a randomized trial of Internet-assisted cognitive behavioural therapy. Behav Res Ther 45(4):649–661, 2007 16899213

Mitchell JE, Crosby RD, Wonderlich SA, et al: A randomized trial comparing the efficacy of cognitive-behavioral therapy for bulimia nervosa delivered via telemedicine versus face-to-face. Behav Res Ther 46(5):581–592, 2008 18374304

Monnier J, Knapp RG, Frueh BC: Recent advances in telepsychiatry: an updated review. Psychiatr Serv 54(12):1604–1609, 2003 14645799

Myers TC, Wonderlich SA, Crosby R, et al: Is multi-impulsive bulimia a distinct type of bulimia nervosa: psychopathology and EMA findings. Int J Eat Disord 39(8):655–661, 2006 16927382

Oorschot M, Kwapil T, Delespaul P, et al: Momentary assessment research in psychosis. Psychol Assess 21(4):498–505, 2009 19947784

Open mHealth: Architecture. 2014. Available at: http://openmhealth.org/architecture/#what-is-open-mhealth. Accessed August 3, 2015.

O'Reilly R, Bishop J, Maddox K, et al: Is telepsychiatry equivalent to face-to-face psychiatry? Results from a randomized controlled equivalence trial. Psychiatr Serv 58(6):836–843, 2007 17535945

Patrick K, Raab F, Adams MA, et al: A text message-based intervention for weight loss: randomized controlled trial. J Med Internet Res 11(1)(e1):e1, 2009 19141433

Paxton SJ, Franko DL: Body image and eating disorders, in Using Technology to Support Evidence-Based Behavioral Health Practices: A Clinician's Guide. Edited by Cucciare MA, Weingardt KR. New York, Routledge, 2010, pp 151–168

Paxton SJ, McLean SA, Gollings EK, et al: Comparison of face-to-face and Internet interventions for body image and eating problems in adult women: an RCT. Int J Eat Disord 40(8):692–704, 2007 17702020

Pew Research Internet Project: Cell phone and smartphone ownership demographics. January 2014. Available at: http://www.pewinternet.org/data-trend/mobile/cell-phone-and-smartphone-ownership-demographics/. Accessed March 18, 2015.

PROMIS Network: PROMIS overview. 2011. Available at: http://www.nihpromis.org/about/overview. Accessed March 18, 2015.

ProYouth: Register with ProYouth self-test [in German]. 2013. Available at: http://www.proyouth.eu/de/join#. Accessed March 18, 2015.

Rao G, Burke LE, Spring BJ, et al; American Heart Association Obesity Committee of the Council on Nutrition, Physical Activity and Metabolism; Council on Clinical Cardiology; Council on Cardiovascular Nursing; Council on the Kidney in Cardiovascular Disease; Stroke Council: New and emerging weight management strategies for busy ambulatory settings: a scientific statement from the American Heart Association endorsed by the Society of Behavioral Medicine. Circulation 124(10):1182–1203, 2011 21824925

Recovery Record: Recovery Record: eating disorder management for bulimia, anorexia, binge eating, EDNOS, and body image concerns (Version 4.5) [software]. 2014. Available at: http://www.recoveryrecord.com. Accessed March 18, 2015.

Recovery Warriors: Rise Up+Recover: an eating disorder monitoring and management tool for anorexia, bulimia, binge eating, and EDNOS (Version 1.3.0) [software]. 2014. Available at: http://recoverywarriors.com. Accessed March 18, 2015.

Robinson P, Serfaty M: Computers, e-mail and therapy in eating disorders. Eur Eat Disord Rev 11:210–221, 2003

Rodgers A, Corbett T, Bramley D, et al: Do u smoke after txt? Results of a randomised trial of smoking cessation using mobile phone text messaging. Tob Control 14(4):255–261, 2005 16046689

Sánchez-Ortiz VC, Munro C, Stahl D, et al: A randomized controlled trial of Internet-based cognitive-behavioural therapy for bulimia nervosa or related disorders in a student population. Psychol Med 41(2):407–417, 2011 20406523

Selby EA, Doyle P, Crosby RD, et al: Momentary emotion surrounding bulimic behaviors in women with bulimia nervosa and borderline personality disorder. J Psychiatr Res 46(11):1492–1500, 2012

Shapiro JR, Bauer S, Andrews E, et al: Mobile therapy: use of text-messaging in the treatment of bulimia nervosa. Int J Eat Disord 43:513–519, 2010 19718672

Shiffman S: Ecological momentary assessment (EMA) in studies of substance use. Psychol Assess 21(4):486–497, 2009 19947783

Shingleton RM, Richards LK, Thompson-Brenner H: Using technology within the treatment of eating disorders: a clinical practice review. Psychotherapy (Chic) 50(4):576–582, 2013 23527906

Smyth J, Wonderlich S, Crosby R, et al: The use of ecological momentary assessment approaches in eating disorder research. Int J Eat Disord 30(1):83–95, 2001 11439412

Smyth JM, Wonderlich SA, Heron KE, et al: Daily and momentary mood and stress are associated with binge eating and vomiting in bulimia nervosa patients in the natural environment. J Consult Clin Psychol 75(4):629–638, 2007 17663616

Smyth JM, Wonderlich SA, Sliwinski MJ, et al: Ecological momentary assessment of affect, stress, and binge-purge behaviors: day of week and time of day effects in the natural environment. Int J Eat Disord 42(5):429–436, 2009 19115371

Spring B, Duncan JM, Janke EA, et al: Integrating technology into standard weight loss treatment: a randomized controlled trial. JAMA Intern Med 173(2):105–111, 2013 23229890

Steinhausen HC: The outcome of anorexia nervosa in the 20th century. Am J Psychiatry 159(8):1284–1293, 2002 12153817

Steinhausen HC, Weber S: The outcome of bulimia nervosa: findings from one-quarter century of research. Am J Psychiatry 166(12):1331–1341, 2009 19884225

Stice E, Rohde P, Durant S, et al: A preliminary trial of a prototype Internet dissonance-based eating disorder prevention program for young women with body image concerns. J Consult Clin Psychol 80(5):907–916, 2012 22506791

Stice E, Durant S, Rohde P, et al: Effects of a prototype Internet dissonance-based eating disorder prevention program at 1- and 2-year follow-up. Health Psychol 33(12):1558–1567, 2014 25020152

Taylor B: 26 fitness trackers ranked from worst to first. TIME, January 9, 2014. Available at: http://time.com/516/26-fitness-trackers-ranked-from-worst-to-first/. Accessed March 18, 2015.

Taylor CB, Bryson S, Luce KH, et al: Prevention of eating disorders in at-risk college-age women. Arch Gen Psychiatry 63(8):881–888, 2006 16894064

Valdagno M, Goracci A, di Volo S, et al: Telepsychiatry: new perspectives and open issues. CNS Spectr 19(6):479–481, 2014 24382055

Wagner G, Penelo E, Wanner C, et al: Internet-delivered cognitive-behavioural therapy v. conventional guided self-help for bulimia nervosa: long-term evaluation of a randomised controlled trial. Br J Psychiatry 202:135–141, 2013 23222037

Weitzel JA, Bernhardt JM, Usdan S, et al: Using wireless handheld computers and tailored text messaging to reduce negative consequences of drinking alcohol. J Stud Alcohol Drugs 68(4):534–537, 2007 17568957

Wonderlich S: Capturing real time, ecologically valid data in eating disorder research: the utility of ecological momentary assessment. Presentation at the annual meeting of the Eating Disorder Research Society, Boston, MA, October 2010

Wonderlich SA, Rosenfeldt S, Crosby RD, et al: The effects of childhood trauma on daily mood lability and comorbid psychopathology in bulimia nervosa. J Trauma Stress 20(1):77–87, 2007 17345648

Wonderlich SA, Peterson CB, Crosby RD, et al: A randomized controlled comparison of integrative cognitive-affective therapy (ICAT) and enhanced cognitive-behavioral therapy (CBT-E) for bulimia nervosa. Psychol Med 44(3):543–553, 2014 23701891

PART IV

Treatment

13 Treatment of Restrictive Eating and Low-Weight Conditions, Including Anorexia Nervosa and Avoidant/Restrictive Food Intake Disorder

Joanna Steinglass, M.D.
Laurel Mayer, M.D.
Evelyn Attia, M.D.

A salient feature at the core of anorexia nervosa (AN) is energy intake that is inadequate with respect to caloric requirements, resulting in significantly low body weight. Restrictive eating may be characterized by food rules, some of which are remarkably similar across individuals (e.g., recurrent selection of low-fat foods) and some of which are idiosyncratic (e.g., eating only at 10 minutes after the hour). Although present across eating disorders, restrictive eating poses particular challenges when it leads to undernourishment, nutrient deficiencies, or frank starvation, as in the cases of AN and avoidant/restrictive food intake disorder (ARFID). Restrictive eating behaviors in these disorders warrant particular attention because they contribute to the severity of illness, including medical morbidity, the need for hospitalization or other intensive treatment, and mortality.

Restrictive intake by individuals with AN has been documented in objective studies of eating behavior, showing caloric intake below caloric needs and a significantly reduced intake of fat specifically (Hadigan et al. 2000; Mayer et al. 2012). In a study of hospitalized patients with AN, measurement of eating in a laboratory setting revealed significantly reduced intake compared with that of healthy control subjects at the time of hospital admission. Although intake increased after normalization of weight, it remained significantly reduced compared with that observed in the control subjects. In addition to their restricted energy intake, patients with AN showed a specific reduction in calories from fat. Patterns of restriction have been shown to be related to longer-term outcome (Schebendach et al. 2008); these patterns include rigid rules, repetitive intake of the same few foods with little variety, and intake of low-energy foods and noncaloric beverages. Ecological momentary assessment studies and laboratory meal studies among individuals who restrict food have demonstrated a relationship between affective state and restriction (Lavender et al. 2013; Steinglass et al. 2010).

AN and ARFID differ in the psychological features that motivate food restriction, and fewer studies have been done of eating behavior in ARFID specifically. Nevertheless, treatments for both have similar components because the common goal is normalization of weight and eating behavior. In this chapter, we outline principles for treating feeding and eating disorders that are characterized by low weight and restrictive eating, including AN and ARFID. The principles of treatment in this chapter are derived from the treatment of AN, with applicability to ARFID. We consider features specific to ARFID at the end of the chapter.

Principles of Treatment for Restrictive Eating and Low Weight

Low-weight disorders are challenging to treat for two notable reasons: First, no treatment has emerged as the clear, empirically supported treatment of choice for all patients. Second, for many individuals, there is a reluctance to utilize treatment, including aspects that emphasize improved eating behavior and improved weight status.

AN and ARFID are different illnesses in their initiating and sustaining factors. AN is characterized by inadequate intake relative to requirements associated with fear of fatness or behavioral interference with weight gain, together with body weight or shape concerns. ARFID is an eating or feeding disturbance that is manifested by failure to meet appropriate nutritional and/or energy needs that is *not* associated with body weight or shape concern but may be associated with anxiety about eating and associated features (e.g., fear of vomiting, fear of choking) or with food avoidance due to the sensory characteristics of food.

Because ARFID is a newly described disorder in DSM-5 (American Psychiatric Association 2013), very little has been written about its treatment. In contrast, much has been described about approaches for AN, but small study sample sizes, high dropout rates, negative findings in randomized clinical trials using particular treatment strategies, and tiny numbers of studies examining more comprehensive, multimodal treatment approaches have limited the evidence base for treatments for AN. Most treatment information regarding AN appears in professional guideline and expert consensus documents, and this information suggests that behavioral management is a core strategy for the achievement of behavioral change in the treatment of AN (American Psychiatric Association 2006; Wilson and Shafran 2005).

Both AN and ARFID are psychiatric conditions with medical as well as psychological features; therefore, treatment needs to include a comprehensive assessment of medical and psychiatric symptoms and a specific assessment of the acute medical and psychiatric risks. This assessment will inform treatment goals and the selection of an appropriate treatment setting. Selection of treatment setting usually includes consideration of the least restrictive setting that is appropriate for the identified goals (Table 13–1). Treatment goals for individuals with restrictive eating and low weight include medical stabilization as needed, nutritional rehabilitation (reversal of nutritional deficiencies and restoration of normal weight), and interruption of eating-disordered behaviors. Strategies for achieving these goals are described in the remainder of this chapter.

Medical Stabilization

Both AN and ARFID are associated with nutritional compromise and physiological changes, many of them severe and some potentially life-threatening. Height and weight assessments are a first step in assessing nutritional status. A clinician's determination of underweight commonly includes assessment of weight in the context of an individual's baseline or highest weight, as well as assessment of physiological disturbances that may be associated with weight status (see Chapter 2, "Eating Problems in Adults"). According to the National Heart, Lung, and Blood Institute (2000) and the World Health Organization (1995), the lower limit of a normal body mass index (BMI) is 18.5 kg/m^2. Notably, the World Health Organization defines moderate thinness as BMI less than 17.0 kg/m^2, severe thinness as BMI less than 16.0 kg/m^2, and extreme thinness as less than 15.0 kg/m^2.

TABLE 13–1. Treatment settings for individuals with eating disorders

Setting	Description	Indications
Outpatient	Individual or group-based sessions are available, and patients often select or are recommended for several treatment components, often offered by clinicians from different clinical disciplines (e.g., psychology, nutrition, medicine). Outpatient treatment is optimized when providers communicate regularly in order to coordinate care, creating a treatment "team."	An outpatient program is the most commonly used setting for eating disorder treatment. Many patients utilize outpatient treatment as they begin engagement in eating disorder treatment or because they are unable to access higher levels of care because of geographic or other resource limitations. Outpatient treatment is most appropriate for individuals who are medically stable and are achieving or maintaining behavioral goals using this level of care.
Intensive outpatient program (IOP)	IOP refers to a routine of outpatient sessions in which visits include several hours of treatment per visit offered at a frequency of several visits (e.g., three) each week. Supervised meals are often available as part of an IOP visit.	An IOP is appropriate for individuals who are medically stable and require small amounts of meal instruction or meal supervision without additional daily programmatic structure. An IOP is often used as a step-down from higher levels of care.
Partial hospital program (PHP)	Also known as day treatment programs, PHPs offer more hours of weekly treatment than do IOPs. A PHP may serve as a transition from inpatient to outpatient care or may help some individuals avoid the need for hospitalization. PHPs generally include 4–7 days of treatment with two or three supervised meals each treatment day.	A PHP is appropriate when meal supervision is needed without requirement for 24-hour supervision. PHP admission generally requires that patients be at or above a minimally acceptable weight (e.g., ≥80% ideal body weight) and maintain other evidence of medical stability. A PHP is often used as a step-down from a higher level of care, or as a step-up from a lower level of care.

TABLE 13–1. Treatment settings for individuals with eating disorders *(continued)*

Setting	Description	Indications
Residential treatment center (RTC)	RTCs offer specialized treatment delivered in a full-time setting; however, they are less structured than hospital programs. They include less medical monitoring and less staffing at night than do hospital-based programs.	An RTC is appropriate for patients with low weight (e.g., <85% ideal body weight) and/or evidence of eating disorder behaviors who are in need of close supervision but not in need of daily medical attention. Patients in an RTC must demonstrate motivation needed for voluntary treatment.
Inpatient program	Psychiatric hospitalization represents the highest level of care and may be necessary for some individuals with eating disorders, especially those at low weights and those with comorbidities. Specialized inpatient programs include medical personnel, such as psychiatrists and nurses.	An inpatient program is appropriate for patients with significantly low weight (e.g., <75% ideal body weight) and/or the presence of other signs of medical or psychiatric instability (e.g., vital sign or electrolyte disturbance; comorbidity, including behavioral dyscontrol and/or suicidality). Inpatient treatment is also appropriate for individuals who have failed to respond to treatment at an RTC.

For children and adolescents, assessments of weight and height require comparison to reference standard data for age and sex. BMI varies greatly in growing children, and BMI-for-age reference standards are important for evaluating healthy and expected growth. BMI assessment for children should be examined in the context of individual growth curves (see Chapter 3, "Eating Problems in Children and Adolescents"). Failure to gain as expected may be as serious an indication of nutritional compromise in a child or adolescent as weight loss is for an adult with a restrictive eating disorder.

Many of the physical consequences of malnourishment that are commonly manifested in AN may be manifested in ARFID as well. Almost every system in the body is affected as part of the physiological responses of the body to being underweight, including cardiac, metabolic, endocrine, skeletal, hematopoietic, gastrointestinal, and dermatological (including skin and hair). Physiological responses to low weight commonly include bradycardia, decreased respiration rates, and low body temperature. Laboratory assessments commonly reflect abnormalities consistent with nutritional deficiencies, dehydration, and purging behaviors (see Chapters 2 and 3 for additional information about medical complications of low weight). Although many of these complications are chronic consequences of starvation and weight loss, others present acute management issues (Trent et al. 2013). As refeeding is initiated, vital signs and laboratory test results should be monitored closely and should improve as energy intake and hydration reach daily requirements.

Nutritional Rehabilitation

Successful treatment of restrictive eating associated with AN or ARFID requires nutritional rehabilitation. Resumption of energy intake adequate for gaining weight to and then maintaining weight within a healthy range is essential. Psychological support can help with motivation to eat and making specific behavioral changes, but formal psychotherapy and other psychosocial interventions may be of limited utility in underweight and nutritionally deficient individuals. Patients are encouraged to restore weight fully (e.g., BMI=20–22 kg/m^2; weight consistent with pre-illness weight range or growth curve, if patient had healthy baseline; or weight consistent with return of normal menstruation for the amenorrheic patient). Better long-term outcomes have been shown to be associated with full weight restoration (Baran et al. 1995; Kaplan et al. 2009).

Initial Refeeding

Nutritional plans for initial weight gain involve reintroducing foods at modest caloric levels (e.g., 1,500–1,800 kcal/day); providing supervision, psychological support, and psychoeducation (Table 13–2); and medical monitoring. Macronutrient composition is prescribed consistent with the standard daily macronutrient requirements per the Institute of Medicine to ensure adequate dietary fat in particular (Marzola et al. 2013). Liver function should be monitored because abnormalities, including paradoxically elevated cholesterol, are common. In addition to the medical monitoring described above, patients may benefit from the nutritional information that their cholesterol will improve with a normal diet. Low-fat diets are not indicated.

Caloric prescription should increase steadily (e.g., by 400 kcal every 48–72 hours), with ongoing monitoring, until a weight gain rate of 1–2 kg per week is consistently achieved. Weight restoration at this rate commonly requires consumption of 3,500–4,000 kcal/day. In addition to food, meals and snacks, nutritional supplements are often needed during weight

TABLE 13–2. Guidelines for engagement of underweight patients

Low-weight patients may benefit from information about the physiological and psychological consequences of low weight and restrictive eating.
For some low-weight individuals, it may be useful to emphasize the identified diagnosis (e.g., anorexia nervosa or avoidant/restrictive food intake disorder), whereas for others, especially those who insist that their eating disturbance has atypical features, it is preferable to begin with the identified risk of low weight or restrictive eating and the need for nutritional change, without one particular diagnostic label.
Individuals with low weight should be informed that many of their symptoms (e.g., anxiety, depression, preoccupation with food) would be expected to improve with weight gain, despite their often strong beliefs that weight gain or changed eating behaviors would worsen their mood or anxiety symptoms.
Obtaining a careful history of cognitive and psychological functioning prior to the onset of restrictive eating may identify baseline strengths that may be used as treatment targets and possible motivators for embarking on weight and eating change.
For individuals with avoidant/restrictive food intake disorder, obtaining a careful history from patient and/or family of symptoms that interfere with normal eating and inform specific food choices is essential. Treatment needs to include individualized goals appropriate for specific symptoms. Discomfort with food sensations may require graded exposure to novel foods; restrictive eating due to fear of choking or vomiting may require exercises that target these concerns.

gain. Vitamin supplements (e.g., daily multivitamin, thiamine, folate) are commonly prescribed. Supportive acknowledgment of the physical discomfort associated with the gastrointestinal sequelae of starvation, including decreased motility and constipation, which may contribute to early fullness and related discomfort after eating, and the sequelae related to laxative use discontinuation (e.g., edema and constipation) is needed. Repeated reassurance that continued intake will lead to improvement in these physical symptoms is often required. Stool softeners (e.g., docusate sodium) and nonstimulant bulking agents (e.g., polyethylene glycol) may also be considered.

Nutritional rehabilitation emphasizes normative eating, with structured meals and snacks that include adequate dietary variety and energy density. Feeding via nasogastric tube may be necessary for individuals resistant to eating voluntarily or for those prescribed exceptionally large doses of liquid intake. Individuals with ARFID may need meal plans that target specific nutrient deficiencies that have developed in the context of the eating disturbance.

Therapeutic meal plans should be designed to improve diet variety and increase energy density. For example, they should include items with higher kilocalories per gram, meals that moderate water consumption, and minimal noncaloric foods and beverages. Although meal plans initially may not offer patients much preference or choice, greater autonomy in food selection is given as patients improve in medical status, weight, and eating behavior. Following weight restoration, nutritional plans should adjust to help patients stay within a healthy weight range.

Nutritional Rehabilitation and Psychological Change

It is important to understand that while nutritional rehabilitation targets weight and physiological change, it also improves psychological symptoms associated with AN and ARFID. Many of the psychological features attributed to these conditions are, in fact, part of the natural sequelae of starvation and being underweight. In their landmark study of semistarvation in previously healthy male subjects who were given restrictive diets, Keys et al. (1950) described depressed mood, restricted affect, heightened anxiety, poor concentration, perfectionism, and obsessionality associated with the underweight and malnourished state. Even in these subjects without an eating disorder, the authors observed increased preoccupation with food, as well as unusual patterns of eating (e.g., eating quickly or dawdling over eating) in the setting of significant weight loss. These historical findings suggest that the psychological symptoms present in low-weight restrictive eaters with AN or ARFID may have developed or intensified as a result of the state of undernutrition.

Other common psychological sequelae of the underweight state in individuals with AN or ARFID include poor sleep, sadness, hopelessness, and anxiety. Anxiety symptoms may include social fears, generalized worry, and physical symptoms of anxiety, as well as eating-related and non-eating-related obsessions and compulsions. Cognitive disturbances, including poor attention, visuospatial deficits, and executive functioning deficits, have been well described in the underweight state among individuals with AN (Steinglass and Glasofer 2011). It is recommended that individuals with AN or ARFID receive psychoeducation about both the physical and psychological consequences of low weight as they are supported through nutritional rehabilitation (see Table 13–2).

Psychiatric Comorbidities

In addition to experiencing psychological change secondary to nutritional depletion, patients with AN or ARFID may have co-occurring psychiatric diagnoses, most commonly mood and anxiety disorders, and these may not resolve with refeeding. In a sample of 172 individuals with AN presenting for treatment, 35% met criteria for comorbid mood disorders and 11% for anxiety disorders (Bühren et al. 2014). In their retrospective study of 173 children and adolescents receiving day treatment for a feeding or eating disorder, Nicely et al. (2014) reported that 72% of the 39 individuals with ARFID met criteria for an anxiety disorder, in contrast to the lower rate of 37% of the 93 individuals with AN. Additionally, the investigators found that 13% of those with ARFID and none of those with AN met criteria for autism spectrum disorder. Also, across many studies, suicidal ideation, suicide attempts and self-injury, and rates of completed suicides were consistently reported to be high in samples of patients with AN (Berkman et al. 2007).

Significant improvement in psychological symptoms is seen with nutritional rehabilitation and weight restoration (Attia et al. 1998; Sysko et al. 2005). Psychological improvement may lag behind physiological change, which can be a challenging situation for patients who seek relief of symptoms. Mood and anxiety symptoms, in particular, may continue to be outside the normal range at the time of acute weight normalization. These symptoms show continued improvement with long-term maintenance of healthy eating and healthy weight (Pollice et al. 1997).

Behavioral Management

Because both AN and ARFID may be associated with reluctance to normalize eating behaviors, behavioral management treatment is commonly employed to reverse or reduce many of the most worrisome features of these eating disorders (Attia and Walsh 2009). Behavioral management programs are those that encourage the achievement of normal weight and eating behavior through the use of reinforcements for healthy behavioral choices. Behavioral management may be delivered as part of inpatient or outpatient treatment; if it is offered as part of outpatient treatment, a frequency of more than once weekly is generally required. Commonly, these treatments include supervised meals and snacks, use multiple treatment modalities, and include clinicians across disciplines. The aim of the meal supervision is to address behaviors at meals that contribute to the perpetuation of eating restriction. Supervision is additionally included after meals to support "having eaten" and to prevent compensatory behaviors, including vomiting, standing, and exercising.

Behavioral programs reinforce healthy eating by offering privileges or activities following the successful completion of eating goals. As an example, the specialty eating disorders treatment program at Columbia University offers off-unit privileges to patients who consume all of prescribed food, offers additional groups and activities for those at healthier weight ranges, and offers opportunities for brief unaccompanied passes to patients once weight gain goals have been achieved. Part of the power of the behavioral treatment comes from the consistency of the program, which sets standards that all participants can achieve. The expectation that all program participants will aim to eat 100% of prescribed food contributes to the likelihood that the goal will be met and to the overall therapeutic effect. Additionally, the treatment milieu provides group reinforcement for healthy choices. Participants often report that they meet their treatment goals to avoid disappointing their peers as much as for any other motivation for change. In addition to the standard reinforcements of the program, individually tailored reinforcements can be introduced. For example, if an individual demonstrates lack of motivation for the privilege of an off-unit pass, contingencies may be adjusted to reinforce healthy eating and weight with opportunities on the unit (e.g., opportunities for food preparation and cooking on the unit).

Behavioral management for ARFID may require more attention to the individualized assessment of restrictive behaviors and a plan that specifically reinforces successful eating of the restricted foods or reversal of some of the avoidant or restrictive behaviors. Patients who avoid foods because of their sensory characteristics (e.g., smells, textures) may need treatments that expose patients to the specific sensations that are associated with their restrictive eating. Treatments for ARFID need to reinforce reversal of specific eating disturbances in addition to generally reinforcing any required increase in food intake, weight restoration, and improvements in identified nutritional deficiencies.

Behavioral management is incorporated into most intensive treatment programs for individuals with low weight and restrictive eating (see Table 13–1). Intensive treatment programs include inpatient, residential, day treatment, and other intensive outpatient programs that generally require several visits weekly. Less intensive outpatient treatment for individuals with these disorders should similarly include firm behavioral goals. Outpatient treatment may be offered by a team of clinicians, including an internist or pediatrician, a therapist, and a nutritionist. Patients in outpatient treatment–and sometimes their families–should participate in setting treatment goals that reinforce healthy and improved eating behaviors and weight change.

Psychotherapeutic Approaches

Several specific psychotherapeutic approaches that emphasize behavioral change, including family-based treatment, cognitive-behavioral therapy

(CBT), and exposure and response-prevention treatment, have been studied in the treatment of AN and are commonly used in outpatient settings. There are no published treatment studies of ARFID, but behavioral strategies used in other eating disorders are commonly applied to the treatment of ARFID and other conditions that include avoidant or restrictive eating.

Also known as the Maudsley approach, family-based treatment for adolescents with AN is a psychological treatment with solid empirical support (Agras et al. 2014; Lock et al. 2010). Family-based treatment emphasizes participation by all family members and empowers parents to refeed their undernourished child. This outpatient approach aims to help adolescents achieve full weight restoration with normal eating behaviors. When successful, the 6- to 12-month treatment terminates with a transition back to developmentally appropriate autonomy regarding eating and food choice for the weight-restored adolescent.

With stronger support for its effectiveness for the treatment of BN than for AN, CBT is, nevertheless, used by eating disorder clinicians treating low-weight conditions (Fairburn 2008). CBT generally begins with education about the medical and psychological effects of being underweight (see Table 13–2). With attention to treatment alliance and goal setting, the clinician encourages the patient to examine and change behaviors that contribute to the restrictive state and to create a plan for regular, healthier eating. As behavioral change is made and nutritional status improves, the treatment examines and addresses the cognitive distortions that contribute to the individual's illness. Food monitoring records are a mainstay of treatment, and close attention is paid to actual eating behavior. Over time, thought records and methods for challenging problematic beliefs (i.e., cognitive distortions) are introduced. These techniques have shown modest benefit, although they are not empirically superior to other outpatient psychotherapies that pay close attention to weight and eating behavior (McIntosh et al. 2005). For individuals who have already achieved full weight restoration, CBT has been shown to be more successful than nutritional counseling alone in preventing relapse of AN (Pike et al. 2003).

Exposure and response prevention is the cornerstone of treatment for many anxiety disorders and obsessive-compulsive disorder and is a behavioral treatment strategy that has shown some promise for individuals with AN. The premise of the technique is that individuals need to confront rather than avoid the anxiety-producing stimuli. With incremental exposure to feared stimuli, patients learn that anxiety dissipates over time and that feared consequences do not occur. With this behavioral learning as the mechanism of change, patients practice resisting avoidance behaviors (i.e., response prevention). In treatment of eating disorders specifically, exposure and response prevention targets eating-related anxiety and aims to support patients in confronting rather than avoiding eating-related fears. In inpatient settings, these techniques successfully supported healthier eating behavior and clinical improvement (Simpson et al. 2013; Steinglass et al. 2014a).

Management of ARFID

Because ARFID is newly described as a distinct diagnosis in DSM-5, no data specific to ARFID are yet available to provide empirical support for treatment. Clinical guidelines suggest that behavioral treatment approaches are likely to be beneficial, because the primary concern is the need to alter behavior. CBT principles are likely to be applicable and successful. CBT, however, is a general therapeutic approach that often needs to be specifically tailored to diagnoses with different features. For example, the CBT manuals for depression differ significantly from those for anxiety disorders. Even within the anxiety disorders category, each diagnosis has its own emphasis for helpful interventions. ARFID is likely a heterogeneous category, and behavioral strategies will need to be tailored differently, depending on the type of illness. The features specific to ARFID, however, suggest particular directions for the development of useful CBT interventions. For example, those individuals whose ARFID symptoms occur within the context of autism spectrum disorder will differ from those whose symptoms are more strongly associated with an anxious temperament or anxiety spectrum. For the anxious patient, interventions may focus on exposure to sensations, whereas for the individual with autism, interventions may focus on consistent meal schedules and positive reinforcement of adequate intake.

Exposure and response prevention, as described in the subsection "Psychotherapeutic Approaches," may be particularly relevant for treating ARFID. Among some individuals with ARFID, symptoms develop as a conditioned negative response to an experience of eating. These cases of ARFID share many features with specific phobias; however, among individuals with ARFID, the avoidant or restrictive eating behavior has become the primary focus of treatment. Principles of exposure therapy suggest that for each individual, a hierarchy of feared situations can be created. Similar to individuals treated for fear of heights who are gradually exposed to higher and higher floors of a building, individuals with ARFID would begin treatment with eating-related activities that generate low levels of anxiety. As the individual becomes increasingly able to engage in these behaviors, the assignments move toward increasingly higher levels of anxiety. When ARFID includes avoidant or restrictive intake associated with heightened sensory awareness or sensitivity around aspects of eating, exposure to various eating sensations may be necessary. Additionally, techniques that promote awareness of internal bodily sensations may be useful for exposure.

Psychopharmacology

Pharmacological trials in patients with AN are few in number. Owing to the lack of information about the neurobiological mechanisms underlying AN, approaches to medication management in patients with AN have by necessity relied on shared features with other psychiatric illnesses. The high levels of depressive and anxiety symptoms that accompany starvation led to consideration of antidepressants, in particular, as potentially helpful for weight restoration treatment. Many medications appeared promising in case reports or case series, only to prove disappointing when compared with placebo treatment in randomized controlled trials (Hay and Claudino 2012). Meta-analyses have attempted to use the available data from small studies to advance understanding of which strategies may or may not hold promise, and these have similarly shown limited utility of medications (de Vos et al. 2014). These studies highlight the need for rigorous testing of medications, including comparison with placebo, for both AN and ARFID. Although current treatment guidelines have emphasized the lack of utility of medications for AN (Aigner et al. 2011; Watson and Bulik 2013), medications continue to be frequently prescribed, contributing to the cost of treatment and the potential for unwanted complications from medication.

Antidepressants

Individuals with AN often present with significant depressive symptoms, including sad mood, hopelessness, and/or anhedonia. Furthermore, early antidepressants were also associated with weight gain as an unwelcome side effect in non–eating disorder populations. Together, these data suggested the potential utility of antidepressant medications for the treatment of AN. Unfortunately, these strategies proved disappointing. Early trials of tricyclic antidepressants showed no benefit for weight gain (indicating no significant impact on eating behavior) (Biederman et al. 1985; Halmi et al. 1986; Lacey and Crisp 1980), and these medications are associated with cardiac side effects that preclude their use in underweight individuals with AN.

Some of the most influential data have come from a study comparing fluoxetine with placebo in patients with AN receiving behavioral treatment for weight restoration (Attia et al. 1998). This study clearly indicated that fluoxetine offered no benefit over placebo when offered together with a comprehensive weight restoration program. Although all study participants showed improvement in weight as well as in mood and anxiety symptoms during the study period, there were no differences between the fluoxetine-treated and placebo-treated groups.

Underweight individuals with AN are associated with profoundly altered physiology. Therefore, the possibility that antidepressants may confer benefit only after nutritional rehabilitation has been accomplished has been studied separately. Unfortunately, these data have been similarly disappointing. The largest randomized clinical trial among weight-restored individuals with AN showed no benefit of fluoxetine compared with placebo (Walsh et al. 2006). These patients were studied for 1 year after hospital discharge, while receiving CBT aimed at relapse prevention. Fluoxetine again conferred no benefit in rate of relapse or in improvement of psychological symptoms.

Together, these data are very convincing that antidepressants do not significantly improve the treatment of AN.

Anxiolytics

Individuals with AN commonly struggle with anxiety, specifically around mealtimes. This may be a prominent feature of ARFID as well (Nicely et al. 2014). Because anxiety has been shown to be related to actual food intake (Engel et al. 2013; Steinglass et al. 2010), medications that may reduce anxiety acutely seem worth consideration, such as for individuals during structured treatment. Benzodiazepines are commonly considered as an option to relieve premeal anxiety, yet there are no randomized controlled trials of the clinical utility of benzodiazepines in restrictive eating. The only available data show no benefit of alprazolam compared with placebo in reducing premeal anxiety among a small group of hospitalized patients with AN or in improving their intake in a laboratory meal (Steinglass et al. 2014b). Similarly, in the treatment of obsessive-compulsive disorder, benzodiazepines have not been shown to reduce symptoms (Hollander et al. 2003).

Antipsychotics

Antipsychotic medications have been considered for the treatment of AN, both for the potential psychological benefits and to capitalize on the weight gain side effects seen in other populations. The concrete, rigid, and near-delusional thought processes seen in AN make this class of medications a compelling possibility for treatment. Early trials were uninformative, because the complications from these medications precluded their use (i.e., seizures, binge and purge symptoms) (Dally and Sargant 1960; Vandereycken 1984; Vandereycken and Pierloot 1982). With the innovation of second-generation antipsychotics and their broad-ranging pharmacology and improved side-effect profile, a new treatment possibility emerged. Initial studies have shown some weight gain benefit of olanzapine among adults with AN (Attia et al. 2011; Bissada et al. 2008), although not in adolescents (Kafantaris et al. 2011). Additionally, it may be that olanzapine relieves some of the obsessionality around eating seen in individuals with AN (Bissada et al. 2008) and thereby may contribute to improved eating. Larger trials will be informative as to whether olanzapine may be a useful treatment for outpatients with AN.

Hormonal Treatments

Bone health issues, osteopenia and osteoporosis, are well documented in individuals with AN, and reduced bone density may be the single medical complication that may not fully normalize with complete weight restoration. Bone issues occur in the context of a low-estrogen state, leading to increased bone resorption and poor nutrition, which, in turn, lead to decreased bone formation. Reductions in bone mineral density can be seen on dual-energy X-ray absorptiometry (DXA) as early as 6–12 months after onset of illness (Castro et al. 2000). Results from a more recent study (Faje et al. 2014) suggest that patients with AN carry an increased fracture risk, even in the absence of identifiable areal bone mineral density deficits. A number of pharmacological interventions have been studied, including oral and transdermal hormone replacement, growth factors (i.e., insulin-like growth factor 1), and bisphosphonates. Only one study in adolescents of transdermal estrogen with cyclic progesterone has shown significant promise (Misra et al. 2011). Studies of bisphosphonates suggest that these drugs may offer modest improvement; however, their long half-life and potential impact on a developing fetus make them inappropriate for use in women of reproductive potential.

Medications for ARFID

No medication trials have been done specifically for the treatment of ARFID. Given the similarities in malnourishment between AN and ARFID, it is certainly plausible that medications will be similarly disappointing for ARFID as they have been for AN. However, there may be significant differences in the underlying psychological and neurobiological mechanisms that differentiate these illnesses. Pharmacological treatment studies for ARFID are needed. The prominence of anxiety symptoms and phobic-like traits among individuals with ARFID suggests that anxiolytic medications–and possibly selective serotonin reuptake inhibitors–may be more useful in this population than they have been for individuals with AN. Given the potential promise of second-generation antipsychotics in treating AN, these are worth studying for the treatment of ARFID as well.

Conclusion

Restrictive eating and low weight, associated with eating disorders such as AN and ARFID, require careful clinical evaluation and management. Low weight is associated with many physiological disturbances and substantial medical risk. Low weight is also associated with psychological symptoms that may worsen in the context of nutritional deficiencies. Nutritional rehabilitation and behavioral management, requiring multimodal treatment, are the core components for reversing low weight and normalizing disturbances in eating behavior. Empirical support for specific treatments is limited for AN and entirely absent for ARFID. Novel treatment approaches need to be developed for AN. Descriptive data as well as preliminary data regarding treatment efforts are sorely needed for the recently identified ARFID category.

Key Clinical Points

- Anorexia nervosa (AN) and avoidant/restrictive food intake disorder (ARFID) differ in identified motivation for restrictive eating, but individuals with either disorder may develop significant psychological and medical symptoms associated with low weight and undernutrition and may benefit from structured, behaviorally focused treatment that reinforces healthy eating and weight.
- Treatment for low weight and restrictive eating commonly includes supervision during meals and snacks, together with a nutritional plan that ensures consistent weight restoration.
- In AN, as nutritional status improves, treatment includes targeting the problematic beliefs that underlie the behaviors. Cognitive interventions ask patients to acknowledge and challenge problematic thoughts about food and about shape and weight.
- For younger patients with AN, family-based treatment engages the family to provide the structure and behavioral interventions that help nourish adolescents back to normal weight.

- In AN and ARFID, restrictive eating may be associated with anxiety. Helpful interventions can include exposure to specific foods, food groups, or somatic experiences (e.g., swallowing exercises in individuals with ARFID with choking fears). These strategies may be helpful in diminishing food-related anxiety symptoms.
- Unfortunately, no medication has emerged as an evidence-based approach to restrictive eating and undernourishment.

References

Agras WS, Lock J, Brandt H, et al: Comparison of 2 family therapies for adolescent anorexia nervosa: a randomized parallel trial. JAMA Psychiatry 71(11):1279–1286, 2014 25250660

Aigner M, Treasure J, Kaye W, et al: World Federation of Societies of Biological Psychiatry (WFSBP) guidelines for the pharmacological treatment of eating disorders. World J Biol Psychiatry 12(6):400–443, 2011 21961502

American Psychiatric Association: Treatment of patients with eating disorders, third edition. Am J Psychiatry 163 (7 suppl):4–54, 2006 1692519

American Psychiatric Association: Diagnostic and Statistical Manual of Mental Disorders, 5th Edition. Arlington, VA, American Psychiatric Association, 2013

Attia E, Walsh BT: Behavioral management for anorexia nervosa. N Engl J Med 360(5):500–506, 2009 19179317

Attia E, Haiman C, Walsh BT, et al: Does fluoxetine augment the inpatient treatment of anorexia nervosa? Am J Psychiatry 155(4):548–551, 1998 9546003

Attia E, Kaplan AS, Walsh BT, et al: Olanzapine versus placebo for out-patients with anorexia nervosa. Psychol Med 41(10):2177–2182, 2011 21426603

Baran SA, Weltzin TE, Kaye WH: Low discharge weight and outcome in anorexia nervosa. Am J Psychiatry 152(7):1070–1072, 1995 7793445

Berkman ND, Lohr KN, Bulik CM: Outcomes of eating disorders: a systematic review of the literature. Int J Eat Disord 40(4):293–309, 2007 17370291

Biederman J, Herzog DB, Rivinus TM, et al: Amitriptyline in the treatment of anorexia nervosa: a double-blind, placebo-controlled study. J Clin Psychopharmacol 5(1):10–16, 1985 3973067

Bissada H, Tasca GA, Barber AM, et al: Olanzapine in the treatment of low body weight and obsessive thinking in women with anorexia nervosa: a randomized, double-blind, placebo-controlled trial. Am J Psychiatry 165(10):1281–1288, 2008 18558642

Bühren K, Schwarte R, Fluck F, et al: Comorbid psychiatric disorders in female adolescents with first-onset anorexia nervosa. Eur Eat Disord Rev 22(1):39–44, 2014 24027221

Castro J, Lázaro L, Pons F, et al: Predictors of bone mineral density reduction in adolescents with anorexia nervosa. J Am Acad Child Adolesc Psychiatry 39(11):1365–1370, 2000 11068891

Dally PJ, Sargant W: A new treatment of anorexia nervosa. BMJ 1(5188):1770–1773, 1960 13813846 de Vos J, Houtzager L, Katsaragaki G, et al: Meta analysis on the efficacy of pharmacotherapy versus placebo on anorexia nervosa. J Eat Disord 2(1):27, 2014 25379181

Engel SG, Wonderlich SA, Crosby RD, et al: The role of affect in the maintenance of anorexia nervosa: evidence from a naturalistic assessment of momentary behaviors and emotion. J Abnorm Psychol 122(3):709–719, 2013 24016011

Fairburn CG: Cognitive Behavior Therapy and Eating Disorders. New York, Guilford, 2008

Faje AT, Fazeli PK, Miller KK, et al: Fracture risk and areal bone mineral density in adolescent females with anorexia nervosa. Int J Eat Disord 47(5):458–466, 2014 24430890

Hadigan CM, Anderson EJ, Miller KK, et al: Assessment of macronutrient and micronutrient intake in women with anorexia nervosa. Int J Eat Disord 28(3):284–292, 2000 10942914

Halmi KA, Eckert E, LaDu TJ, et al: Anorexia nervosa: treatment efficacy of cyproheptadine and amitriptyline. Arch Gen Psychiatry 43(2):177–181, 1986 3511877

Hay PJ, Claudino AM: Clinical psychopharmacology of eating disorders: a research update. Int J Neuropsychopharmacol 15(2):209–222, 2012 21439105

Hollander E, Kaplan A, Stahl SM: A double-blind, placebo-controlled trial of clonazepam in obsessive-compulsive disorder. World J Biol Psychiatry 4(1):30–34, 2003 12582975

Kafantaris V, Leigh E, Hertz S, et al: A placebo-controlled pilot study of adjunctive olanzapine for adolescents with anorexia nervosa. J Child Adolesc Psychopharmacol 21(3):207–212, 2011 21663423

Kaplan AS, Walsh BT, Olmsted M, et al: The slippery slope: prediction of successful weight maintenance in anorexia nervosa. Psychol Med 39(6):1037–1045, 2009 18845008

Keys A, Brozek J, Henschel A, et al: The Biology of Human Starvation. Minneapolis, University of Minnesota Press, 1950

Lacey JH, Crisp AH: Hunger, food intake and weight: the impact of clomipramine on a refeeding anorexia nervosa population. Postgrad Med J 56 (suppl 1):79–85, 1980 6994086

Lavender JM, De Young KP, Wonderlich SA, et al: Daily patterns of anxiety in anorexia nervosa: associations with eating disorder behaviors in the natural environment. J Abnorm Psychol 122(3):672–683, 2013 23647124

Lock J, Le Grange D, Agras WS, et al: Randomized clinical trial comparing family based treatment with adolescent-focused individual therapy for adolescents with anorexia nervosa. Arch Gen Psychiatry 67(10):1025–1032, 2010 20921118

Marzola E, Nasser JA, Hashim SA, et al: Nutritional rehabilitation in anorexia nervosa: review of the literature and implications for treatment. BMC Psychiatry 13:290, 2013 24200367

Mayer LE, Schebendach J, Bodell LP, et al: Eating behavior in anorexia nervosa: before and after treatment. Int J Eat Disord 45(2):290–293, 2012 21495053

McIntosh VV, Jordan J, Carter FA, et al: Three psychotherapies for anorexia nervosa: a randomized, controlled trial. Am J Psychiatry 162(4):741–747, 2005 15800147

Misra M, Katzman D, Miller KK, et al: Physiologic estrogen replacement increases bone density in adolescent girls with anorexia nervosa. J Bone Miner Res 26(10):2430–2438, 2011 21698665

National Heart, Lung, and Blood Institute: The Practical Guide: Identification, Evaluation, and Treatment of Overweight and Obesity in Adults (NIH Publ No 00-4084), Bethesda, MD, National Heart, Lung, and Blood Institute, 2000.

Nicely TA, Lane-Loney S, Masciulli E, et al: Prevalence and characteristics of avoidant/restrictive food intake disorder in a cohort of young patients in day treatment for eating disorders. J Eat Disord 2(1):21, 2014 25165558

Pike KM, Walsh BT, Vitousek K, et al: Cognitive behavior therapy in the posthospitalization treatment of anorexia nervosa. Am J Psychiatry 160(11):2046–2049, 2003 14594754

Pollice C, Kaye WH, Greeno CG, et al: Relationship of depression, anxiety, and obsessionality to state of illness in anorexia nervosa. Int J Eat Disord 21(4):367–376, 1997 9138049

Schebendach JE, Mayer LE, Devlin MJ, et al: Dietary energy density and diet variety as predictors of outcome in anorexia nervosa. Am J Clin Nutr 87(4):810–816, 2008 18400701

Simpson HB, Wetterneck CT, Cahill SP, et al: Treatment of obsessive-compulsive disorder complicated by comorbid eating disorders. Cogn Behav Ther 42(1):64–76, 2013 23316878

Steinglass JE, Glasofer DR: Neuropsychology, in Eating Disorders and the Brain. Edited by Lask B, Frampton I. Chichester, UK, Wiley, 2011, pp 106–121

Steinglass JE, Sysko R, Mayer L, et al: Pre-meal anxiety and food intake in anorexia nervosa. Appetite 55(2):214–218, 2010 20570701

Steinglass JE, Albano AM, Simpson HB, et al: Confronting fear using exposure and response prevention for anorexia nervosa: a randomized controlled pilot study. Int J Eat Disord 47(2):174–180, 2014a 24488838

Steinglass JE, Kaplan SC, Liu Y, et al: The (lack of) effect of alprazolam on eating behavior in anorexia nervosa: a preliminary report. Int J Eat Disord 47(8):901–904, 2014b 25139178

Sysko R, Walsh BT, Schebendach J, et al: Eating behavior among women with anorexia nervosa. Am J Clin Nutr 82(2):296–301, 2005 16087971

Trent SA, Moreira ME, Colwell CB, et al: ED management of patients with eating disorders. Am J Emerg Med 31(5):859–865, 2013 23623238

Vandereycken W: Neuroleptics in the short-term treatment of anorexia nervosa: a double-blind placebo-controlled study with sulpiride. Br J Psychiatry 144:288–292, 1984 6367876

Vandereycken W, Pierloot R: Pimozide combined with behavior therapy in the short-term treatment of anorexia nervosa: a double-blind placebo-controlled cross-over study. Acta Psychiatr Scand 66(6):445–450, 1982 6758492

Walsh BT, Kaplan AS, Attia E, et al: Fluoxetine after weight restoration in anorexia nervosa: a randomized controlled trial. JAMA 295(22):2605–2612, 2006 16772623

Watson HJ, Bulik CM: Update on the treatment of anorexia nervosa: review of clinical trials, practice guidelines and emerging interventions. Psychol Med 43(12):2477–2500, 2013 23217606

Wilson GT, Shafran R: Eating disorders guidelines from NICE. Lancet 365(9453):79–81, 2005 15639682

World Health Organization: The Use and Interpretation of Anthropometry (Report of a WHO Expert Committee, WHO Technical Report Series 854). Geneva, Switzerland, World Health Organization, 1995.

14 Treatment of Binge Eating, Including Bulimia Nervosa and Binge-Eating Disorder

Loren Gianini, Ph.D.
Allegra Broft, M.D.
Michael Devlin, M.D.

In this chapter, we provide an overview of the general approach to treating binge eating that is typically seen in the context of bulimia nervosa (BN) or binge-eating disorder (BED). We discuss evidence-based psychotherapeutic and pharmacological treatments for BN and BED, as well as other promising treatment approaches. The reader is encouraged to view Video 2 for sample questions regarding the preliminary assessment of binge eating and compensatory behaviors by a general practitioner.

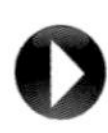

Video Illustration 2: Assessing eating problems in the primary care setting (3:24)

General Approach to the Treatment of Binge Eating

Normalization of Eating

The primary goal of treatment for individuals with either BN or BED is the normalization of eating behavior. The common behavior shared by these conditions is binge eating, and an important focus of interventions for BN and BED is to eliminate both *objective binge episodes* (i.e., episodes during which abnormally large amounts of food are consumed with a sense of loss of control) and *subjective binge episodes* (i.e., episodes in which a normal amount is consumed with a sense of loss of control) (see also Chapter 2, "Eating Problems in Adults" and Chapter 5, "Assessment of Eating Disorders and Problematic Eating Behavior in Bariatric Surgery Patients"). For individuals with BN, an additional goal is to eliminate inappropriate behaviors undertaken to compensate for binge episodes or for other forms of eating; these behaviors include vomiting, use of laxatives or diuretics, and excessive or compulsive exercise. Some individuals with BED and the majority with BN engage in some type of dietary restraint or rigid dietary rules, although success in adhering to these rules may be sporadic, especially for those with BED (Carrard et al. 2012). Restriction may consist of attempts to eat very little throughout the day or strict rules about what can and cannot be eaten (e.g., no sweets, no high-fat foods), and it has been linked to the maintenance of binge eating. Thus, a common goal of treatment is to increase dietary flexibility and ensure that individuals eat on a regular basis and in a manner that meets their daily caloric needs.

Overvaluation of Shape and Weight

In addition to targeting maladaptive eating behaviors, another common goal in treating binge eating is reducing the overvaluation of body shape and weight. This overvaluation is typically defined as self-evaluation that is unduly influenced by an individual's perception of his or her body shape or weight. *Body shape* may refer to the overall shape and size of the body or of a particular body area (e.g., stomach, buttocks), whereas *body weight* refers to the number on the scale. The self-evaluation of individuals with BN, by definition, is influenced by shape and weight to an impairing degree; however, this presentation is also seen in a significant portion of individuals with BED, and it is associated with heightened eating pathology, depression, and worsened treatment outcomes (Grilo et al. 2012b). Overvaluation of shape and weight is often entrenched and difficult to change during the course of treatment, although significant inroads can be made in this area. Treatment follow-up studies in BN have also demonstrated that when body image disturbance is high following treatment, individuals are at heightened risk of poor outcomes and relapse (Keel et al. 2005).

Weight Management

Many individuals with BED, and a smaller subset of individuals with BN, who present for treatment in clinical settings have a body mass index

(BMI) in the overweight or obese range (≥25 kg/m^2; Bulik and Reichborn-Kjennerud 2003; Masheb and White 2012). These individuals are at increased risk for presenting with obesity-related medical complications such as hypertension and type 2 diabetes. Furthermore, some evidence suggests that in the 12 months prior to entering treatment, a significant portion of individuals with BED report gaining upward of 15 pounds (Blomquist et al. 2011). Therefore, weight management may be included as a component of treatment for binge eating; however, caution should be observed so as not to reinforce preoccupation with shape or weight.

Evidence-Based Treatments for Bulimia Nervosa and Binge-Eating Disorder

Cognitive-Behavioral Therapy

Cognitive-behavioral therapy (CBT) is a brief, present-focused treatment with a strong evidence base for both BN and BED. CBT is considered the treatment of choice for BN, with a Cochrane Review demonstrating the superiority of CBT over no treatment, wait-list control, and other psychotherapies with regard to reductions in binge eating, purging, and depression (Hay et al. 2009). CBT can effectively eliminate binge eating and purging behaviors in 30%–50% of patients with BN. A large portion of patients who are not abstinent from binge eating or vomiting experience meaningful reductions in symptoms, including improvements in dietary restraint, eating, and weight and shape concerns, at the end of treatment and in long-term follow-up (Fairburn et al. 1995). Similarly, CBT reduces or eliminates binge eating in 50%–60% of patients with BED, and it is superior to behavioral weight loss treatment and pharmacological interventions (Grilo et al. 2005, 2012a).

CBT for BN and BED, as manualized by Fairburn (2008), is rooted in the hypothesis that individuals' eating disorders are maintained by maladaptive thoughts and beliefs (i.e., overvaluation of shape and weight) that lead to maladaptive behaviors (i.e., binge eating, compensatory behaviors, restrictive eating) and vice versa. An important first step in treatment is creating an individualized "formulation" in which the clinician and patient work together to visually diagram the reinforcing relationship between the eating-disordered thoughts and behaviors experienced by the patient (Figure 14–1). Creation of this formulation is intended to increase the patient's interest in and understanding of the mechanisms maintaining the disorder. It can also help direct the patient to what thoughts and behaviors will be targeted in the treatment and why.

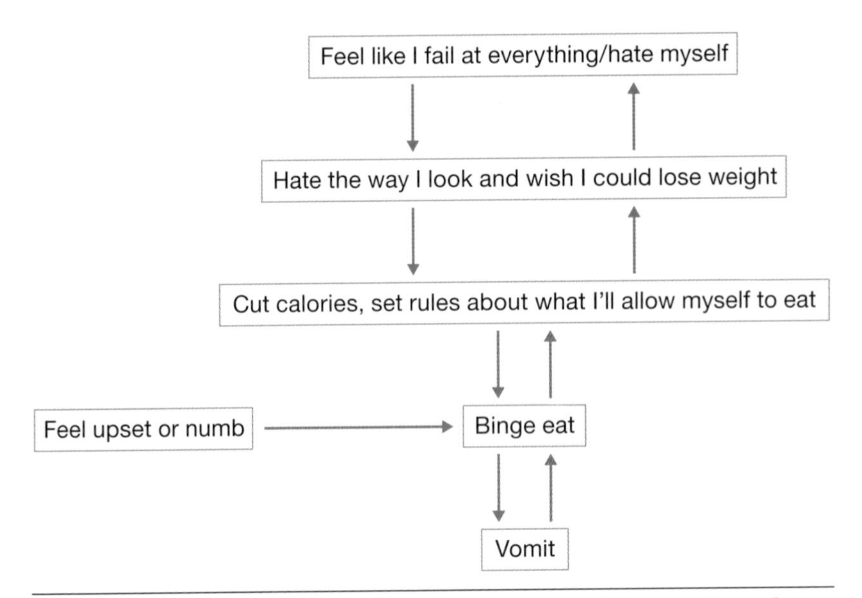

FIGURE 14–1. Individualized cognitive-behavioral therapy formulation of bulimia nervosa (patient's wording).

Self-monitoring of eating behavior is a cornerstone of CBT for BN and BED. Traditionally, clinicians provide patients with preprinted self-monitoring forms that allow for tracking of food consumed; the presence of binge eating, purging, or other eating-disordered behaviors; and the context (time, place, thoughts) of the eating episode. Electronic applications with self-monitoring capabilities for smartphones and/or computers are also now available (see Chapter 12, "Application of Modern Technology in Eating Disorder Assessment and Intervention"). Patients are encouraged to monitor for the duration of treatment in real time and to record what they have eaten as closely to the eating episode as possible (Figure 14–2). Self-monitoring has two purposes: First, it allows the clinician and patient to work together to identify and effectively target maladaptive eating patterns; they can also use monitoring logs to track progress and identify what is going well for the patient. Second, the act of monitoring eating behavior in real time may have the effect of reducing eating-disordered behaviors. It is thought that having to write down and share details of eating-disordered episodes may dissuade patients from engaging in these behaviors in the moment. It is also possible that real-time monitoring leads to heightened self-awareness of one's actions, and patients may feel they have more agency over their decisions in the moment and may opt out of eating-disordered behaviors.

Time	Food & Drink	Location	Binge	Vomit	Comments
6:45	Orange juice Oatmeal with blueberries	Kitchen			Very hungry from restricting yesterday. Trying to get back on track today.
1:00	1 small container Greek yogurt Salad: lettuce, tomato, cucumber, carrot, chickpeas, crushed walnuts, 1 tablespoon nonfat dressing Seltzer water	Desk at work			Brought lunch from home. I know it's small, but I worry that if I eat more, I won't be able to stop and I'll have a binge.
3:00	2 seltzer waters	Break room at work			I am getting hungry, and it's hard to concentrate on work. Hoping these seltzers will fill me up so that I don't eat more.
6:00	Bagel with cream cheese Twix bar Bag of potato chips Ice cream sandwich	Walking to the bus after work	X	V	Went into different shops on my way to the bus, buying food. Feel like I can't stop myself.
	Macaroni and cheese Medium pizza Pint of ice cream	Living room	X	V	After getting off the bus near home, I went into the deli and bought the rest of my binge food. I'm so ashamed of myself. I promised myself I wouldn't do this today.
10:00	Glass of water	Kitchen			Today was awful. I'm exhausted and just want to go to bed. I'm worried I haven't gotten rid of all the calories from my binges.

FIGURE 14–2. Example of eating behavior self-monitoring form.

Following successful self-monitoring, patients are typically prescribed a pattern of "regular eating," or three meals and two to three snacks per day. Patients are encouraged to eat every few hours and to let no more than 4 hours elapse between eating episodes. Regular, frequent meals and snacks reduce disordered eating behaviors because significant dietary restriction (e.g., going more than 4 hours without eating) increases food craving and binge eating. Aberrant eating patterns among individuals with BN and BED may result in abnormal sensations of hunger and satiety, along with other physiological signals that would typically help initiate or terminate eating (e.g., slowed gastric emptying in BN; Devlin et al. 1997). Often, the maintenance of a pattern of regular eating will greatly reduce the frequency of binge episodes. For residual binges, techniques such as stimulus control, *urge surfing* (a strategy for systematic delay of disordered behavior such as binge eating or purging), or use of distraction are often implemented.

Patients are asked to weigh themselves once weekly at treatment sessions. Those weighing themselves more often are educated about the deleterious effects of frequent weighing, namely, the manner by which this behavior reinforces preoccupation with weight, and about normative fluctuations in weight even while weight is stable. Weighing provides both the patient and the clinician with objective information about the effect of regular eating on the patient's weight. CBT clinicians also provide patients with psychoeducation regarding the typical nature of dieting, binge eating, and compensatory behaviors (and their relative ineffectiveness as weight-control strategies) within the context of BN and BED.

The initial focus of CBT for BN and BED is behavioral, and after the disordered eating behaviors are better managed, the treatment shifts to addressing thoughts. To start, the cognitive distortions that are targeted are those that relate to eating behavior and dietary rules (e.g., "Eating carbohydrates will make me fat"). Next, thoughts (and related behaviors) that maintain an overvaluation of shape and weight are tackled. The clinician may target beliefs, such as "If I feel fat, it means that I *am* fat," or behaviors, such as body checking and body comparisons, that reinforce maladaptive shape- and weight-related thoughts. Patients are encouraged to increase participation in activities not focused on shape and weight to expand the number of options the patients have for self-evaluation and ultimately to detract from the prominence of body weight and shape in determining self-worth.

CBT typically concludes with a progress-maintenance/relapse-prevention phase focused on short-term and long-term maintenance plans. This phase includes 1) steps to minimize the likelihood that a relapse will occur, 2) identification of warning signs that the patient is beginning to slip back into eating-disordered thoughts and behaviors, and

3) development of specific, actionable plans for what the patient can do if this occurs.

Fairburn (2008) also developed an enhanced version of CBT (CBT-E) that can be applied transdiagnostically across eating disorders. CBT-E allows for broad and focused treatment courses. The focused treatment strictly addresses reducing core eating disorder psychopathology, whereas the broad treatment addresses other issues that may help maintain eating pathology, such as perfectionism, low self-esteem, and interpersonal difficulties. Interpersonal difficulties are addressed through the simultaneous implementation of CBT and an abbreviated version of interpersonal psychotherapy (IPT; discussed in more detail in the section "Interpersonal Psychotherapy"). Studies assessing the efficacy of CBT-E in treating BN and BED are limited. For individuals with binge-eating behavior, one randomized controlled trial (RCT) found significant improvements in eating pathology with both the broad and focused versions of CBT-E in a sample of patients with BN and eating disorder not otherwise specified, with the broad version potentially being more effective for individuals with complex psychopathology (Fairburn et al. 2009).

CBT for BN and BED can be delivered in either pure or guided self-help formats. In the pure version, patients typically follow a treatment book without clinical interaction, whereas patients receiving guided self-help typically have at least brief meetings with a clinician to implement the treatment. Evidence suggests that self-help treatments are significantly more effective than wait-list control conditions in reducing binge-eating and purging behaviors; however, it is unclear whether pure self-help and guided self-help are equally efficacious, and evidence suggests that self-help interventions may be less potent than more intensive face-to-face treatments (Sysko and Walsh 2008).

Interpersonal Psychotherapy

IPT was originally developed as a brief, time-limited intervention for the treatment of depression and was subsequently modified for the treatment of both BN and BED (Murphy et al. 2012). IPT focuses primarily on helping patients identify and address current interpersonal problems that are hypothesized to maintain and perpetuate their eating disorders; healthy interpersonal functioning is posited as necessary for psychological well-being. Because individuals with BN and BED report a significant number of interpersonal difficulties, including deficits in social problem solving, loneliness, and poor self-esteem (Ansell et al. 2012), this approach may be particularly appealing to patients. Within the IPT framework, binge eating is theorized to occur as a response to interpersonal disturbances (e.g., social isolation) and consequent negative mood (Fairburn et al. 1993).

A distinguishing feature of IPT is the assignment of the "sick role" to the patient. This process involves presenting patients with a formal diagnosis of an eating disorder and emphasizing the importance of focusing their efforts on treatment and recovery, as one would with any medical illness, even if this means that other responsibilities take a backseat during the duration of treatment. In contrast to CBT, IPT does not so overtly focus on the modification of disturbed eating behaviors or overvaluation of shape and weight.

During the course of IPT, clinicians work with patients to identify typical types of interpersonal problems and determine what the patient can do to effectively address these issues. As a first step toward identifying interpersonal difficulties, the clinician takes an extensive interpersonal history, including an inventory of the patient's significant relationships. The patient is requested to reflect on how the development of eating disorder symptoms interacted with relationships in the past. The clinician also assesses current interpersonal functioning and the effect of the eating disorder on current relationships. Through this assessment process, one or more primary problem areas are identified and become an area of focus in treatment; these areas include role transitions, interpersonal role disputes, grief, and interpersonal deficits. *Role transitions* frequently include such situations as beginning new employment, graduation, marriage, or the dissolution of an intimate relationship; *role disputes* might include conflicts an individual has about what is expected given a particular role (e.g., at work, as a family member); *grief* may be related to the loss of a person, relationship, or an important piece of one's identity; and *interpersonal deficits* usually refers to instances when an individual lacks significant relationships, which may be due to poor social skills. Clinicians encourage mastery of current social roles as well as adjustment to evolving interpersonal situations (Wilfley et al. 2002). A primary goal of treatment is to help mitigate or resolve these interpersonal difficulties in a way that in turn promotes the abstinence from eating-disordered behaviors. To this end, eating disorder symptoms can be linked consistently back to their role in the perpetuation or maintenance of the patient's interpersonal domain of focus (Tanofsky-Kraff and Wilfley 2010).

IPT is effective in the reduction and elimination of binge eating and purging in BN, although it is somewhat less effective than CBT (Agras et al. 2000). In a multisite trial comparing CBT with IPT in 220 individuals with BN, 45% of individuals in the CBT treatment condition had attained abstinence from binge eating and purging at the end of treatment, compared with 8% of individuals in the IPT treatment arm (Agras et al. 2000). At 12-month follow-up assessment, 40% of the individuals who had completed CBT had achieved abstinence, compared with 27% of those completing IPT, a difference that was not statistically significant.

Although the existing evidence indicates that CBT is superior to IPT in the treatment of BN, CBT and IPT appear to be equally efficacious in the treatment of BED, both immediately following treatment and in longer-term follow-up (Wilfley et al. 2002; Wilson et al. 2010). For example, a large study comparing CBT and IPT in the treatment of patients with BED found that 73% of individuals in the IPT condition achieved remission from binge eating at the end of treatment, compared with 79% of individuals in the CBT condition (Wilfley et al. 2002). At the time of a 12-month follow-up, 62% of individuals in the IPT condition reported abstinence from binge eating, compared with 59% in the CBT condition. Subgroup analyses suggest that individuals with BED are heterogeneous, which may affect overall treatment outcome. Patients with BED experiencing the most mood symptoms and high shape and weight concerns appeared to derive more benefit from IPT, and patients with increased eating disorder pathology experienced greater improvements from CBT (Sysko et al. 2010).

Pharmacotherapy

Bulimia Nervosa

Although several medications are efficacious for the treatment of BN, the role of pharmacotherapy is often best viewed as adjunctive. Some evidence suggests that the combination of pharmacotherapy and psychotherapy may be more efficacious than either intervention alone, but pharmacotherapy alone may be inferior to psychotherapy alone (Hay et al. 2001). Therefore, pharmacotherapy should be considered as a standalone treatment for BN primarily when evidence-based psychotherapy is not feasible or has not been successful. The mechanism by which pharmacological interventions produce clinical improvement in BN is unknown.

Antidepressant medications, including selective serotonin reuptake inhibitors (SSRIs), tricyclic antidepressants (TCAs), and monoamine oxidase inhibitors (MAOIs), are the most commonly studied classes of medications for the treatment of BN. Comprehensive reviews of placebo-controlled RCTs indicate that each of these classes of medications is significantly more effective than placebo in reducing binge eating, purging, and depression (Flament et al. 2012). Although MAOIs and TCAs alleviate symptoms in BN, both classes of medication have a number of problematic side effects and the potential for fatal overdose; therefore, they are not recommended as first-line treatments for BN and are not typically used. Furthermore, use of MAOIs involves maintaining a tyramine-free diet, which places several restrictions on types of foods that can be safely consumed, and thus may be especially problematic for individuals with disordered eating (Schatzberg et al. 2010).

The SSRI fluoxetine is the most widely studied medication for BN and was approved by the U.S. Food and Drug Administration (FDA) for this diagnosis. Therefore, it is considered to be the pharmacological intervention of choice for individuals with BN. Fluoxetine is typically prescribed at a dosage of 20 mg/day for the treatment of depression; however, a 60-mg/day dosage is significantly more effective in reducing binge eating, purging, weight and shape concerns, and depression among patients with BN. Therefore, this higher dosage is typically recommended (Fluoxetine Bulimia Nervosa Collaborative Study Group 1992; Romano et al. 2002). The common side effects of fluoxetine and other SSRIs are milder and better tolerated by patients than those of MAOIs and TCAs. Other SSRIs that produce meaningful reductions in symptoms (albeit in fewer trials than with fluoxetine) include citalopram (Leombruni et al. 2006), fluvoxamine (Fichter et al. 1997), and sertraline (Milano et al. 2004). One additional non-antidepressant medication option for BN is the anticonvulsant topiramate. Topiramate acts as a γ-aminobutyric acid (GABA) receptor agonist and glutamate receptor antagonist and may alleviate symptoms by improving regulation of appetite and impulsive behaviors. In placebo-controlled RCTs, frequency of binge eating and purging decreased significantly more in the topiramate condition than in the placebo condition (Nickel et al. 2005). Furthermore, individuals in the topiramate condition experienced significant reductions in weight compared with individuals in the placebo group. Therefore, before prescribing topiramate for BN, it may be important to consider the BMI of a patient and the potential implications (both positive and negative) of weight loss.

Most RCTs examining the efficacy of medications in the treatment of BN have been relatively short in duration (e.g., approximately 8 weeks). Of the few trials that have followed patients for significantly longer periods of time, dropout rates have been high (Romano et al. 2002), and therefore the ideal length of pharmacotherapy for BN is unknown. (A minimum of 6–12 months of treatment is consistent with evidence-based recommendations for the pharmacological treatment of depression and is often recommended for patients with BN in the absence of other clarifying data.)

Of note, there has been one placebo-controlled RCT using the antidepressant bupropion, and this trial was discontinued prematurely after 4 of 55 patients taking bupropion experienced grand mal seizures (Horne et al. 1988). As a result, use of bupropion is currently contraindicated in the treatment of BN.

Binge-Eating Disorder

Lisdexamfetamine dimesylate, a dextroamphetamine prodrug, has recently received FDA approval for the treatment of BED (McElroy et al. 2015). Long-term efficacy of this medication has not yet been assessed.

Whereas several antidepressant medications have been associated with short-term reduction in binge eating, no particular antidepressant medication has been found to be superior to others. A 2008 meta-analysis analyzing seven studies of SSRIs (i.e., citalopram, fluoxetine, fluvoxamine, sertraline) and a TCA (imipramine) in short-term trials indicated that significantly more participants experienced remission from binge eating in the active medication conditions than in the placebo condition (40.5% vs. 22.2%; Stefano et al. 2008). Although these results are promising, no long-term studies of the efficacy of antidepressants in BED have been conducted, and the durability of these short-term improvements remains untested.

Many individuals with BED have BMIs in the overweight or obese range, and most seeking treatment for their binge eating identify weight loss as a goal of treatment. For this reason, the efficacy of the anticonvulsants topiramate and zonisamide, both of which can have the side effect of weight loss, has been examined in the treatment of BED. Topiramate has been studied in three trials (Claudino et al. 2007; McElroy et al. 2003, 2007). When topiramate was employed in the absence of psychotherapy, intent-to-treat analyses showed superior rates of binge-eating remission in the topiramate groups (58%–64%) compared with the placebo groups (29%–30%; McElroy et al. 2003, 2007). Furthermore, the active medication groups experienced significantly greater reductions in weight than did the placebo groups (5.9 kg vs. 1.2 kg). In a study comparing topiramate and CBT with placebo and CBT, 83.3% of those in the topiramate group and 61.1% of those in the placebo group achieved binge-eating remission during the 21-week trial (Claudino et al. 2007). Despite these benefits, the side effects associated with topiramate can be difficult to tolerate, and treatment adherence can be a problem with this medication. In an open-label extension trial of topiramate lasting 42 weeks, McElroy et al. (2004) found that 68% of study participants failed to complete the trial, with adverse events and nonadherence to treatment being among the primary reasons cited for discontinuation. Similarly, one RCT used zonisamide and found it to be associated with significant reductions in both binge eating and weight. Side effects were similar to those seen with topiramate and were not well tolerated by study participants (McElroy et al. 2006).

Currently, there are four FDA-approved medications for weight loss: lorcaserin, naltrexone-bupropion, orlistat, and phentermine-topiramate. Of these, only orlistat, a pancreatic lipase inhibitor, has been studied in individuals with BED; in these studies, the medication was combined with either a guided self-help version of CBT (Grilo et al. 2005) or a very low calorie diet (Golay et al. 2005). Orlistat does not appear more effective than placebo in achieving remission from binge eating, but there is some evidence that compared with placebo, it causes greater weight loss and that the loss is better maintained after a 3-month follow-up period (Golay et al. 2005; Grilo et al. 2005).

Other Promising Psychotherapies

Dialectical Behavior Therapy

Dialectical behavior therapy (DBT) is a behaviorally focused outpatient intervention that is efficacious in the treatment of borderline personality disorder (Linehan 1993). DBT is based on a model that views maladaptive behaviors, such as self-injury, as attempts to regulate distressing emotions. Because negative affect often precedes binge eating and other eating-disordered behaviors, affect regulation has been hypothesized as a maintaining mechanism, and therefore a treatment such as DBT may be indicated (Haedt-Matt and Keel 2011). DBT was adapted for BED and BN by Safer et al. (2009), and it directly targets binge eating, purging, mindless eating, and any other behaviors that appear to interfere with progress in psychotherapy. As currently manualized, DBT for BED and BN includes modules devoted to teaching and developing mindfulness skills, including eating mindfully, distress tolerance, and emotion regulation skills. A strong emphasis is placed on daily monitoring of eating-disordered behaviors, concurrent mood states, and use of skills taught during sessions via diary cards.

Although there have been few trials of DBT in treating BN and BED, the results of extant studies have been promising. In a small trial comparing DBT with a wait-list control condition for patients with BED, 89% (16 of 18) of those in the DBT group experienced remission from binge eating and improvements in general eating pathology, compared with 12% (2 of 16) of those on the wait list (Telch et al. 2001). In a larger trial, 101 adults with BED were randomly assigned to 20 group sessions of either DBT or supportive psychotherapy (Safer et al. 2010). At posttreatment, 64% of patients in the DBT group had achieved abstinence from binge eating, compared with 36% in the supportive psychotherapy group, which was a significant difference. At 12-month follow-up, this significant difference had disappeared, with 64% of DBT patients and 56% of supportive psychotherapy patients maintaining abstinence. Notably, attrition for DBT was lower, in that only 4% of those receiving DBT dropped out of treatment, whereas 33.3% of patients in the supportive psychotherapy condition prematurely discontinued treatment. In patients with BN, a smaller trial comparing 20 weeks of individual DBT to a wait-list control condition found that by the end of treatment, 29% of participants (4 of 14) in the DBT condition had achieved abstinence from bingeing and purging, whereas none of the 15 patients in the wait-list control condition experienced remission, representing a statistically significant difference (Safer et al. 2001).

Integrative Cognitive-Affective Therapy

Integrative cognitive-affective therapy (ICAT) is a brief, present-focused therapy developed for the outpatient treatment of BN (Wonderlich et al. 2008). ICAT is similar in many ways to other therapies such as CBT and DBT; for example, patients are instructed to engage in a regular pattern of eating meals and snacks throughout the day and to track this behavior for analysis during sessions, although meal planning may be more prescriptive and detailed in nature than in these other therapies. In addition, ICAT emphasizes the role of interpersonal patterns in the maintenance of disordered eating, especially through the activation of negative affective states, which may, in turn, lead to emotionally driven disordered eating behaviors. Maladaptive interpersonal styles and negative emotions are first identified and then addressed through the use of targeted interventions. The use of electronic technologies, such as personal digital assistants, is integrated into treatment so that patients can track their emotions and use of skills taught during treatment sessions.

In the first RCT studying ICAT for patients with BN, Wonderlich et al. (2014) compared 21 sessions of ICAT with CBT-E among 80 adults with BN. At the end of treatment, 37.5% of individuals randomly assigned to the ICAT condition and 22.5% of those in the CBT-E condition had achieved abstinence from binge eating and purging; the difference was not statistically significant. At the 4-month follow-up assessment, 32.5% of individuals randomly assigned to ICAT and 22.5% of individuals randomly assigned to CBT-E reported abstinence from these behaviors; again, this was not a statistically significant difference. These results are promising and suggest that ICAT is an intervention worthy of further study.

Conclusion

The primary objective of the treatment of BN and BED is the normalization of eating. Reduction of overvaluation of shape and weight is often an additional target of treatment. Weight management is sometimes an additional treatment target. Because of the strong evidence base for the use of CBT in the treatment of BN, CBT should be considered the treatment of choice. IPT and pharmacotherapy (SSRIs, fluoxetine in particular) should be considered as viable alternatives when CBT is not available. CBT and IPT both have very strong evidence supporting their efficacy in the treatment of BED, and although no individual medication has emerged as superior, pharmacotherapy may also confer significant benefit and reductions in binge eating in this group.

Key Clinical Points

- The primary goal of treatment for binge eating is to normalize eating behavior and eliminate objective and subjective binge episodes. Additional goals may include the reduction of overvaluation of shape and weight and weight management.
- Cognitive-behavioral therapy (CBT) is considered the treatment of choice for bulimia nervosa (BN). CBT has also demonstrated significant effectiveness in eliminating binge eating in binge-eating disorder (BED) and has demonstrated superiority to behavioral weight loss treatment and pharmacological interventions.
- Interpersonal psychotherapy (IPT) is effective in the reduction and elimination of binge eating and purging in BN, although it is less effective than CBT and slower to produce improvements. CBT and IPT appear to be equally efficacious in the treatment of BED.
- Fluoxetine, at a dosage of 60 mg/day, is the pharmacological intervention of choice for BN. Use of other selective serotonin reuptake inhibitors also results in meaningful reductions in symptoms. The combination of pharmacotherapy and psychotherapy may be more efficacious than either intervention alone; however, pharmacotherapy alone may be inferior to psychotherapy alone. Use of bupropion is contraindicated in the treatment of BN.
- Antidepressant medications may be effective for reducing binge eating in BED, although no one medication has emerged as superior to others. For those patients who can tolerate its side effects, topiramate may also be effective in the treatment of BED.
- Two promising psychotherapeutic interventions worthy of further study include dialectical behavior therapy, which has been adapted for BN and BED, and integrative cognitive-affective therapy, developed for the treatment of BN.

References

Agras WS, Walsh T, Fairburn CG, et al: A multicenter comparison of cognitive-behavioral therapy and interpersonal psychotherapy for bulimia nervosa. Arch Gen Psychiatry 57(5):459–466, 2000 10807486

Ansell EB, Grilo CM, White MA: Examining the interpersonal model of binge eating and loss of control over eating in women. Int J Eat Disord 45(1):43–50, 2012 21321985

Blomquist KK, Barnes RD, White MA, et al: Exploring weight gain in year before treatment for binge eating disorder: a different context for interpreting limited weight losses in treatment studies. Int J Eat Disord 44(5):435–439, 2011 20635382

Bulik CM, Reichborn-Kjennerud T: Medical morbidity in binge eating disorder. Int J Eat Disord 34(suppl):S39–S46, 2003 12900985

Carrard I, Crépin C, Ceschi G, et al: Relations between pure dietary and dietary-negative affect subtypes and impulsivity and reinforcement sensitivity in binge eating individuals. Eat Behav 13(1):13–19, 2012 22177390

Claudino AM, de Oliveira IR, Appolinario JC, et al: Double-blind, randomized, placebo-controlled trial of topiramate plus cognitive-behavior therapy in binge-eating disorder. J Clin Psychiatry 68(9):1324–1332, 2007 17915969

Devlin MJ, Walsh BT, Guss JL, et al: Postprandial cholecystokinin release and gastric emptying in patients with bulimia nervosa. Am J Clin Nutr 65(1):114–120, 1997 8988922

Fairburn CG: Cognitive Behavior Therapy and Eating Disorders. New York, Guilford, 2008

Fairburn CG, Jones R, Peveler RC, et al: Psychotherapy and bulimia nervosa: longer-term effects of interpersonal psychotherapy, behavior therapy, and cognitive behavior therapy. Arch Gen Psychiatry 50(6):419–428, 1993 8498876

Fairburn CG, Norman PA, Welch SL, et al: A prospective study of outcome in bulimia nervosa and the long-term effects of three psychological treatments. Arch Gen Psychiatry 52(4):304–312, 1995 7702447

Fairburn CG, Cooper Z, Doll HA, et al: Transdiagnostic cognitive-behavioral therapy for patients with eating disorders: a two-site trial with 60-week follow-up. Am J Psychiatry 166(3):311–319, 2009 19074978

Fichter MM, Leibl C, Krüger R, et al: Effects of fluvoxamine on depression, anxiety, and other areas of general psychopathology in bulimia nervosa. Pharmacopsychiatry 30(3):85–92, 1997 9211569

Flament MF, Bissada H, Spettigue W: Evidence-based pharmacotherapy of eating disorders. Int J Neuropsychopharmacol 15(2):189–207, 2012 21414249

Fluoxetine Bulimia Nervosa Collaborative Study Group: Fluoxetine in the treatment of bulimia nervosa: a multicenter, placebo-controlled, double-blind trial. Arch Gen Psychiatry 49(2):139–147, 1992 1550466

Golay A, Laurent-Jaccard A, Habicht F, et al: Effect of orlistat in obese patients with binge eating disorder. Obes Res 13(10):1701–1708, 2005 16286517

Grilo CM, Masheb RM, Salant SL: Cognitive behavioral therapy guided self-help and orlistat for the treatment of binge eating disorder: a randomized, double-blind, placebo-controlled trial. Biol Psychiatry 57(10):1193–1201, 2005 15866560

Grilo CM, Crosby RD, Wilson GT, et al: 12-month follow-up of fluoxetine and cognitive behavioral therapy for binge eating disorder. J Consult Clin Psychol 80(6):1108–1113, 2012a 22985205

Grilo CM, Masheb RM, Crosby RD: Predictors and moderators of response to cognitive behavioral therapy and medication for the treatment of binge eating disorder. J Consult Clin Psychol 80(5):897–906, 2012b 22289130

Haedt-Matt AA, Keel PK: Revisiting the affect regulation model of binge eating: a meta-analysis of studies using ecological momentary assessment. Psychol Bull 137(4):660–681, 2011 21574678

Hay PP, Claudino AM, Kaio MH: Antidepressants versus psychological treatments and their combination for bulimia nervosa. Cochrane Database Syst Rev 4(4):CD003385, 2001

Hay PP, Bacaltchuk J, Stefano S, et al: Psychological treatments for bulimia nervosa and binging. Cochrane Database Syst Rev 4(4):CD000562, 2009 19821271

Horne RL, Ferguson JM, Pope HG Jr, et al: Treatment of bulimia with bupropion: a multicenter controlled trial. J Clin Psychiatry 49(7):262–266, 1988 3134343

Keel PK, Dorer DJ, Franko DL, et al: Postremission predictors of relapse in women with eating disorders. Am J Psychiatry 162(12):2263–2268, 2005 16330589

Leombruni P, Amianto F, Delsedime N, et al: Citalopram versus fluoxetine for the treatment of patients with bulimia nervosa: a single-blind randomized controlled trial. Adv Ther 23(3):481–494, 2006 16912031

Linehan M: Cognitive-Behavioral Treatment of Borderline Personality Disorder. New York, Guilford, 1993

Masheb R, White MA: Bulimia nervosa in overweight and normal-weight women. Compr Psychiatry 53(2):181–186, 2012 21550028

McElroy SL, Arnold LM, Shapira NA, et al: Topiramate in the treatment of binge eating disorder associated with obesity: a randomized, placebo-controlled trial. Am J Psychiatry 160(2):255–261, 2003 12562571

McElroy SL, Shapira NA, Arnold LM, et al: Topiramate in the long-term treatment of binge-eating disorder associated with obesity. J Clin Psychiatry 65(11):1463–1469, 2004 15554757

McElroy SL, Kotwal R, Guerdjikova AI, et al: Zonisamide in the treatment of binge eating disorder with obesity: a randomized controlled trial. J Clin Psychiatry 67(12):1897–1906, 2006 17194267

McElroy SL, Hudson JI, Capece JA, et al; Topiramate Binge Eating Disorder Research Group: Topiramate for the treatment of binge eating disorder associated with obesity: a placebo-controlled study. Biol Psychiatry 61(9):1039–1048, 2007 17258690

McElroy SL, Hudson JI, Mitchell JE, et al: Efficacy and safety of lisdexamfetamine for treatment of adults with moderate to severe binge-eating disorder: a randomized clinical trial. JAMA Psychiatry 72(3):235–246, 2015 25587645

Milano W, Petrella C, Sabatino C, et al: Treatment of bulimia nervosa with sertraline: a randomized controlled trial. Adv Ther 21(4):232–237, 2004 15605617

Murphy R, Straebler S, Basden S, et al: Interpersonal psychotherapy for eating disorders. Clin Psychol Psychother 19(2):150–158, 2012 22362599

Nickel C, Tritt K, Muehlbacher M, et al: Topiramate treatment in bulimia nervosa patients: a randomized, double-blind, placebo-controlled trial. Int J Eat Disord 38(4):295–300, 2005 16231337

Romano SJ, Halmi KA, Sarkar NP, et al: A placebo-controlled study of fluoxetine in continued treatment of bulimia nervosa after successful acute fluoxetine treatment. Am J Psychiatry 159(1):96–102, 2002 11772696

Safer DL, Telch CF, Agras WS: Dialectical behavior therapy for bulimia nervosa. Am J Psychiatry 158(4):632–634, 2001 11282700

Safer DL, Telch CF, Chen EY: Dialectical Behavior Therapy for Binge Eating and Bulimia. New York, Guilford, 2009

Safer DL, Robinson AH, Jo B: Outcome from a randomized controlled trial of group therapy for binge eating disorder: comparing dialectical behavior therapy adapted for binge eating to an active comparison group therapy. Behav Ther 41(1):106–120, 2010 20171332

Schatzberg AF, Cole JO, DeBattista C: Manual of Clinical Psychopharmacology, 7th Edition. Washington, DC, American Psychiatric Association, 2010

Stefano SC, Bacaltchuk J, Blay SL, et al: Antidepressants in short-term treatment of binge eating disorder: systematic review and meta-analysis. Eat Behav 9(2):129–136, 2008 18329590

Sysko R, Walsh BT: A critical evaluation of the efficacy of self-help interventions for the treatment of bulimia nervosa and binge-eating disorder. Int J Eat Disord 41(2):97–112, 2008 17922533

Sysko R, Hildebrandt T, Wilson GT, et al: Heterogeneity moderates treatment response among patients with binge eating disorder. J Consult Clin Psychol 78(5):681–690, 2010 20873903

Tanofsky-Kraff M, Wilfley DE: Interpersonal psychotherapy for bulimia nervosa and binge-eating disorder, in The Treatment of Eating Disorders: A Clinical Handbook. Edited by Grilo CM, Mitchell JE. New York, Guilford, 2010, pp 271–293

Telch CF, Agras WS, Linehan MM: Dialectical behavior therapy for binge eating disorder. J Consult Clin Psychol 69(6):1061–1065, 2001 11777110

Wilfley DE, Welch RR, Stein RI, et al: A randomized comparison of group cognitive-behavioral therapy and group interpersonal psychotherapy for the treatment of overweight individuals with binge-eating disorder. Arch Gen Psychiatry 59(8):713–721, 2002 12150647

Wilson GT, Wilfley DE, Agras WS, et al: Psychological treatments of binge eating disorder. Arch Gen Psychiatry 67(1):94–101, 2010 20048227

Wonderlich SA, Engel SG, Peterson CB, et al: Examining the conceptual model of integrative cognitive-affective therapy for BN: two assessment studies. Int J Eat Disord 41(8):748–754, 2008 18528869

Wonderlich SA, Peterson CB, Crosby RD, et al: A randomized controlled comparison of integrative cognitive-affective therapy (ICAT) and enhanced cognitive-behavioral therapy (CBT-E) for bulimia nervosa. Psychol Med 44(3):543–553, 2014 23701891

15 Treatment of Other Eating Problems, Including Pica and Rumination

Eve Khlyavich Freidl, M.D.
Evelyn Attia, M.D.

In this chapter, we describe the evidence-based and evidence-informed treatments of several of the feeding and eating disorders about which there has been limited research and clinical description: pica, rumination disorder, night eating syndrome, purging disorder, and atypical anorexia nervosa (AN). With the publication in 2013 of DSM-5 (American Psychiatric Association 2013), pica and rumination disorder have joined the more commonly recognized eating disorders in the feeding and eating disorders diagnostic classification, and several other conditions, including night eating syndrome, purging disorder, and atypical AN, have been categorized under "other specified feeding or eating disorder." We briefly review diagnosis, prevalence, associated symptoms, and assessment for pica, rumination disorder, night eating syndrome, and purging disorder in order to provide context to the therapeutic approaches reviewed. We also briefly discuss therapeutic approaches for atypical AN.

Pica

Pica is defined in DSM-5 as persistent eating of nonnutritive, nonfood substances inappropriate to developmental level and not in the context of culturally or socially normative practice. The term originated from the Latin word for magpie, a bird thought to have a diet of edible and nonedible items, and medical case reports date back to the sixteenth century (Parry-Jones and Parry-Jones 1992). Despite the behavior's long history, epidemiological studies of pica are limited and its prevalence remains unclear, perhaps in part because cases may only reach clinical attention when complications require medical or surgical treatment. Pica is seen across all ages and genders but most commonly in individuals with developmental disabilities, in pregnant women, and in children at lower socioeconomic levels (Rose et al. 2000). Geophagia, or dirt and clay ingestion, is believed to have medicinal purposes in some cultures, in which case it does not meet criteria for a diagnosis of pica.

Pica has been described in the context of nutritional deficiency, especially iron deficiency, although it remains unclear if the nutritional deficiency is a cause or a result of pica. Pica is associated with many serious complications, including toxicity; intestinal obstruction from foreign body ingestion, as well as from bezoars that develop from hair ingestion; excessive calorie intake; nutritional deprivation; parasitic infections; and dental injury (Rose et al. 2000). Physical examination and clinical assessments with attention to these complications are important in the clinical evaluation of pica. Laboratory tests for pica commonly include complete blood count with peripheral smear; iron, ferritin, and lead levels; general chemistry panel (including electrolytes and liver function tests); stool studies for ova and parasites; and an abdominal radiograph to evaluate for foreign objects, bezoars, and parasites.

Because pica is most prevalent among individuals with developmental disabilities, much of the empirical evidence for behavioral treatment for pica has focused on this population (Matson et al. 2013). Behavioral treatments, especially those combining reinforcement and response reduction procedures, are well-established treatments for pica (Hagopian et al. 2011).

Earlier treatments relied on behavioral techniques that limited opportunities to engage in the eating disturbances that characterize pica and often applied punitive measures. Although some of the older research utilized methods that may not be considered socially or ethically appropriate at this time, we review these techniques, including aversive or noxious stimuli, restraint, overcorrection, and response blocking and interruption. Because the risk of serious physical harm due to pica may be quite high in certain populations, the consideration of procedures with aversive elements may be warranted.

Aversive stimuli that have been studied in case reports include lemon juice, aromatic ammonia, and water mist; taste aversion; and auditory stimulation. In these studies, the aversive stimuli were employed when pica behaviors were attempted, and the technique resulted in pica suppression (Bell and Stein 1992). Restraint, including mechanical restraint and physical restraint, has been shown to be effective both when applied contingently to target behavior and when used protectively in a noncontingent manner. Mechanical restraints include mittens, arm splints, helmets with mouth coverings, and fencing masks. Physical restraint has been used contingently, with brief holds used after attempted or actual ingestions (Paniagua et al. 1986). In more dangerous situations, longer-duration restraints have been required. Restraint is usually considered justified only when the risk of serious physical harm is high, when lesser restrictions are unsuccessful, and when restraint is used as one of the strategies in a comprehensive treatment plan (Hagopian et al. 2011).

Overcorrection is a technique considered to have high validity because it requires restitution and then engages the individual in practicing a new, more appropriate behavior. For example, when an individual who ingests feces is discovered to have feces or the traces of feces on his or her mouth or hand, a trainer guides the patient to the toilet and encourages him or her to spit the feces into the toilet bowl. Then the patient is given oral hygiene training that includes brushing the mouth, teeth, and gums with a toothbrush soaked in a mild antiseptic; is directed to wash hands and scrub fingernails with a nailbrush in warm soapy water for 10 minutes; and is required to clean his or her anal area and repeat brief hand washing. Finally, the patient is guided to the area where he or she was discovered to be engaged in pica and is required to mop the floor with disinfectant. When used with two cognitively impaired young adults, this 30-minute overcorrection procedure reduced target behaviors to zero (Singh and Bakker 1984).

Response blocking and interruption, a commonly used intervention for challenging behaviors in persons with developmental disabilities, may be promising in pica. However, there is limited research regarding its specific use in pica. Response blocking alone has been shown to produce aggression, but when paired with an interruption with alternatively preferred foods, it has been shown to reduce pica. This technique involves training in which the patient is offered the inedible objects typically ingested and is blocked from ingesting these but simultaneously given an alternative preferred food item (Hagopian and Adelinis 2001).

More contemporary behavioral procedures, including reinforcement, habit reversal, stimulus control, and environmental changes, are considered preferred methods to the older techniques just discussed. These newer, less restrictive methods allow individuals to have a more normalized routine and stimulating environment.

Differential reinforcement techniques include reinforcing lower rates of pica, reinforcing behavior other than pica, and reinforcing habits incompatible with pica. Several studies using these techniques with small numbers of individuals had positive results (Donnelly and Olczak 1990; Smith 1987). Habit reversal includes awareness training, competing response training, and social support. Awareness training, also called discrimination training, involves teaching the patient to differentiate between food and nonfood times (e.g., "What is this?" "Should you eat it?"). Then, the patient is instructed to do a competing behavior that is incompatible with eating, such as pursing lips, and is praised for doing this alternative behavior (Madden et al. 1981). Stimulus control, by definition, is any method used to increase the amount of effort required to do the undesired behavior. For pica, this includes placement of desired inedible objects in more difficult to reach places or in containers that require time to open.

Environmental changes, including the creation of a safe and enriched environment, also have an important role in treating pica. Safety measures may include special attention to garbage collection systems, such as safe containers for disposal of latex gloves, especially in an institutional setting (Williams and McAdam 2012). Other safety measures may include ensuring that nuts and bolts are tightly fastened in furniture, securing of cleaning and medical materials in locked cabinets, and maintaining clean areas. The rationale for an enriched environment is informed by high rates of lead poisoning and mouthing of objects observed in impoverished settings. The environment may be enriched with toys (Madden et al. 1981) and the intervention further strengthened by reinforcement or praise for play with toys (rather than engaging in pica). Increases in leisure activities and time for special attention from a caregiver are other techniques for enrichment.

In practical terms, functional behavioral analysis of the pica is an appropriate first step to determine which behavioral components should be part of an individual's treatment plan. Functional behavioral analysis aims to define variables that maintain a target behavior. This assessment includes operationalizing the target behavior by describing its mode (e.g., cognitive, affective, motor components) and defining the parameters of frequency, duration, and intensity. A clear definition of the pica allows for the identification of an objectively measurable behavior and then allows for examination of the contextual variables that are related to the behavior, including social contingencies and internal reinforcement. Pica appears predominantly to be a motor behavior that is reinforced by an individual's sensory responses. Specific details of this process allow for the development of a unique treatment plan that is likely to combine stimulus control, training in alternative or incompatible behaviors, and reinforcement.

Nutritional supplementation has limited support for the treatment of pica. Even in cases in which a specific nutritional deficiency is identified by laboratory examination, results have been variable. Iron supplementation seems to have the most benefit for individuals with iron deficiency who ingest ice, whereas in other cases of pica associated with iron deficiency, iron repletion has had limited effect on the behavior (Khan and Tisman 2010).

Psychopharmacological interventions should target comorbid conditions that may exacerbate pica. No studies to date support the use of psychopharmacological agents specifically for pica (Matson et al. 2013).

Rumination Disorder

DSM-5 defines *rumination* as a disorder of repeated regurgitation in which the regurgitated food may be re-chewed, re-swallowed, or spit out. Rumination disorder has been observed across the age span for many centuries, but in earlier editions of DSM, it was defined as an illness only of infancy or early childhood (Olden 2001). Epidemiological studies indicate that infants, children, and adults with developmental delay, as well as individuals with normal cognitive abilities, may have rumination disorder. Prevalence rates are uncertain, and they are difficult to ascertain because care providers do not often screen for this disorder, even in the context of other feeding or eating problems, and because many affected individuals consider this an embarrassing problem that they are reluctant to disclose.

Rumination disorder has been associated with weight loss, malnutrition, dental erosion, halitosis, electrolyte abnormalities, and gastroesophageal reflux disease (GERD), and it may be associated with high morbidity in pediatric patients (O'Brien et al. 1995).

Rumination as a symptom may occur in association with eating disorders, including AN and bulimia nervosa (BN). According to the DSM-5 definition for rumination disorder, individuals with AN or BN do not meet criteria for rumination disorder because they have another disorder, but they may, nonetheless, warrant specific treatments to target this behavior.

The diagnosis of rumination disorder is made on the basis of patient history and physical examination by a clinician; however, some authors suggest that supporting diagnostic tests are indicated. Because rumination occurs via the relaxation of the lower esophageal sphincter accompanied by increased intra-abdominal pressures, a characteristic pattern is seen on upper gastrointestinal manometry. Kessing et al. (2014) suggest that this testing, which reveals a different profile from GERD, is indicated because behavioral treatments for rumination disorder are costly and time-consuming. In contrast, Chial et al. (2003) reviewed medical records of pediatric patients and found that only 40% had the characteristic pattern on manometry, and therefore they do not recommend the monitoring because it is invasive and is typically performed only at tertiary care centers. Furthermore, Chial et al. (2003) suggest that invasive tests have often led to misdiagnosis of GERD or gastroparesis. Other groups have also recommended against diagnostic testing to rule out medical conditions such as GERD or gastroesophageal motility disorders, because these procedures are invasive and the diagnosis can be made based on clinical observation alone (O'Brien et al. 1995).

Behavioral approaches for treatment of rumination disorder are supported by a number of case reports; however, no controlled trials have been reported to date. A brief review of the proposed physiological mechanism of rumination is helpful to understand the most common treatment interventions. Although animals that ruminate as part of their digestive process use reverse peristalsis, this mechanism is not observed in the human esophagus. It appears that regurgitation in humans is made possible by an increase in intragastric pressure (voluntary or otherwise) at the same time as a lowering of lower esophageal sphincter tone (again, voluntary or otherwise), which seems to occur by tonic contraction of the diaphragm (via contracting abdominal muscles). Thus, diaphragmatic breathing has been shown to be an effective treatment for rumination to disrupt this mechanism (Chitkara et al. 2006).

Diaphragmatic breathing is described as both a relaxation technique and a strategy of simple habit reversal; however, this distinction is mostly semantic because the implementation of the technique varies minimally. Diaphragmatic breathing is taught by asking a patient to place one hand on the upper chest and one hand on the abdomen and to take a deep inspiration and allow only the hand on the abdomen to move while the hand on the chest stays still (Chial et al. 2003). Patients are trained to breathe diaphragmatically throughout a meal, with the goal that they will begin to unconsciously breathe diaphragmatically during events that precipitate regurgitation (Chitkara et al. 2006). Diaphragmatic breathing as a habit reversal technique is considered to be a behavior incompatible with regurgitation, and training includes awareness training of regurgitation, practice of the incompatible behavior, and social support (Wagaman et al. 1998).

Some case reports note the importance of education about regurgitation and its consequences as part of the treatment plan (Khan et al. 2000). Levine et al. (1983) described several patients who experienced relief of symptoms when they learned that their habit was typically harmless. Biofeedback and gum chewing have also been reported as useful techniques (Fredericks et al. 1998; Weakley et al. 1997). Operant conditioning, in which attention is withdrawn in response to rumination and additional attention is demonstrated in response to appropriate feeding behavior, has been reported to be helpful for infants and for individuals with developmental disabilities (Olden 2001).

As mentioned earlier in this section, studies have shown a relationship between eating disorders and rumination symptoms (Blinder 1986; Fairburn and Cooper 1984). There are special considerations for treatment of patients who ruminate following recovery from an eating disorder and patients who ruminate in the context of AN or BN because these symptoms may go unnoticed or may not be assessed by the clinician. In these patients, it may be more common that regurgitated food is spit out in an attempt to avoid absorbing calories, consistent with the fear of gaining weight or becoming fat. For these patients, psychoeducation about rumination and its possible medical sequelae, as well as about the physiology of digestion, may be important to emphasize. Additionally, strategies aimed at vomiting prevention may be useful in prevention of spitting out regurgitated food.

Pharmacological strategies have limited utility for rumination disorder. Proton pump inhibitors may be considered to protect the esophagus, oropharynx, and teeth. Gastric motility agents should be considered only if a specific motility disorder is identified. Antidepressant or anxiolytic medications may be considered to target comorbid disorders that may contribute to rumination disorder. In the past, surgical procedures that targeted the lower esophageal sphincters were used, but there is little evidence to support these interventions; although rumination reportedly resolved following surgery, complications, including gas bloat syndrome and gastroparesis secondary to vagal nerve damage, were reported (Olden 2001).

Night Eating Syndrome

Night eating syndrome is one of the DSM-5 other specified feeding or eating disorders. Night eating syndrome is described in DSM-5 as "recurrent episodes of night eating, as manifested by eating after awakening from sleep or by excessive food consumption after the evening meal" (p. 354). A key feature of this disorder is that the individual has awareness and recall of the eating; in contrast, in sleep-related eating disorder, the individual has no conscious awareness of the nocturnal behavior (Winkelman 1998).

Prevalence of night eating syndrome is estimated at 1.5% of the general population, with a higher prevalence among obese patients seeking weight loss treatment, including bariatric surgery, and among patients with other eating disorders, especially binge-eating disorder (Colles et al. 2007). Although the prevalence of night eating syndrome increases with body mass index in patient populations, several studies have demonstrated that night eating syndrome is not correlated with obesity in the general population (Rand et al. 1997; Striegel-Moore et al. 2006). Night eating syndrome affects men and women in comparable proportions, although more women seek weight loss treatment, which may contribute to the impression that the disorder predominantly affects women.

Screening for night eating syndrome should be part of the diagnostic assessment when evaluating disordered eating behavior. In addition, because night eating may interfere with weight loss and with glucose management in patients with diabetes, clinicians should also assess for the presence of this behavior in overweight and obese individuals and patients with diabetes (Vander Wal 2012). Night eating syndrome is associated with morning anorexia, insomnia, and other sleep disturbances.

Studies support both psychotherapy and pharmacotherapy as effective treatment strategies for night eating syndrome (Allison et al. 2010; O'Reardon et al. 2006; Pawlow et al. 2003). Abbreviated progressive muscle relaxation and cognitive-behavioral therapy (CBT) have shown promise as treatment approaches for night eating syndrome. In a randomized controlled trial comparing abbreviated progressive muscle relaxation with sitting quietly, Pawlow et al. (2003) found that patients trained in abbreviated progressive muscle relaxation showed significant improvement in anxiety, relaxation, and morning and evening hunger patterns. Nonsignificant improvements in the number of breakfasts eaten, awakenings from sleep, and weight were also demonstrated. In the abbreviated progressive muscle relaxation used in this trial, subjects were instructed to establish a consistent bedtime routine, listen to a soothing tape, and monitor mood and food intake, indicating that sleep hygiene instruction and self-monitoring may be important elements of an effective treatment. In an uncontrolled pilot study, Allison et al. (2010) demonstrated that patients who received CBT specifically developed for night eating syndrome had significant decreases in caloric intake after dinner, number of nocturnal ingestions, weight, and scores on the Night Eating Symptom Scale (NESS; O'Reardon et al. 2004). The core components of this CBT treatment included psychoeducation, self-monitoring, relaxation strategies, sleep hygiene, cognitive restructuring, and implementation of a regular eating schedule of structured meals. Case reports also support the use of additional daytime calories (Aronoff et al. 1994) and of bright light therapy for night eating syndrome that presents together with comorbid depression (Friedman et al. 2004). Several studies support the use of selective serotonin reuptake inhibitors for night eating syndrome. In one double-blind placebo-controlled trial, sertraline was associated with significant improvements in the number of nighttime awakenings, nocturnal ingestions, and post-evening-meal caloric intake (O'Reardon et al. 2006). Furthermore, overweight patients in the sertraline group lost more weight than those in the control group.

Purging Disorder

Purging disorder is described in DSM-5 as a disorder of "recurrent purging behavior to influence weight or shape…in the absence of binge eating" (p. 353). Purging behaviors include self-induced vomiting and misuse of laxatives, diuretics, and other medications.

Lifetime prevalence rates for purging disorder ranged from 1% to 5% in several epidemiological studies (Favaro et al. 2003; Machado et al. 2007; Wade et al. 2006). Patients with purging disorder are within a normal weight range. This disorder differs from BN, which requires recurrent episodes of objective binge eating, although patients with purging disorder may report subjective binge episodes in which they experience loss of control but do not consume more food than what most people would eat under similar circumstances. Purging disorder is associated with dietary restraint, depression, and anxiety (Keel et al. 2005).

Assessment of individuals with purging disorder should include physical examination and laboratory studies recommended for patients with BN. Patients should be assessed for parotid gland enlargement, gastroesophageal reflux symptoms, dental erosion, and electrolyte imbalance, because individuals who engage in self-induced vomiting are at risk for esophageal damage and electrolyte abnormalities (e.g., hypokalemia, hypochloremic metabolic acidosis).

No treatment trials have been reported for purging disorder; therefore, treatment strategies are best informed by evidence-based approaches for other eating disorders, especially BN, because of the overlap of some treatment targets, such as purging, dietary restraint, and overvaluation of shape and weight. Evidence-based treatments for BN include psychotherapy (CBT, interpersonal psychotherapy) and pharmacotherapy (Shapiro et al. 2007) (for details, see Chapter 14, "Treatment of Binge Eating, Including Bulimia Nervosa and Binge-Eating Disorder").

Very strong evidence supports the use of CBT for the reduction and remission of purging episodes in BN. In multiple comparison trials, CBT has been shown to be more effective than behavioral treatment alone, exposure with response prevention, supportive therapy, nutritional counseling, and wait list (Shapiro et al. 2007). Interpersonal psychotherapy has been shown to be as effective as CBT at 1-year follow-up, but CBT has much more rapid symptom relief (Fairburn et al. 1991).

A transdiagnostic CBT approach that was evaluated in a longitudinal trial showed similar benefit to that associated with CBT for BN (Fairburn et al. 2009). Transdiagnostic CBT, also called enhanced CBT (CBT-E), utilizes a dimensional approach to treatment and focuses on the shared clinical features of several eating disorders and the common mechanisms that are involved in the persistence of disordered eating behavior. In addition to the core elements of CBT for BN (e.g., attempts to normalize eating, prevention strategies to decrease binge and purge episodes, techniques to address overvaluation of shape and weight), CBT-E has specific models to address clinical perfectionism, core self-esteem issues (e.g., negative self-evaluation that extends beyond body image), mood intolerance, and interpersonal difficulties. The transdiagnostic approach may be particularly well suited for purging disorder, with the rationale that a dimensional view of eating disorders places purging disorder somewhere in the middle of the continuum, so a broader strategy may be more helpful than one aimed specifically at BN.

Atypical Anorexia Nervosa

DSM-5 suggests that the term *atypical anorexia nervosa* be used if an individual meets all criteria for AN, except that despite a significant weight loss, his or her weight is within or above the normal range. Although this presentation has been recognized for some time, minimal research data are available regarding its prevalence, presentation, or course to inform clinical care. Patients with atypical AN may present for treatment because of clear functional impairment and may benefit from strategies used in the treatment of other eating disorders (Wade and O'Shea 2014). In addition, this eating disorder profile has been described in patients who have undergone bariatric surgery (Conceição et al. 2013).

The primary treatment goals for typical AN patients are refeeding and restoring normal weight. In patients in a malnourished state, specific psychotherapeutic interventions have little empirical support (Bulik et al. 2007), but in weight-restored patients, CBT has more promising results, especially for relapse prevention (Pike et al. 2003). Furthermore, as described in the section on purging disorder, there is very strong evidence that CBT is effective in treating BN. Thus, for normal-weight or overweight patients with restricted diet, intense fear of gaining weight, and disturbance in body image, CBT is an obvious first choice for therapeutic approach. The behavioral management must be targeted at normalizing eating, because these individuals often fast, restrict food variety, and avoid forbidden foods. Stimulus control and coping strategies may need to be aimed at excessive exercise behavior, which appears to be common in individuals with atypical AN. Strategies to prevent vomiting and other purging behaviors may also be necessary. Finally, cognitive and exposure work focused on body image distortion are crucial. For adolescent patients with atypical AN, family-based treatment should also be considered (Le Grange et al. 2005).

Although psychopharmacological interventions have not been shown to be helpful in weight gain for patients with AN (Bulik et al. 2007), medication has been shown to reduce target eating disorder symptoms in BN (Levine 1992). Therefore, a trial of fluoxetine may be a reasonable approach for atypical AN, especially if binge and/or purge symptoms are present.

Rapid weight loss has been associated with medical complications, possibly including hormonal changes similar to those seen in AN (Pi-Sunyer 1993). Therefore, even though patients with atypical AN have normal or above-normal weights, medical assessment and monitoring remain important for this group of patients.

Conclusion

Patients with pica, rumination disorder, and other specified feeding or eating disorder, including purging disorder, night eating syndrome, and atypical AN, may benefit from treatment approaches that have been better studied in the formally classified feeding and eating disorders. The inclusion in DSM-5 of these specified categories of subthreshold and other conditions hopefully will encourage clinicians and researchers to collect and report data about these groups and thereby create a useful evidence base.

Key Clinical Points

- Pica is best treated with a combination of stimulus control, habit reversal, and reinforcement.
- Environmental safety and enrichment are important components of a successful treatment plan for pica.
- Diaphragmatic breathing (as a relaxation strategy or simple habit reversal technique) is a promising treatment approach for rumination disorder.
- Clinical trials support the use of abbreviated progressive muscle relaxation, cognitive-behavioral therapy, and selective serotonin reuptake inhibitors for night eating syndrome.

- Treatments for purging disorder should be based on treatments of known effectiveness for bulimia nervosa.
- Although patients with atypical anorexia nervosa have normal or above-normal weight, medical assessment and monitoring are important.

References

Allison KC, Lundgren JD, Moore RH, et al: Cognitive behavior therapy for night eating syndrome: a pilot study. Am J Psychother 64(1):91–106, 2010 20405767

American Psychiatric Association: Diagnostic and Statistical Manual of Mental Disorders, 5th Edition. Arlington, VA, American Psychiatric Association, 2013

Aronoff NJ, Geliebter A, Hashim SA, et al: The relationship between daytime and nighttime food intake in an obese night-eater. Obes Res 2(2):145–151, 1994 16353615

Bell KE, Stein DM: Behavioral treatments for pica: a review of empirical studies. Int J Eat Disord 11(4):377–389, 1992

Blinder BJ: Rumination: a benign disorder? Int J Eat Disord 5(2):385–386, 1986

Bulik CM, Berkman ND, Brownley KA, et al: Anorexia nervosa treatment: a systematic review of randomized controlled trials. Int J Eat Disord 40(4):310–320, 2007 17370290

Chial HJ, Camilleri M, Williams DE, et al: Rumination syndrome in children and adolescents: diagnosis, treatment, and prognosis. Pediatrics 111(1):158–162, 2003 12509570

Chitkara DK, Van Tilburg M, Whitehead WE, et al: Teaching diaphragmatic breathing for rumination syndrome. Am J Gastroenterol 101(11):2449–2452, 2006 17090274

Colles SL, Dixon JB, O'Brien PE: Night eating syndrome and nocturnal snacking: association with obesity, binge eating and psychological distress. Int J Obes (Lond) 31(11):1722–1730, 2007 17579633

Conceição E, Orcutt M, Mitchell J, et al: Eating disorders after bariatric surgery: a case series. Int J Eat Disord 46(3):274–279, 2013 23192683

Donnelly DR, Olczak PV: The effect of differential reinforcement of incompatible behaviors (DRI) on pica for cigarettes in persons with intellectual disability. Behav Modif 14(1):81–96, 1990 2294903

Fairburn CG, Cooper PJ: Rumination in bulimia nervosa. Br Med J (Clin Res Ed) 288(6420):826–827, 1984 6423100

Fairburn CG, Jones R, Peveler RC, et al: Three psychological treatments for bulimia nervosa: a comparative trial. Arch Gen Psychiatry 48(5):463–469, 1991 2021299

Fairburn CG, Cooper Z, Doll HA, et al: Transdiagnostic cognitive-behavioral therapy for patients with eating disorders: a two-site trial with 60-week follow-up. Am J Psychiatry 166(3):311–319, 2009 19074978

Favaro A, Ferrara S, Santonastaso P: The spectrum of eating disorders in young women: a prevalence study in a general population sample. Psychosom Med 65(4):701–708, 2003 12883125

Fredericks DW, Carr JE, Williams WL: Overview of the treatment of rumination disorder for adults in a residential setting. J Behav Ther Exp Psychiatry 29(1):31–40, 1998 9627823

Friedman S, Even C, Dardennes R, et al: Light therapy, nonseasonal depression, and night eating syndrome (letter). Can J Psychiatry 49(11):790, 2004 15633866

Hagopian LP, Adelinis JD: Response blocking with and without redirection for the treatment of pica. J Appl Behav Anal 34(4):527–530, 2001 11800195

Hagopian LP, Rooker GW, Rolider NU: Identifying empirically supported treatments for pica in individuals with intellectual disabilities. Res Dev Disabil 32(6):2114–2120, 2011 21862281

Keel PK, Haedt A, Edler C: Purging disorder: an ominous variant of bulimia nervosa? Int J Eat Disord 38(3):191–199, 2005 16211629

Kessing BF, Smout AJ, Bredenoord AJ: Current diagnosis and management of the rumination syndrome. J Clin Gastroenterol 48(6):478–483, 2014 24921208

Khan S, Hyman PE, Cocjin J, et al: Rumination syndrome in adolescents. J Pediatr 136(4):528–531, 2000 10753253

Khan Y, Tisman G: Pica in iron deficiency: a case series. J Med Case Rep 4:86, 2010 20226051

Le Grange D, Binford R, Loeb KL: Manualized family based treatment for anorexia nervosa: a case series. J Am Acad Child Adolesc Psychiatry 44(1):41–46, 2005 15608542

Levine DF, Wingate DL, Pfeffer JM, et al: Habitual rumination: a benign disorder. Br Med J (Clin Res Ed) 287(6387):255–256, 1983 6409271

Levine LR: Fluoxetine in the treatment of bulimia nervosa: a multicenter, placebo-controlled, double-blind trial. Arch Gen Psychiatry 49(2):139–147, 1992 1550466

Machado PP, Machado BC, Gonçalves S, et al: The prevalence of eating disorders not otherwise specified. Int J Eat Disord 40(3):212–217, 2007 17173324

Madden NA, Russo DC, Cataldo MF: Behavioral treatment of pica in children with lead poisoning. Child Fam Behav Ther 2(4):67–81, 1981

Matson JL, Hattier MA, Belva B, et al: Pica in persons with developmental disabilities: approaches to treatment. Res Dev Disabil 34(9):2564–2571, 2013 23747942

O'Brien MD, Bruce BK, Camilleri M: The rumination syndrome: clinical features rather than manometric diagnosis. Gastroenterology 108(4):1024–1029, 1995 7698568

Olden KW: Rumination. Curr Treat Options Gastroenterol 4(4):351–358, 2001 11469994

O'Reardon JP, Stunkard AJ, Allison KC: Clinical trial of sertraline in the treatment of night eating syndrome. Int J Eat Disord 35(1):16–26, 2004 14705153

O'Reardon JP, Allison KC, Martino NS, et al: A randomized, placebo-controlled trial of sertraline in the treatment of night eating syndrome. Am J Psychiatry 163(5):893–898, 2006 16648332

Paniagua FA, Braverman C, Capriotti RM: Use of a treatment package in the management of a profoundly mentally retarded girl's pica and self-stimulation. Am J Ment Defic 90(5):550–557, 1986 3953688

Parry-Jones B, Parry-Jones WL: Pica: symptom or eating disorder? A historical assessment. Br J Psychiatry 160(3):341–354, 1992 1562860

Pawlow LA, O'Neil PM, Malcolm RJ: Night eating syndrome: effects of brief relaxation training on stress, mood, hunger, and eating patterns. Int J Obes Relat Metab Disord 27(8):970–978, 2003 12861239

Pike KM, Walsh BT, Vitousek K, et al: Cognitive behavior therapy in the posthospitalization treatment of anorexia nervosa. Am J Psychiatry 160(11):2046–2049, 2003 14594754

Pi-Sunyer FX: Short-term medical benefits and adverse effects of weight loss. Ann Intern Med 119(7 Pt 2):722–726, 1993

Rand CS, Macgregor A, Stunkard AJ: The night eating syndrome in the general population and among postoperative obesity surgery patients. Int J Eat Disord 22(1):65–69, 1997

Rose EA, Porcerelli JH, Neale AV: Pica: common but commonly missed. J Am Board Fam Med 13(5):353–358, 2000

Shapiro JR, Berkman ND, Brownley KA, et al: Bulimia nervosa treatment: a systematic review of randomized controlled trials. Int J Eat Disord 40(4):321–336, 2007 17370288

Singh NN, Bakker LW: Suppression of pica by overcorrection and physical restraint: a comparative analysis. J Autism Dev Disord 14(3):331–341, 1984 6480550

Smith MD: Treatment of pica in an adult disabled by autism by differential reinforcement of incompatible behavior. J Behav Ther Exp Psychiatry 18(3):285–288, 1987 3667957

Striegel-Moore RH, Franko DL, Thompson D, et al: Night eating: prevalence and demographic correlates. Obesity (Silver Spring) 14(1):139–147, 2006 16493132

Vander Wal JS: Night eating syndrome: a critical review of the literature. Clin Psychol Rev 32(1):49–59, 2012 22142838

Wade TD, O'Shea A: DSM-5 unspecified feeding and eating disorders in adolescents: what do they look like and are they clinically significant? Int J Eat Disord May 22, 2014 [Epub ahead of print] 24854848

Wade TD, Bergin JL, Tiggemann M, et al: Prevalence and long-term course of lifetime eating disorders in an adult Australian twin cohort. Aust N Z J Psychiatry 40(2):121–128, 2006 16476129

Wagaman JR, Williams DE, Camilleri M: Behavioral intervention for the treatment of rumination. J Pediatr Gastroenterol Nutr 27(5):596–598, 1998 9822330

Weakley MM, Petti TA, Karwisch G: Case study: chewing gum treatment of rumination in an adolescent with an eating disorder. J Am Acad Child Adolesc Psychiatry 36(8):1124–1127, 1997 9256592

Williams DE, McAdam D: Assessment, behavioral treatment, and prevention of pica: clinical guidelines and recommendations for practitioners. Res Dev Disabil 33(6):2050–2057, 2012 22750361

Winkelman JW: Clinical and polysomnographic features of sleep-related eating disorder. J Clin Psychiatry 59(1):14–19, 1998 9491060

Index

Page numbers printed in **boldface** type refer to figures and tables.